Social Work and Neoliberalism

Social work educators and practitioners are grappling with many difficulties confronting the profession in the context of an increasingly neoliberal world.

The contributors of this book examine how neoliberalism—and the modes with which it structures the world—has an impact on, and shapes, social work as a disciplinary 'field'. Drawing on new empirical work, the chapters in this book highlight how neoliberalism is affecting social work practices 'on the ground'. The book seeks to stimulate international debate on the totalizing effects of neoliberalism, and in so doing, also identify various ways through which it can be resisted both locally and globally.

The chapters in this book were originally published as a special issue of the *European Journal of Social Work*.

Edgar Marthinsen is Professor at the Norwegian University of Science and Technology, Trondheim, Norway.

Nina S. Skjefstad is Associate Professor at the Norwegian University of Science and Technology, Trondheim, Norway.

Anne Juberg is Associate Professor at the Norwegian University of Science and Technology, Trondheim, Norway.

Paul Michael Garrett works at NUI Galway, Republic of Ireland.

Social Work and Neoliberalism

Edited by
Edgar Marthinsen, Nina S. Skjefstad,
Anne Juberg, and Paul Michael Garrett

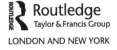

Routledge
Taylor & Francis Group

LONDON AND NEW YORK

First published 2022
by Routledge
2 Park Square, Milton Park, Abingdon, Oxon OX14 4RN

and by Routledge
605 Third Avenue, New York, NY 10158

Routledge is an imprint of the Taylor & Francis Group, an informa business

Introduction, Chapters 1, 2, 4–12 and 14 © 2022 Taylor & Francis
Chapter 3 © 2018 Jessica H. Jönsson. Originally published as Open Access.
Chapter 13 © 2018 Marcus Lauri. Originally published as Open Access.

British Library Cataloguing in Publication Data
A catalogue record for this book is available from the British Library

ISBN: 978-0-367-69548-4 (hbk)
ISBN: 978-0-367-69549-1 (pbk)
ISBN: 978-1-003-14222-5 (ebk)

DOI: 10.4324/9781003142225

Typeset in Myriad Pro
by Newgen Publishing UK

Publisher's Note
The publisher accepts responsibility for any inconsistencies that may have arisen during the conversion of this book from journal articles to book chapters, namely the inclusion of journal terminology.

Disclaimer
Every effort has been made to contact copyright holders for their permission to reprint material in this book. The publishers would be grateful to hear from any copyright holder who is not here acknowledged and will undertake to rectify any errors or omissions in future editions of this book.

Contents

Citation Information

The chapters in this book were originally published in the *European Journal of Social Work*, volume 22, issue 2 (2019). When citing this material, please use the original page numbering for each article, as follows:

Chapter 13

Mind your own business: technologies for governing social worker subjects
Marcus Lauri
European Journal of Social Work, volume 22, issue 2 (2019), pp. 338–349

Chapter 14

Neoliberalisation, the social investment state and social work
Edgar Marthinsen
European Journal of Social Work, volume 22, issue 2 (2019), pp. 350–361

For any permission-related enquiries please visit:
www.tandfonline.com/page/help/permissions

Notes on Contributors

Cristina Pinto Albuquerque, Faculty of Psychology and Educational Sciences/Social Work, University of Coimbra, Coimbra, Portugal.

Uschi Bay, Department of Social Work, Monash University, Melbourne, Australia.

Marion Bogo, Factor-Inwentash Faculty of Social Work, University of Toronto, Toronto, Ontario, Canada.

Helen Charnley, Department of Sociology, Durham University, Durham, UK.

Alexandra Ciocănel, Faculty of Sociology and Social Work, University of Bucharest, Bucharest, Romania.

Konstantina Dionysopoulou, School of Social Sciences, Education and Social Work, Queen's University Belfast, Belfast, Northern Ireland.

Daniela Gaba, Faculty of Sociology and Social Work, University of Bucharest, Bucharest, Romania.

Paul Michael Garrett, works at NUI Galway, Republic of Ireland.

Jessica Herschman, Child Development Institute in Toronto, Ontario, Canada.

Anne Juberg, Department of Social Work, Norwegian University of Science and Technology, Trondheim, Norway.

Kirsi Juhila, SOC/Faculty of Social Sciences, University of Tampere, Finland.

Marjorie Johnstone, School of Social Work, Dalhousie University, Halifax, Nova Scotia, Canada.

Jessica H. Jönsson, Department of Social work, Mid Sweden University, Östersund, Sweden.

Marcus Lauri, Department of Social Work, Mid Sweden University, Östersund, Sweden.

Florin Lazăr, Faculty of Sociology and Social Work, University of Bucharest, Bucharest, Romania.

Eunjung Lee, Factor-Inwentash Faculty of Social Work, University of Toronto, Toronto, Ontario, Canada.

Ana I. Lima Fernandez, Trabajo Social y Servicios Sociales, National University of Distance Education, Madrid, Spain; Trabajo Social y Servicios Sociales, Complutense Madrid University, Madrid, Spain.

Edgar Marthinsen, Deputy Head of Department for Research, Norwegian University of Science and Technology, Faculty of Social and Educational Sciences, Department of Social Work, Trondheim, Norway.

María Inés Martínez Herrero, School of Health and Social Care, University of Essex, Southend-on-Sea, UK.

Anca Mihai, Faculty of Sociology and Social Work, University of Bucharest, Bucharest, Romania.

Shari Munch, School of Social Work, Rutgers, The State University of New Jersey, New Brunswick, New Jersey, USA.

Gianinna Muñoz Arce, Department of Social Work, Alberto Hurtado University, Santiago, Chile.

Enrique Pastor Seller, Trabajo Social y Servicios Sociales, Universidad de Murcia, Murcia, Spain.

Maria Pentaraki, School of Social Sciences, Education and Social Work, Queen's University Belfast, Belfast, Northern Ireland.

Suvi Raitakari, SOC/Faculty of Social Sciences, University of Tampere, Finland.

Jenni-Mari Räsänen, SOC/Faculty of Social Sciences, University of Tampere, Finland.

Georgiana Rentea, Faculty of Sociology and Social Work, University of Bucharest, Bucharest, Romania.

Nina S. Skjefstad, Department of Social Work, Norwegian University of Science and Technology, Trondheim, Norway.

A. Ka Tat Tsang, Factor-Inwentash Faculty of Social Work, University of Toronto, Toronto, Ontario, Canada.

Carmen Verde Diego, Departamento de Análise e Intervención PsicoSocioEducativa, Universidad de Vigo, Galicia, Spain.

Introduction

Social work and neoliberalism

In November 2018, *The Guardian* newspaper reported that vulnerable children were being 'treated like cattle' since many councils, responsible for their care, were inviting private companies to compete for contracts to look after them through an online bidding system (Greenfield & Marsh, 2018, p. 5). This online tendering process was associated with one council publishing adverts including the personal details of children: dates of birth, family histories and even accounts of sexual abuse. The same newspaper later revealed that around three-quarters of English children's homes are now run for profit. More fundamentally, confided an editorial column, local councils, having to deal with the crisis generated by a lack of adequate funding from central government are having to reinvent themselves as shoppers 'seeking a bargain' (*The Guardian*, 13 November, 2018). Within this framework, social work values dissolve and children become mere commodities to be traded.

Perhaps the UK reflects more pervasive international trends, with this instance helping to illuminate some of the focal concerns and preoccupations in this themed issue. Reflecting on neoliberalism's dominance, social activity and exchange become 'judged on their degree of conformity to market culture' with 'business thinking migrating to all social activities' (Holborow, 2015, pp. 34–35). More theoretically, building on Foucault's analysis, Brown (2015, p. 10) maintains that neoliberalism 'transmogrifies every human domain and endeavour, along with humans themselves according to a specific image of the economic. All conduct is economic conduct; all spheres of existence are framed and measured in economic terms and metrics'.

However, in recent years, neoliberalism has become a contested term across a range of academic disciplines (Dunn, 2017). Indeed, as core concept, it has been suggested to have 'failed analytically' and to be 'hopelessly confused' (Mair in Venkatesan, Laidlaw, Eriksen, Mair, & Martin, 2015, p. 917). Some commentators even assert that the term constitutes an obstacle and should simply be dropped (Laidlaw in Venkatesan et al., 2015). More recently, it has been suggested that that neoliberalism is in ruins. According to Nancy Fraser, as a 'hegemonic project, neoliberalism is finished; it may retain its capacity to dominate, but it has lost its ability to persuade' (in Fraser & Jaeggi, 2018, p. 222). Certainly the articles in this issue suggest that neoliberalism – able to 'persuade' or not – continues to adversely impact on social work.

Moreover, as revealed in the scathing report by the United Nations (UN) Special Rapporteur on extreme poverty and human rights, the UK furnishes a paradigmatic example of how mass impoverishment is now found in even in the most prosperous parts of Western Europe:

> 14 million people, a fifth of the population, live in poverty. Four million of these are more than 50% below the poverty line, 1 and 1.5 million are destitute, unable to afford basic essentials. The widely respected Institute for Fiscal Studies predicts a 7% rise in child poverty between 2015 and 2022, and various sources predict child poverty rates of as high as 40%. For almost one in every two children to be poor in twenty-first century Britain is not just a disgrace, but a social calamity and an economic disaster, all rolled into one (Alston, 2018, p. 1).

In having regard to such statistics, it is now important to recall that the UK is the world's fifth largest economy and that the hardship reported by the UN official is wholly avoidable and a direct consequence of a bundle of political and economic choices now governed by an encompassing neoliberal rationality. Furthermore, being in employment does not magically overcome poverty. In-work poverty is increasingly common and almost 60% of those in poverty in the UK are in families where someone works. There are 2.8 million people living in poverty in families where all adults work full time. (Alston, 2018, p. 17; see also Dukelow & Kennett, 2018)

Readers of the UN report are presented with a striking tableau of a country in which there has been an

immense growth in foodbanks and the queues waiting outside them, the people sleeping rough in the streets, the growth of homelessness, the sense of deep despair that leads even the Government to appoint a Minister for suicide prevention and civil society to report in depth on unheard of levels of loneliness and isolation. (Alston, 2018, p. 1)

This is also an economic and social landscape in which the social work profession is charged with promoting the 'empowerment and liberation of people' with the principle of 'social justice' being foregrounded (International Federation of Social Workers, 2014; see also Hyslop, 2016, 2018).

Troubled by the inroads made by neoliberalism within social work, the idea for this themed issue was sparked by an international seminar taking place at the Norwegian University of Science and Technology in Trondheim in April 2016. A number of social educators and practitioners began to grapple with some of the difficulties confronting the profession. Indeed, Trondheim provided a welcoming and critically reflective foundational space for our ensuing project. In short, we envisioned a special themed issue as a forum to encourage contributions that would:

- Examine how neoliberal imperatives are continuing to impact on, and shape, social work as a disciplinary 'field';
- Draw on new empirical work to highlight how neoliberal imperatives are impacting on social work practices 'on the ground';
- Stimulate international debate on toxic impact of neoliberalism and social work;
- Prompt practitioners and educators to consider ways in which neoliberalism can be resisted.

This resulting themed issue of the *EJSW* brings together a rich array of authors from Europe, North and South America and Australasia. We are, of course, immensely grateful for their participation in our project. We recognise, however, that the issue does not include contributions from Africa and Asia and does not engage with relevant core concerns, such as forced migration and the coercive, neoliberal management of displaced populations (see Garrett, 2015), or the rise of the neo-Fascism. These and possibly other important matters are unfortunately beyond the scope of this issue. What, then, will readers find in the following pages?

In the first article, Paul Michael Garrett maintains that neoliberalism remains an analytically useful concept if social work educators and practitioners are prepared to try and define it, teasing out its complex meaning (see also Schram & Pavlovskaya, 2018). He suggests that those aiming to comprehend neoliberalism should take into account six intermeshed facets: the overturning of 'embedded liberalism'; the re-configuration of the state in order to better serve the interests of capital; new patterns of income and wealth distribution to benefit the rich and super-rich; insecurity and precariousness; the rise in mass incarceration; a strategic pragmatism. In conclusion, Garrett, tentatively proposes that we may be witnessing the emergence, in some quarters, of what he terms 'rhetorically recalibrated neoliberalism' (RRN).

Next, located in Australia, Uschi Bay also dwells on theoretical questions related to neoliberalism. Drawing on the work of Foucault, she argues that neoliberalism constitutes a specific 'art of government' (see also Garrett, 2018). Central to this 'art' is the notion that individuals are governed through – in Foucauldian terms – technologies of self-responsibilisation and the freedom to choose. Social work practitioners can be perceived as part of 'enabling' networks assisting individuals who are considered self-excluded due to their irresponsible choices to work on themselves so as to constitute 'entrepreneurial' selves. However, this does not rule out forms of oppositional activities and forms of 'counter conduct'.

Sweden was formerly something of a social democratic beacon with one of the most developed welfare states in the world. Nevertheless, retrogressive neoliberal transformations are occurring. In the next contribution, Jessica H. Jönsson usefully explores the impact of this development on social work. Crucially, she argues, that the traditional 'solidary role' fulfilled by practitioners is being undermined. Grounded in empirical work, the article points to the growing and widespread worry about 'new' professional roles and the neoliberal organisation of public social work. Importantly, it is argued that social workers are far from passive actors, but have the ability to craft their roles in order to foster solidarity amongst themselves and with those for whom they provide services.

Having 'visited' northern Europe, the fourth article takes readers to England and Spain with María Inés Martínez Herrero and Helen Charnley furnishing empirical research exploring social work educators' understandings of, and strategies used in, learning and teaching human rights and social justice. Their findings show that prevailing neoliberal ideology has pervaded social work in both countries (more pervasively in England), placing pressure on social work educators to convey narrow understandings of human rights and social justice and to adopt bureaucratic and 'distant relationships' with students. Nevertheless, spaces remain for bolstering a human rights and social justice orientation (see also Fenton, 2018).

Our fifth article, is a collective contribution from Eunjung Lee and her colleagues located in Canada. It examines how governing forms of neoliberal rationality serve to generate the specific ways in which social workers interact with 'clients' in moment-to-moment interactions. This fascinating article is part of a more encompassing project exploring cross-cultural social work practice in outpatient community mental health settings in one particular city. In the sixth article, Anne Juberg and Nina Schiøll Skjefstad focus on how 'substance misuse' disorder and youth unemployment are discursively assembled in contemporary Norwegian policy documents. Their specific interest is the situation of young adults (18–30) who are not in employment, education and training (NEET) and who have problems with alcohol or other drugs. Three predominant discourses tend to be to the fore: a medicalisation discourse, a stigma discourse and one circulating around a social investment discourse. Significantly, all of these can be associated with the neoliberal tendency to individualise and medicalise 'social problems'. However, there appears to be little evidence in epidemiology and other research that substance abuse determines the NEET status among young people. Neither is there any manifest evidence that problems with alcohol and drugs among young adults will, in the long run, negatively impact on their capacity to work. Nonetheless, the three identified discourses are still likely to perpetuate myth-making.

Remaining in northern Europe, Suvi Raitakari, Kirsi Juhila and Jenni-Mari Räsänen focus on Finland in order to analyse two state-level policy documents preoccupied with an 'activation' initiative called inclusive social security (ISS). The authors are interested in how social workers and clients are constructed as 'responsible subjects' within this documentation. Here, they argue that an advanced liberal mode of governmentality aims to strengthen citizens' abilities to self-govern through various techniques including enmeshed elements of surveillance and 'empowerment'. Enrique Pastor Seller and his colleagues next shift the focus to Spain revealing that neoliberal policies have led to sizable cuts in the public social welfare systems, prompting an increase in demand and unwarranted public hardship. The article summarises the glaringly adverse impact on families. Concerned by social services' limited capacity to respond to this ongoing crisis, the General Council of Social Work carried out research illuminating the serious consequences that so-called 'austerity' measures have had on the population, social welfare systems and social workers.

For anyone wanting to comprehend the neoliberal project, the events in Chile are of major significance (see also Grugel & Riggirozzi, 2018). In an important article, Gianinna Muñoz Arce reminds readers that the right-wing dictatorship (1973–1990) implemented the first neoliberal 'experiment' in the world. More than 40 years after the coup, the legacy of the dictatorship continues to function as an obstacle to discussion and to the expression of critical perspectives in social work. The introduction of the Social Protection System in 2000 has served to embed depoliticised and individually oriented approaches within the profession. Despite this, practices of resistance to this apparent hegemonic order can still be identified (see also Ishkanian & Glasius, 2018).

In the more recent past, the Greek working class has been targeted for a 'gigantic disciplining operation – a huge experiment in violent downward social mobility and neoliberal adjustment and restructuring' (Stavrakakis, 2013, p. 315). In the tenth article of the issue, Maria Pentaraki and Konstantina Dionysopoulou refer to a qualitative study of mental health social workers working in the non-profit sector. Their findings evoke a picture of social workers experiencing precarious conditions as they also become part of the growing working poor. On occasions, many practitioners are even unable to pay for their commuting expenses to and from work.

Remaining in southern Europe, Cristina Pinto Albuquerque's article dwells on the neoliberal induced transformation of social work in Portugal (see also Papadopoulos & Roumpakis, 2018). Potentially, can this development create a 'phoenix' 'moment' or is the profession destined to be enclaved in a 'black hole'? In order to examine this question, the author investigates data derived from interviews with social workers. Florin Lazăr and his colleagues next explore the trajectory of the profession in Romania. The ruling Communist administration disbanded the profession in 1968, but it was reinstated after in 1989. Subsequently, social work has evolved within a neoliberal paradigm which has promoted both state withdrawal from welfare provision and individuals taking responsibility for their own welfare. Utilising a qualitative approach, the article explores how practitioners risk being left with little room for manoeuvre in creating more progressive forms of policy and practice.

In our penultimate article, Marcus Lauri investigates some of the ways in which neoliberalisation may be sustained by shaping social workers' subjectivity so as to render them compliant with neoliberal endeavours. From interviews with social workers in Sweden, it is suggested that governing technologies aim to create practitioners lacking the capacity to stand 'shoulder to shoulder' with both co-workers and clients. Fittingly, the special issue concludes with an article from Edgar Marthinsen, the convenor of the Trondheim initiative, in which he focuses on the challenges facing social work. The author also furnishes an outline of the history of resistance in social work against neoliberalism and goes onto analyse the coupling of neoliberal policy and social investment policy (see also Laruffa, 2018).

We hope that you will welcome this special themed issue – Now read, organise and resist!

References

Alston, P. (2018, November 16). Statement on Visit to the United Kingdom, by Professor Philip Alston, United Nations Special Rapporteur on extreme poverty and human rights, London.
Brown, W. (2015). *Undoing the Demos*. New York: Zone Books.
Dukelow, F. & Kennett, P. (2019). Discipline, debt and coercive communication: Post-crisis neoliberalism and the welfare state in Ireland, the UK and the USA. *Critical Social Policy*, 38(3), 482–504.
Dunn, B. (2017). Against neoliberalism as a concept. *Capital & Class*, 41(3), 435–454.
Fenton, J. (2018). Putting old heads on young shoulders: helping social work students uncover the neoliberal hegemony. *Social Work Education*, 37, 941–954. doi:10.1080/02615479.2018.1468877.
Fraser, N., & Jaeggi, R. (2018). *Capitalism: A Conversation in Critical Theory*. Cambridge: Polity.
Garrett, P. M. (2015). 'Constraining and confining ethnic minorities: impoverishment and the logics of control in neoliberal Ireland. *Patterns of Prejudice*, 49(4), 414–434.
Garrett, P. M. (2018). Revisiting "The Birth of Biopolitics": Foucault's account of neoliberalism and the remaking of social policy. *Journal of Social Policy*, 1–19. Published online: 17 September, doi:10.1017/S0047279418000582.
Greenfield, P., & Marsh, S. (2018, November 10). Vulnerable children "auctioned online" in care-home system, experts warn. *The Guardian*, 7.
Grugel, J., & Riggirozzi, P. (2018). Neoliberal disruption and neoliberalism's afterlife in Latin America: What is left of post-neoliberal? *Critical Social Policy*, 38(3), 547–566.
Holborow, M. (2015). *Language and Neoliberalism*. London: Routledge.
Hyslop, I. (2016). Social work in the teeth of a gale: a resilient counter-discourse in neoliberal times. *Critical and Radical Social Work*, 4(1), 21–37.

Hyslop, I. (2018). Neoliberalism and social work identity. *European Journal of Social Work, 21*(1), 20–31.

International Federation of Social Workers. (2014). *Global definition of social Work*. http://ifsw.org/get-involved/global-definition-of-social-work/

Ishkanian, A., & Glasius, M. (2018). Resisting neoliberalism? Movements against austerity and for democracy in Cairo, Athens and London. *Critical Social Policy, 38*(3), 527–546.

Laruffa, F. (2018). Social investment: Diffusing ideas for redesigning citizenship after neoliberalism? *Critical Social Policy, 38*(4), 688–707.

Papadopoulos, T., & Roumpakis, A. (2018). Rattling Europe's ordoliberal "iron cage": the contestation of austerity in Southern Europe. *Critical Social Policy, 38*(3), 505–526.

Schram, S. F., & Pavlovskaya, M. (Eds.). (2018). *Rethinking Neoliberalism*. New York, USA: Routledge.

Stavrakakis, Y. (2013). Dispatches from the Greek lab. *Psychoanalysis, Culture & Society, 18*(3), 313–324.

Venkatesan, S., Laidlaw, J., Eriksen, T. H., Mair, J., & Martin, K. (2015). Debate: "The concept of neoliberalism has become an obstacle to the anthropological understanding of the twenty-first century. *Journal of the Royal Anthropological Institute, 21*, 911–923.

Edgar Marthinsen

Anne Juberg

Nina S. Skjefstad

Paul Michael Garrett

What are we talking about when we talk about 'Neoliberalism'?

Paul Michael Garrett

ABSTRACT
Based on a review of the critical literature, the article provides readers with an overview of neoliberalism's main dimensions. In this sense, it furnishes an accessible conceptual foundation for a number of the articles in the themed issue. It is suggested that those seeking to comprehend neoliberalism should take into account six intermeshed facets: the overturning of 'embedded liberalism'; the re-configuration of the state in order to better serve the interests of capital; new patterns of income and wealth distribution to benefit the rich and super-rich; insecurity and precariousness; the rise in mass incarceration; a strategic pragmatism. The article briefly dwells on the capitalist crisis which began in 2007 and goes on to suggest that we may be witnessing the emergence of what is termed 'rhetorically recalibrated neoliberalism' (RRN).

Introduction

The word 'neoliberalism' is frequently used in a casual way as 'shorthand for a prevailing dystopian zeitgeist' (Venugopal, 2015, p. 168; see also Gray, Dean, Agllias, Howard, & Schubert, 2015). However, underpinning the exploration in this article is the understanding that neoliberalism is an historically specific form of capital accumulation deliberately conceived as a 'counter-revolution against welfare capitalism' (Fairclough & Graham, 2002, p. 221). What follows aims, therefore, to furnish readers with an accessible synthesis of some of neoliberalism's main dimensions. Drawing on mostly Anglo-American and critical sources, it provides an introductory resource for social work educators, practitioners and students keen to bring into view the 'bigger picture' which, on occasions, risks being elided or obscured in social work and associated fields. The article also briefly refers to the economic crisis which began in 2007 and identifies what I refer to as the emergence of 'rhetorically recalibrated neoliberalism' (RRN).

Those seeking to grasp the meaning of neoliberalism should be attentive to six overlapping dimensions: the overturning of 'embedded liberalism' (Harvey, 2005); the re-configuration of the state in order to better serve the interests of capital; new patterns of income and wealth distribution to benefit the rich and super-rich; insecurity and precariousness; the rise in mass incarceration; a strategic pragmatism. Each of these dimensions will now be briefly examined.

Six dimensions of neoliberalism

Overturning 'embedded liberalism'

Neoliberalism, for Bourdieu (2001, p. 35), is best perceived as a 'conservative revolution' that 'ratifies and glorifies the reign of ... the financial markets, in other words the return of the kind of radical capitalism, with no other law than the return of maximum profit, an unfettered capitalism ...

pushed to the limits'. More theoretically, we can perhaps comprehend neoliberalism as seeking to succeed the type of 'embedded liberalism' largely dominant in most of the industrial West from the end of the Second World War into the 1970s. During this period 'market processes and entrepreneurial and corporate activities were surrounded by a web of social and political constraints and a regulatory environment that sometimes restrained … economic and industrial strategy'. In contrast, the neoliberal project seeks to 'disembed capital from these constraints' (Harvey, 2005, p. 11). Thus, to different degrees, depending on the specific cultural and national context, neoliberalism endeavours to 'strip away the protective coverings that embedded liberalism allowed and occasionally nurtured' (Harvey, 2005, p. 168).

This process is illustrated by circumstances surrounding the major fire occurring at Grenfell Tower, on 14 June 2017, which resulted in the deaths over seventy people. Completed in 1974, Grenfell Tower was a 24-storey residential tower block in North Kensington, London, England. It was often referred to as the 'Moroccan tower' because many residents came from the local Moroccan immigrant community. Prior to the catastrophic fire, a residents' organisation, the Grenfell Action Group (GAG), had highlighted fire safety issues and poor maintenance (GAG, 2016). In *The Guardian*, passionately castigating the 'violence of neoliberal "austerity"', Chakrabortty (2017, p. 25) drew comparisons between contemporary social and economic conditions and the not entirely dissimilar circumstances concerning Marx and Engels in Victorian Britain (Garrett, 2018a). This was period, of course, before liberalism had been partly 'embedded' within a constraining network of relationships aiming to promote values at odds with, or existing in tension with, those of market rationality. Nevertheless, over

> 170 years later, Britain remains a country that murders its poor … What happened last week [at Grenfell Tower] wasn't a 'terrible tragedy' or some other studio-sofa platitude: it was social murder … Spectacular examples of social violence, such as Grenfell, are thankfully rare. They usually occur out of public sight. This decade of austerity has been a decade of social violence … Austerity is at the heart of the Grenfell story … Spending cuts, deregulation, outsourcing: between them they have turned a state supposedly there to protect and support citizens into a machine to make money for the rich while punishing the poor. It's never described like that, of course. Class warfare is passed off as book-keeping. Accountability is tossed aside for 'commercial confidentiality', while profiteering is dressed up as economic dynamism.

Appropriately seeking to make the connections to social work, the Social Work Action Network (SWAN, 2017) concluded

> The fire at Grenfell was not a random event; it was a disaster waiting to happen. It was the result of cuts, of austerity, of privatisation of council housing, of deregulation, of out-sourcing and of inequality … The fire, and the deaths, stand as a symbol of all that is wrong with new-liberal social policy … [The] unnecessary deaths of ordinary working people by a system skewed to meet the interests of the wealthy … SWAN denounces the system of cuts, privatisation and deregulation that led to the catastrophe.

Although the inquiry announced by Prime Minister Theresa May in late June 2017 is still to produce findings and all relevant details are not – and probably will never be – known, sufficient evidence is already available to suggest that the process of eroding 'embedded liberalism' by incrementally stripping away solidaristic forms of 'protective coverings' contributed to the fire and the ensuing fatalities at Grenfell Tower.

This dis-embedding of liberalism can also be associated with a fresh and reinvigorated emphasis on competition across all areas of society, including those previously perceived as outside the parameters of commodification (Brown, 2015). For example, within the university sector, tuition fees of up to £9,000 a year in the UK have, of course, also created immense financial difficulties for students and their families. Similarly, the 'de-funding of "public" US colleges and universities means that, as of 2015, students pay nearly 50% of the costs of their education at these institutions, up from 20% just 25 years ago' (Myers, 2017, p. 304).

As Therborn (2007, p. 75) put it, the 'survival of the fittest and Social Darwinism have been given a new impetus by neoliberal globalization, after their post-Fascist quarantine'. Relatedly, neoliberalisation is a process entailing much 'creative destruction' (Harvey, 2005, p. 3). Moreover, the aim has been to install a new 'common sense' to try and ensure that people are led to *think* and *act* in a manner conducive to neoliberalism. Indeed, it has been argued that neoliberalism

> has been ingested into the body politic so successfully that it has become the prevailing commonsense of every-day life … Just as in the aftermath of the Second World War we all became 'social democratic subjects' in one way or another, we may have now become similarly constituted as "neoliberal subjects", in ways that we do not fully recognise. (Thompson, 2008, p. 68)

In this way, neoliberalisation can be perceived as bound up with an individual's sense of self, setting in motion and sustaining a multiplicity of 'identity projects' that are compatible with capitalism. Related to this, in terms of working practices, neoliberalism favours 'flexibility' and is hostile to all forms of social solidarity and identification that can potentially restrain capital accumulation.

Neoliberals endeavour to *remake* work and workscapes and alter the aims, aspirations and affiliations of a range of professional groups (Garrett, 2005, 2009, 2014a). However, across different fields, this project is likely to prompt resistance. For example, people involved in social work – be they the providers or users (and these categories are, moreover, fluid) – are apt to 'find ways of surviving, negotiating, accommodating, refusing and resisting' and do not merely 'act like automatons envisaged in the governmental plans and strategies of the powerful' (Clarke, 2005, p. 159).

Putting the state to work for capital

The core function of the neoliberal state is to furnish an 'apparatus whose fundamental mission [is to] facilitate conditions for profitable capital accumulation on the part of both domestic and foreign capital' (Harvey, 2005, p. 7). Pervasively, the remaking of state apparatuses involves a 'dramatic shift in government commitments from securing the welfare of citizens to facilitating the flow of global capital' with this 'accomplished through a depoliticizing discourse of deficits, competitiveness, and balanced budgets, surrounded by an aura of technocratic neutrality' (Baker, 2009, p. 70). Significant in this respect is the drive toward corporatisation, commodification, and privatisation of hitherto public assets. This entails the opening up of 'new fields for capital accumulation in domains hitherto regarded off-limits to the calculus of profitability' (Harvey, 2005, p. 160). Moreover, the state

> once neoliberalized, becomes a prime agent of retributive policies, *reversing* the flow from the upper classes that had occurred during the era of embedded liberalism. It does this in the first instance through the pursuit of privatization schemes and cutbacks in those state expenditures that support the social wage. (Harvey, 2005, p. 163, emphasis added)

A misguided perspective maintains that neoliberalism heralds an irrepressible 'rolling back' of the state with the 'market' and 'market mechanisms' being *entirely* left to 'take over' society. However, within the neoliberal paradigm, the state continues to play an active role in that it creates and preserves an 'institutional framework' for capital (Brenner & Theodore, 2002). Writing in a US context, Myers (2017, p. 307) observes:

> Regarding the neoliberalization of American society, the language of 'deregulation', for example, obscures as much as it reveals, with the result that even critics may unwittingly reinscribe a key tenet of neoliberal ideology, the myth of non-intervention. It is crucial, then, to specify that the neoliberal social settlement was the result of proactive, inventive measures to *re*regulate the social order.

In his prescient examination of the 'German' roots of neoliberalism, Foucault correctly argues that it is entirely erroneous to simply perceive this body of ideas as simply 'Adam Smith revived' or the type of 'market society' that Marx unpicked and denounced in *Capital* (Foucault, 2008, p. 130). The economy and society mapped by the initial prompters of neoliberalism did not merely replicate or transpose the capitalist models of the past. On the contrary, central to this new 'art of government' is a rejection of nineteenth century *laissez-faire* capitalism in favour of a more regulated approach. The evocative metaphor Foucault uses to describe this shift is that of the 'Highway Code', which dictates that 'vehicles' will no longer be 'allowed to circulate in any direction, according to whim, with avoidable "endless congestion and accidents'" (Foucault, 2008, p. 162). To prevent such mishaps, traffic will be strictly monitored with 'fixed hours', 'routes' and speeds imposed. Hence, at a time of 'faster means of transport this code will not necessarily be the same as in the time of stagecoaches' (Foucault, 2008, p. 162).

Neoliberal 'governmental intervention is no less dense, frequent, active and continuous than in any other system' (Foucault, 2008, p. 145). What occurs, however, is a reconstitution or *remaking* of the state which becomes more vigilant and active in promoting the market economy (Garrett, 2018b). Within this perspective, an unemployed person should never be perceived as a 'social victim' (Foucault, 2008, p. 139). Foreshadowing the later lexicon on so-called 'jobseekers', the unemployed person was better understood as a 'worker in transit ... in transit between an unprofitable activity and more profitable activity' (Foucault, 2008, p. 139) – hence, the emphasis, from the 1990s onwards, on 'positive' or 'proactive' state interventions evident in policies pivoting on 'activating' the unemployed (or 'jobseekers') and in discourses and practices focused on 'social inclusion' and 'prevention'. Specifically in relation to social work, recent years have also witnessed something of a 'boom' with the profession becoming a 'growth industry even in countries that ideologically would rather do without it' (Lorenz, 2005).

In line with this analysis, despite the 'anti-big government' rhetoric often associated with neoliberalism, there has been little diminution in the actual size of many governments in the West. Indeed 'big government' has not gone away even in a world supposedly governed by neoliberal rules. For example, despite the attacks on welfare that have occurred, the data on state expenditure reveals a complex picture. Whilst, the discrepancy between the neoliberal rhetoric and actual spending patterns may appear 'puzzling' (Eagleton-Pierce, 2016, p. 178), there is a need to note that wholesale welfare retrenchment is difficult to achieve. Drastic public spending cuts are likely to be counterproductive and risk generating unmanageable political opposition and resistance. In terms of the social administration of welfare provision, previous 'political and legal legacies can "lock-in" current government spending patterns' limiting the room for control and manoeuvre' (Eagleton-Pierce, 2016, p. 178). More fundamentally, capitalism requires substantial state financial outlays, not only to maintain a measure of stability and social harmony but help to pacify and engineer the smooth social reproduction of the workforce.

Capitalism – even in its neoliberal form – can 'no more do without the state today that it could do in the Keynesian period' (Harman, 2008, p. 97). This was, of course, illustrated during the Northern Rock crisis in the UK, in 2007 at the outset of the 'crash', and in the subsequent response of the US administration to the collapse of the investment banks the following year (Jacques, 2008).

Redistributing from the poor to the rich

Whatever local shape it may take, neoliberalism is an overarching philosophy and series of practices universally aspiring to restore class power through vast transfers of income to the richest groups in society. In short, the chief 'substantive achievement' of neoliberalism has been to 'redistribute, rather than to generate, wealth and income' (Harvey, 2005, p. 159). 'Despite a period of heightened geopolitical uncertainty', the world's ultrawealthy are flourishing' given the wealth of billionaires 'rose 17% in 2016' (UBS/PWC, 2017, p. 5). In the US, for example, the six-member Walton family, heirs to the Walmart fortune, have 'as much wealth as the bottom 41.5% of American families'. Income inequality in recent years, as 'measured by the share of income held by the top 1% and bottom 90% of Americans, rivals that of 1928' (Myers, 2017, p. 304).

Restructuring and reorganising capital, to the disadvantage the majority of the world's inhabitants, neoliberalism has produced an enormous cleavage between the super-rich and the rest. In 2016, according to Oxfam America (2016, p. 1):

> The gap between rich and poor is reaching new extremes. The richest 1% has accumulated more wealth than the rest of the world put together. Meanwhile, the wealth owned by the bottom half of humanity has fallen by a

trillion dollars in the past five years. Just 62 individuals now have the same wealth as 3.6 billion people – half of humanity.

The following year, Oxfam (2017) reported that the concentration in wealth had intensified further with the world's eight richest billionaires now controlling the same wealth between them as the poorest half of the earth's population. Moreover, the 'world's 10 biggest corporations – a list that includes Wal-Mart, Shell and Apple – have a combined revenue greater than the government revenue of 180 "poorest" countries combined' (Oxfam, 2017, p. 16).

Returning to London and echoing facets of the earlier discussion on Grenfell Tower, redistribution in favour of the rich is palpably apparent. In the UK capital, 2.3 million people are in poverty: 37% of London's children, in fact, are poor (Trust for London [TFL], 2017). In terms of the distribution of wealth, the bottom 50% of households 'own just over 5% of London's wealth, whereas the top 10% owns over half' (TFL, 2017). Between 2012 and 2014, a period of supposedly shared 'austerity', those 'in the top 10% saw their wealth grow by 25%' in London (TFL, 2017). In Great Britain, as a whole, the top 10% increased their wealth by 15% (TFL, 2017).

Financialisation refers to the 'significance of financial markets and institutions in the economy and a dramatic increase in the volume, velocity, complexity, and connectedness of financial flows' that has taken place during the neoliberal period (Mahmud, 2012, pp. 474–475). This can also be associated with a tremendous increase in indebtedness. Linked to a mix of factors, including the decline in wages and the socially predatory and reckless practices of lending agencies, by the end of 2008 '70 percent of U.S. families held credit cards, with the total credit card debt reaching $972.73 trillion' (Mahmud, 2012, p. 476). In the UK, the Financial Conduct Authority (FCA, 2017) revealed the scale of indebtedness with 50% of UK adults (25.5 million) displaying 'one or more characteristics' signalling potential financial vulnerability. Particular groups are especially vulnerable: single parents (aged 18–34) are three times more likely than others to use high cost loans (17% to the UK average of 6%). Within the 25–34 year-old population, some 13% are described as being in 'difficulty' because they have missed paying domestic bills or meeting credit commitments in 3 or more of the last 6 months' (FCA, 2017). Indeed, it is increasingly through debt that capital 'cannibalizes labour, disciplines states, transfers wealth from periphery to core and sucks value from households, families, communities and nature' (Fraser, 2016, p. 113).

'Accumulation by dispossession' also encompasses reneging on key commitments negotiated with trade unions in relation to wages and the terms and conditions of employment, including pensions. The 'fundamental mission' is to 'create a "good business climate" and therefore to optimize conditions for capital accumulation no matter what the consequences for employment or social well-being' (Harvey, 2006, p. 25). Thus, the

> neo-liberal state is particularly assiduous in seeking the privatization of assets as a means to open up fresh fields for capital accumulation. Sectors formerly run or regulated by the state (transportation, telecommunications, oil and other natural resources, utilities, social housing, education) are turned over to the private sphere or deregulated. (Harvey, 2006, p. 25)

In January 2018, the disastrous impact of this process was illustrated by the financial collapse of Carillion, the giant construction company, which had benefited from the outsourcing of services from the public sector in the UK (Hutton, 2018).

Poverty and precariousness

A fourth defining characteristic of neoliberalism can be associated with the aspiration to inject new forms of insecurity into people's working lives (Garrett, 2014b). This new insecurity, impinging on social workers and on the lives of many of those engaging with them, is frequently discussed in terms of 'precariousness' (Standing, 2011). As Good Gingrich (2010, p. 109) observes, in the past three

> decades workers across the globe have been confronted by a general deterioration and narrowing of their employment options. Research shows such trends are resulting in deepening poverty, widening income and wealth inequalities, and a rise in part-time, low-wage, unregulated, and temporary work.

Again, London provides a good illustration of the argument that work does not provide a route out of poverty despite the rhetoric of Conservative politicians. In the capital city, the majority of the 2.3 million confronting

> poverty (58%) are living in a working family, the highest this figure has ever been; it was 44% a decade earlier and 28% two decades ago. Around 70% of children in poverty in London are in a working family. In the rest of England 55% of people in poverty are in working families. (TFL, 2017)

Moreover, for many, work is less secure and more precarious with, in 2016, the number of workers in London on temporary contracts at an 'all-time high' (TFL, 2017).

According to Harvey (2005, p. 169), the figure of the 'disposable worker' has emerged as 'proto-typical upon the world stage'. His analysis stresses how this development relates to what Marx called the 'industrial reserve army' and the usefulness for capital of workers who remain 'accessible, socialised, disciplined and of the requisite qualities (i.e. flexible, docile, manipulable and skilled when necessary)' (Harvey, 2010, p. 58). Moreover, unemployment seeks to 'rediscipline labour to accept a lower wage rate' and inferior terms and conditions of employment (Harvey, 2010, p. 60).

A good deal of the 'welfare reform' and the wider *remaking* of welfare undertaken across a range of jurisdictions is founded on this neoliberal perspective. Thus, the neoliberal rationality 'reaches beyond the market, extending and disseminating market values to all institutions and social action so that individuals are conceptualized as rational, entrepreneurial actors whose moral authority is determined by their capacity for autonomy and self-care' (Baker, 2009, p. 277). The role of 'welfare reform' and 'welfare-to-work' initiatives becomes that of installing mechanisms that serve to orientate the unwaged into the low-wage zones of employment market. Thus a panoply of employment 'acti-vation' programmes introduces new means of surveillance to monitor and track 'job-seeking' activi-ties, to mentor, coach and compel. Such programmes 'serve to discipline the whole workforce' in that they operate to, for example, 'support and sustain the secondary, low-wage labour market through the steady supply of suitably flexible and compliant workers who have learned, out of necessity, to contend with instability, uncertainty and vulnerability' (Good Gingrich, 2010, p. 131). In this way, the unemployed are subjected – at a micro level – to 'structural adjustments' to their lifestyles, hopes and aspirations. In many countries, social workers are also becoming incorporated into the management of 'labour market training programmes' targeted at particular groups, such as those with 'mental health problems' (see, for example, Roets et al., 2012).

The rise of mass incarceration

Since about the year 2000 the world prison population total has grown by almost 20%, which is slightly above the estimated 18% increase in the world's general population over the same period (Garrett, 2015a, 2016). The female prison population total has increased by 50% since about 2000, while the equivalent figure for the male prison population is 18% (Walmsley, 2017, p. 3). The recorded total of prisoners is 10.35 million, but the actual number may be in 'excess of 11 million' (Walmsley, 2017, p. 3). The US has the highest proportion of prisoners per 100,000 in the world apart from the Seychelles. It has more than 2.2 million prisoners; 698 prisoners per 100,000 of the national population (Walmsley, 2017, p. 3). In England and Wales the rate is 148 prisoners per 100,000 (Walmsley, 2017, p. 10). Perhaps the enormous size of the US prison popu-lation comfortably outstrips the *national population* size of a number of European States including Estonia (1.31 million), Latvia (1.99 million), Kosovo (1.81 million), Macedonia (2.07 million) and Slo-venia (2.06 million) (extrapolated from Walmsley, 2017).

One of Wacquant's (2009) chief assertions is that those intent on analysing the evolution of neo-liberalism often fail to take into account mass incarceration. For example, the irruption of the penal state in America has gone 'virtually unnoticed' by those academics focusing on the 'crisis of the welfare state' (Wacquant, 2009, p xiii). Arguably, key definers of neoliberalism on the political Left have furnished defective analyses because of this lacuna. For example, Harvey's (2005) respected contributions on the rise of neoliberalism are 'woefully incomplete' because he has 'barely a few passing mentions of the prison' (Wacquant, 2009, p. 309).

Today, Wacquant (2009, p. 99) maintains, it should no longer be intellectually tenable to analyse the 'implementation of welfare policy at ground level without taking into account the overlapping operations of the penal institution'. Welfare offices, for instances, are borrowing the 'stock-in-trade techniques of the correctional institutions ... a constant close-up monitoring, strict spatial assignments and time constraints, intensive record-keeping and case management, periodic interrogation and reporting, and a rigid system of graduated sanctions for failing to perform properly' (Wacquant, 2009, pp. 101–102). Such practices are undergirded by a

> paternalist conception of the role of the state in respect to the poor, according to which the conduct of disposed and dependent citizens must be closely supervised and, whenever necessary, corrected through rigorous protocols of surveillance, deterrence and sanction, very much like those routinely applied to offenders under criminal justice supervision. (Wacquant, 2009, pp. 59–60)

In this context, the 'new punitive organization of welfare programs operates in the manner of a labor parole program designed to push its "beneficiaries" into the sub poverty jobs' (Wacquant, 2009, p. 43).

In the US, on account of concern about the escalating costs of prison during a period of financial cutbacks, various measures have been considered including – outlandishly – using Mexico as a quasi-prison colony. Counties within California are also experimenting with various neoliberal ways to reduce costs and increase revenues. Riverside County, for example, decided to charge inmates $140 per night with prisoner debts recouped from post-prison earnings. In Fremont, inmates are provided with the opportunity to relocate to a safer and quieter area of the prison with such 'upgrades' resulting in a $155 additional charge per night (Aviram, 2016, pp. 270–271).

A more socially pervasive 'new punitiveness' (Pratt, Brown, Brown, Hallsworth, & Morrison, 2005) is also central to neoliberalism's mode of social regulation. This can be associated with the tendency to locate particular sections of the population (those regarded as ambiguously 'troublesome' or ambiguously out of place) within enclosures that may not in the ordinary sense of the word be 'prisons' but remain zones of varying degrees of confinement and supervision (Garrett, 2015b). What is more, there is a related aspiration to use technology to track the troublesome in the 'community'. Indeed, it is now possible to detect a 'whole variety of paralegal forms of confinement ... including pre-emptive or preventive detention prior to a crime being committed' (Rose, 2000, p. 335). These are targeted at, for example, *potential* paedophiles and *potential* terrorists – 'monstrous individuals', the 'incorrigibly anti-social' and others representatives of a 'new human kind' (Rose, 2000, p. 333).

Strategic pragmatism

Finally, there is a need to be cautious and distinguish between 'neoliberalism as a system of thought and actually existing neoliberalism' (Munck, 2005, p. 60). Certainly a 'disjuncture' or discrepancy is detectable between the theory and rhetoric of neoliberalism and its pragmatics. First, the state has not been driven back in the way desired by ideologues such as Friedrich Hayek (Klein, 2007). Second, we are 'dealing here less with a coherently bounded "ism" or "end-state" than with a process ... neoliberalization' (Brenner & Theodore, 2002, p. 6). It is also important to remember that supporters of the neoliberal agenda are rarely presented with a bare landscape on which to operate free of constraints. However, after 'natural' disasters or in post war and post-invasion scenarios, we can observe what Klein (2007) calls neoliberal inspired 'disaster capitalism' and the rolling out of 'neoliberal disaster governance' processes (Pyles, Svistova, & Ahn, 2017). The responses to the Hurricane Katrina, in 2005 and the earthquake in Haiti five years later provide examples of this phenomenon. More frequently, however, neoliberal 'transformation' projects are 'path-dependent' and are apt to falter due to their forced engagement with those ingrained cultural legacies and expectations, those ways of *seeing* and *doing* that are averse to neoliberal 'common sense', its values and dominant orientations (Brenner & Theodore, 2002, p. 3). Nevertheless, neoliberalism is resilient, has a 'dogged dynamism' and 'fails forward' (Peck, 2010).

The willingness to be pragmatic was, of course, in response to the so-called credit crunch triggered on 9 August 2007 by 'the French bank BNP Paribas [suspending] three of its investment funds that had been dabbling in US sub-prime mortgages' ('State of Emergency': Editorial, *The Guardian*, 5 August, 2011). This soon evolved into the 'most serious crisis of the capitalist system since 1929-33' (Hobsbawm, 2008).

A crisis for neoliberal capitalism

In urging Congressional leaders to pass the $700 billion bailout plan ten days after the Lehman collapse, on 15 September 2008, President George W Bush was reported to have confided: 'If money isn't loosened up, this sucker could go down' (in Callinicos, 2010, pp. 93–94). In short, if Congress did not make available this massive package of aid to respond to the liquidity crisis, then the entire capital banking and financial system risked total collapse. The state had to act decisively and quickly to respond to an unprecedented crisis. At the 'epicentre of the problem was the mountain of "toxic" mortgage-backed securities held by banks or marketed to unsuspecting investors all around the world' (Harvey, 2010, p. 2): The 'crash' began, therefore, as the bursting of a speculative bubble in the US housing market associated with the rapid growth of 'predatory lending' during the 1990s and 2000s. However, the expansion of the subprime market had deeper structural roots symbolising the process of financialisation in 'advanced capitalist societies, as even the poorest became identified as worthwhile – that is, profitable – people to lend money to' (Callinicos, 2010, p. 24).

By the autumn of 2008 the crisis had resulted – through change of status, forced mergers or bankruptcy – in the demise of all the major Wall Street investment banks. Most of the world was engulfed as the crisis 'cascaded from one sphere to another and from one geographical location to another, with all manner of knock-on and feedback effects that seemed almost impossible to bring under control, let alone halt and turn back' (Harvey, 2010, p. 38).

The outgoing administration of Bush enacted the Emergency Economic Stabilisation Act 2008. In the UK, the Banking (Special Provisions) Act 2008 provided the government with the power to acquire failing banks and this legislation has been used to bring about the part-nationalisation of a number of banks and associated financial institutions. In France, President Sarkozy declared: 'Laissez faire is finished. The all-powerful market which is always right is finished' (in Callinicos, 2010, p. 5). Such statements and the measures introduced to respond to the crisis seemed to run entirely counter to the rhetoric of neoliberalism and would have been viewed as outlandish by the political mainstream only months previously. The 'very governments at the heart of the deregulated global markets organized mammoth rescues of institutions bankrupted   These amounted to the greatest nationalizations in world history' (Callinicos, 2010, p. 8).

The dominant approach to the 'crisis' evolved into one of 'macro-Keynesianism and micro-neoliberalism' (Callinicos, 2010, p. 129). That is to say, states were mostly willing to intervene financially to safeguard and prop up the corporate banking sector, but workers, the unemployed and other marginalised groups continued to be targeted for punitive and coercive interventions. Indeed, it has been Greece that has faced the most 'radical' experimentation in this regard. The Greek working class has been the targeted for a 'gigantic disciplining operation – a huge experiment in violent downward social mobility and neoliberal adjustment and restructuring' (Stavrakakis, 2013, p. 315). It prompted Dimitris Christoulas, a seventy-seven year-old retired pharmacist, to shoot himself in the head in front of the Parliament building in April 2012. Opposition to vengeful neoliberal economic and social policies also gave rise to the Syriza left coalition. However, after a 'no' vote in the July 2015 referendum rejecting an EU austerity package, the beleaguered Syriza administration simply disregarded it and set about implementing further 'austerity' measures adversely impacting on a range of social work concerns (Pentaraki, 2016). Symbolic also in this respect is the acronym 'PIIGs' (Portugal, Italy, Ireland, Greece and Spain), which has been deployed on one level merely as a shorthand for the

EU's most indebted national economies toward the end of the 2000s, on the other as an insidiously dehumanising metaphor, justifying the use of large number of disenfranchised citizens, as 'guinea pigs' in the EU neoliberal lab (Stavrakakis, 2013, p. 315).

Elsewhere in Europe, the rise in 'welfare chauvinism' has been commented on (Keskinen, Norocel, & Jørgensen, 2016). This refers to the ways in which neo-nationalist and culturally racist parties make use of the welfare state and welfare benefits to draw 'the distinction between "us" and "them" – the natives that are perceived to deserve the benefits and the racialised "others" who are portrayed as undeserving and even exploiting the welfare system at the cost of the "rightful" citizens' (Keskinen et al., 2016, p. 322). Manifestly linked to the material hardships prompted by neoliberalism, 'new forms of hostility' towards migrants and ethnic minorities, observable in many parts of Europe, 'build on and gain their power from the exclusionary nationalist and racialising ideologies, policies and practices that are part of European history' (Keskinen et al., 2016, p. 326). This development might also be connected to the rise of Marine Le Pen and the Front National in France and the AfD in Germany. It is also echoed in the Nordic countries by political formations such as (True) Finn Party, the Danish People's Party and the Sweden Democrats (Norocel, 2016). To differing degrees, such ideological currents and toxic analytics are now lodged within the political mainstream and they cannot solely be discussed in terms of the 'fringe' parties on the political Right.

However, more progressive forces are also mobilising with parties, such as the Bloco de Esquerda – or Left Bloc – in Portugal challenging neoliberal rationality. In the UK, ongoing crisis generated by neoliberalism galvanised groups such as the People's Assembly Against Austerity, the Occupy movement and UK Uncut, as well as more established groups. Jeremy Corbyn's election as Labour Party leader and the party's subsequent performance in the General Election in the summer of 2017 highlight the depth of public antipathy toward the post-'crash' neoliberal agenda and the aspiration to create an alternative socialist 'common sense' (Corbyn, 2018). In the US, the rise Bernie Sanders, the radical US senator who nearly won the Democratic presidential nomination in 2016, also illuminated the growth of a mass movements seeking change (Schram & Pavlovskaya, 2017).

What next? Rhetorically recalibrated neoliberalism (RRN)

Currently, some commentators are claiming that the neoliberal 'moment' has ended (Jacques, 2016). At this current conjuncture, it is certainly possible to identify a discursive reshaping and the emergence of what I refer to as Rhetorically Recalibrated Neoliberalism or RRN. (For a fuller account, see Garrett, 2018c). Essentially, this is a short-hand term to describe attempts to discursively 'repackage' neoliberalism; it is, therefore, a communication or 'messaging' strategies that aspires to disguise the continuing and true intent of the neoliberal project. In this sense, following Bourdieu and Wacquant, we could say it amounts to a politically distracting 'screen discourse' that attempts to mask the brutalism of neoliberalism by providing a new, less harsh, vocabulary and foigned resolve to tackle inequalities (Bourdieu & Wacquant, 2001, p. 4).

In May 2014, this approach was apparent at a high profile conference, organised by the Inclusive Capitalism Initiative, taking place in London. Speakers included key figures, such as Carney (2014) (the Governor of the Bank of England) and Christine Lagarde (the Managing Director of the IMF). This event was co-hosted by Lady Lynn Forester de Rothchild, a member of the famous Rothchild banking dynasty and one of the world's wealthiest families. In attendance were luminaries such Prince Charles and former US president Bill Clinton. A neo-conservative pressure group, the Henry Jackson Society (HJS), was the initiator of the conference and it stated that the 'urgency of the London riots and the on-going effects of the financial crisis, austerity cuts and the Occupy Wall Street movement' had first prompted it to promulgate the notion of 'inclusive capitalism' (Brading, 2012).

In seeking to articulate a new narrative on 'inclusive capitalism' and criticising the concentration of wealth in the hands of a few, Lagarde (2014) referred to the 'need to ingrain a greater social consciousness' that would 'seep into the financial world and forever change the way it does business'.

Carney's contribution was the most extensive mapping of the construct. Setting his ideas against those of 'market fundamentalism', he asserted that only by 'returning to true markets ... can we make capitalism more inclusive' (Carney, 2014, pp. 3–4). However, within this new paradigm, 'business ultimately needs to be seen as a vocation, an activity with high ethical standards, which in turn conveys certain responsibilities' (Carney, 2014, p. 8). If such moves were made, it would lead to the return of a 'more trustworthy, inclusive capitalism ... in which individual virtue and collective prosperity can flourish' (Carney, 2014, p. 10).

Since then, in the UK, it has been maintained that the Brexit vote and the associated 'ructions of 2016 may signal a pivot from punitive to compensatory neoliberalism, as spending cuts and monetary policy reach their political and economic limits' (Watkins, 2016, p. 27). Shifts are clearly detectable in the tonality of policy as this relates to questions pertaining to welfare provision and, more broadly, the role of governments (Elliott & Stewart, 2017). Seemingly, a longing for earlier forms of *nationally* 'embedded liberalism' (Harvey, 2005) has started to seep into the rhetoric deployed by primary definers, such as the UK Prime Minister, Theresa May (2016a). Enunciating the 'new centre ground' of British politics at the Conservative Party conference in October 2016, May (2016b) contended that this was the time for

> a new approach that says while government does not have all the answers, government can and should be a force for good; that the state exists to provide what individual people, communities and markets cannot; and that we should employ the power of government for the good of the people.

If this politics was pursued it would serve to maintain and nurture a 'country of decency, fairness and quiet resolve ... a Great Meritocracy' (May, 2016b). This rhetorical positioning is partly a reaction to challenges from the nationalist Right, within her own party and UKIP, and the insurgent Left within the Labour Party. However, in some respects, this perspective was foreshadowed by some of the narratives circulating around 'inclusive capitalism' in 2014.

In the US, not entirely dissimilar shifts are detectable with the emergence of what Fraser (2016) ironically terms 'progressive' neoliberalism 'celebrating "diversity", meritocracy and "emancipation" while dismantling social protections and re-externalizing social reproduction. The result is not only to abandon defenceless populations to capital's predations, but also to redefine emancipation in market terms' (Fraser, 2016, p. 113). At the level of electoral politics, this form of neoliberalism was embodied, during the 2016 presidential election, by the vapid campaign of the defeated Hillary Clinton (Bernal, Gallegos, McCann, & Solomon, 2017): economically business-as-usual, hawkish overseas, but keen to pursue a liberal social agenda particularly in terms of issues pertaining to gender and sexuality. In Ireland, Prime Minister Leo Varadkar fulfils a similar role; young, from an ethnic minority and gay, his politics are stridently neoliberal and virulently anti-socialist.

Others, however, suggest that neoliberalism is being recalibrated in rather different ways with Davies (2016), for example, arguing that neoliberalism has passed through three stages. A form of 'combative' or insurgent neoliberalism (1979–1989), followed by the 'normative' neoliberalism that began with the fall of the Berlin Wall in 1989 and culminated in the 'crash' of 2008. Since then, neoliberalism can be perceived as entering an unfinished 'punitive' phase in which debt and punishment become more prominent. Perhaps capturing something of the subsequent 'spirit' of the rebarbative and erratic Trump administration, Davies (2016, p. 130) interprets this development as related to the evolution of a 'melancholic condition in which governments and societies unleash hatred and violence'. Moreover, integral to 'punitive' neoliberalism is the decline in mental health, and a public vocabulary inculcating self-blaming.

Conclusion

Some of the developments examined in this article, as is made clear throughout this themed issue inescapably impact on a range of social work concerns. We can certainly make the connections between the abstract theorisation of neoliberalism and what is actually happening in practice, on the ground, in workplaces, homes and communities. As we have seen, this was apparent in terms of the circumstances connected with the Grenfell Tower fire. In this context, the message contained in the SWAN (2017) statement, mentioned earlier, is vital. Practitioners and social work educators should try to 'critique policy, not simply deliver it'. This implies that those located within the field of social work should not simply act as technicians and functionaries merely transmitting pre-package neoliberal policies and practices. Rather, the aspiration should be to critique and challenge them: both within workplaces and as part of the more encompassing movements that are continuing to evolve in opposition to the faltering neoliberal social and economic order.

Disclosure statement

No potential conflict of interest was reported by the author.

References

Aviram, H. (2016). The correctional hunger games. *The ANNALS of the American Academy of Political and Social Science, 664* (1), 260–279.

Baker, J. (2009). Young mothers in late modernity: Sacrifice, respectability and the transformation of the neoliberal subject. *Journal of Youth Studies, 12*(3), 275–288.

Bernal, K., Gallegos, P., McCann, S., & Solomon, N. (2017). *Autopsy: The Democratic Party in crisis.* Retrieved from https://democraticautopsy.org/wp-content/uploads/Autopsy-The-Democratic-Party-In-Crisis.pdf

Bourdieu, P. (2001). *Acts of resistance: Against the new myths of our time.* Cambridge: Polity.

Bourdieu, P., & Wacquant, L. (2001). New liberal speak. *Radical Philosophy, 105,* 2–6.

Brading, F. (2012). *Is the time ripe for a transatlantic response to the crisis in capitalism?* Henry Jackson Society. Retrieved from http://henryjacksonsociety.org/2012/08/10/is-the-time-ripe-for-a-transatlantic-response-to-the-crisis-in-capitalism/

Brenner, N., & Theodore, N. (2002). *Spaces of neoliberalism.* Oxford: Blackwell.

Brown, W. (2015). *Undoing the demos.* New York: Zone Books.

Callinicos, A. (2010, June 20). *Bonfire of illusions.* Cambridge: Polity.

Carney, M. (2014, May 27). *Inclusive capitalism.* Speech at the Conference on Inclusive Capitalism. Retrieved from http://www.bankofengland.co.uk/publications/Documents/speeches/2014/speech731.pdf

Chakrabortty, A. (2017). Over 170 years after Engels, Britain is still a country that murders its poor. *The Guardian,* p. 25.

Clarke, J. (2005). New labour's citizens: Activated, empowered, responsibilized, abandoned?. *Critical Social Policy, 25*(4), 447–463.

Corbyn, J. (2018). Speech at the Labour Party Conference. Retrieved September 26 from https://labour.org.uk/press/jeremy-corbyn-speaking-labour-party-conference-today/

Davies, W. (2016). Neoliberalism 3.0. *New Left Review, 101,* 121–137.

Eagleton-Pierce, M. (2016). *Neoliberalism: Key concepts.* London: Routledge.

Elliott, L., & Stewart, H. (2017, October 12). Time to tax the rich to help the poor, says IMF. *The Guardian,* pp. 1–2.

Fairclough, N., & Graham, P. (2002). Marx as a critical discourse analyst. *Estudios de Sociolinguistica, 3*(1), 185–229.

Financial Conduct Authority. (2017). *FCA reveals findings from its first Financial Lives Survey.* Press release, 18 October. Retrieved from https://www.fca.org.uk/news/press-releases/fca-reveals-findings-from-first-financial-lives-survey

Foucault, M. (2008). *The birth of biopolitics: Lectures at the college de France, 1978-79.* Houndsmill: Palgrave Macmillan.

Fraser, N. (2016). Capital and care. *New Left Review, 100,* 99–119.

Garrett, P. M. (2005). Social work's 'electronic turn': Notes on the deployment of information and communication technologies in social work with children and families. *Critical Social Policy, 25*(4), 529–554.

Garrett, P. M. (2009). *Transforming' children's services? Social work, neoliberalism and the 'modern' world.* Maidenhead: McGraw Hill.

Garrett, P. M. (2014a). Re-enchanting social work? The emerging 'spirit' of social work in an age of economic crisis. *British Journal of Social Work*, 44(3), 503–521.

Garrett, P. M. (2014b). Confronting the 'work society': New conceptual tools for social work. *British Journal of Social Work*, 44(7), 1682–1699.

Garrett, P. M. (2015a). Neoliberalism and 'welfare'. In the shadow of the prison'. In R. Sheehan and J. Ogloff (Eds.), *Working with the forensic paradigm: Cross-discipline approaches for policy and practice* (pp. 85–98). Abingdon: Routledge.

Garrett, P. M. (2015b). Constraining and confining ethnic minorities: Impoverishment and the logics of control in neoliberal Ireland. *Patterns of Prejudice*, 49(4), 414–434.

Garrett, P. M. (2016). Confronting neoliberal penality: Placing prison reform and critical criminology at the core of social work's social justice agenda. *Journal of Social Work*, 16(1), 83–103.

Garrett, P. M. (2018a). Social work and Marxism: A short essay on the 200th anniversary of the birth of Karl Marx. *Critical and Radical Social Work*, 6(2), 179–196.

Garrett, P. M. (2018b). Revisiting 'The Birth of Biopolitics': Foucault's account of neoliberalism and the remaking of social policy. *Journal of Social Policy*. Published online on 17 September. doi:10.1017/S0047279418000582

Garrett, P. M. (2018c). *Welfare words: Critical social work and social policy*. London: Sage.

Good Gingrich, L. (2010). Single mothers, work(fare), and managed precariousness. *Journal of Progressive Human Services*, 21, 107–135.

Gray, M., Dean, M., Agllias, K., Howard, A., & Schubert, L. (2015). Perspectives on neoliberalism for the human service professions. *Social Service Review*, 89(2), 368–392.

Grenfell Action Group. (2016). *KCTMO – Playing with fire! Post on 20 November*. Retrieved from https://grenfellactiongroup.wordpress.com/2016/11/20/kctmo-playing-with-fire/

Harman, C. (2008). Theorising neoliberalism. *International Socialism*, 117, 25–49.

Harvey, D. (2005). *A brief history of neoliberalism*. Oxford: Oxford University.

Harvey, D. (2006). *Spaces of global capitalism*. London: Verso.

Harvey, D. (2010). *The enigma of capital*. London: Verso.

Hobsbawm, E. (2008, October 9). The £500bn question. *The Guardian*, p. 28.

Hutton, W. (2018, January 21). Capitalism's new crisis: After Carillion, can the private sector ever be trusted?. *The Observer*. Retrieved from https://www.theguardian.com/politics/2018/jan/21/capitalism-new-crisis-can-private-sector-be-trusted-carillion-privatisation

Jacques, M. (2008, January 18). Northern Rock's rescue is part of a geopolitical sea change. *The Guardian*, p. 23.

Jacques, M. (2016, August 21). The death of neoliberalism and the crisis in western politics. *The Observer*. Retrieved from https://www.theguardian.com/commentisfree/2016/aug/21/death-of-neoliberalism-crisis-in-western-politics

Keskinen, S., Norocel, O. C., & Jørgensen, M. B. (2016). The politics and policies of welfare chauvinism under the economic crisis. *Critical Social Policy*, 36(3), 321–329.

Klein, N. (2007). *The shock doctrine: The rise of disaster capitalism*. London: Allen Lane.

Lagarde, C. (2014, May 27). *Economic inclusion and financial integrity*. Speech at conference on Inclusive Capitalism. Retrieved from https://www.imf.org/external/np/speeches/2014/052714.htm

Lorenz, W. (2005). Social work and a new social order – challenging neo-liberalism's erosion of solidarity. *Social Work & Society*, 3(1), Retrieved from http://socwork.net/Lorenz2005.pdf

Mahmud, T. (2012). Debt and discipline. *American Quarterly*, 64(3), 469–494.

May, T. (2016a, July 13). *Speech on becoming Prime Minister*. Retrieved from https://www.gov.uk/government/speeches/statement-from-the-new-prime-minister-theresa-may

May, T. (2016b, October 5). *The good that government can do: Speech to the Conservative Party Conference*. Retrieved from http://press.conservatives.com/

Munck, R. (2005). Neoliberalism and politics, and the politics of neoliberalism. In A. Saad-Filho, & D. Johnston (Eds.), *Neoliberalism: A critical reader* (pp. 60–70). London: Pluto.

Myers, E. (2017). The non-scandal of American oligarchy. *Theory & Event*, 20(2), 296–328.

Norocel, O. C. (2016). Populist radical right protectors of the *folkhem*: Welfare chauvinism in Sweden. *Critical Social Policy*, 36(3), 371–390.

Oxfam. (2017). *An economy for the 99%*. Retrieved from https://www.oxfam.org/sites/www.oxfam.org/files/file_attachments/bp-economy-for-99-percent-160117-en.pdf

Oxfam America. (2016, April 14). *Broken at the top*. Media Briefing. Retrieved from http://www.oxfamamerica.org/static/media/files/Broken_at_the_Top_FINAL_EMBARGOED_4.12.2016.pdf

Peck, J. (2010). *Constructions of neoliberal reason*. Oxford: Oxford University.

Pentaraki, M. (2016). I am in a constant state of insecurity trying to make ends meet, like our service users. *British Journal of Social Work*. doi:10.1093/bjsw/bcw099

Pratt, J., Brown, D., Brown, M., Hallsworth, S., & Morrison, W. (2005). Introduction. In J. Pratt, D. Brown, M. Brown, S. Hallsworth, & W. Morrison (Eds.), *The new punitiveness: Trends, theories and perspectives* (pp. xi–1). Devon: Willan.

Pyles, L., Svistova, J., & Ahn, A. (2017). Securitization, racial cleansing, and disaster capitalism: Neoliberal disaster governance in the US gulf coast and Haiti. *Critical Social Policy*, 37(4), 582–603.

Roets, G., Roose, R., Claes, L., Vandekinderen, C., Van Hove, G., & Vadnerplasschen, W. (2012). Reinventing the employable citizen: A perspective for social work. *British Journal of Social Work, 42*(1), 94–110.

Rose, N. (2000). Government and control. *British Journal of Criminology, 40,* 321–339.

Schram S. F., & Pavlovskaya, M. (Eds.) (2017). *Rethinking neoliberalism.* New York: Routledge.

Social Work Action Network. (2017, July 4). *SWAN statement on the Grenfell disaster: Social work must critique policy not simply deliver it.* Retrieved from http://socialworkfuture.org/articles-resources/uk-articles/567-swan-statement-on-the-grenfell-disaster-social-work-must-critique-policy-not-simply-deliver-it

Standing, G. (2011). *The precariat.* London: Bloomsbury Academic.

Stavrakakis, Y. (2013). Dispatches from the Greek lab: Metaphors, strategies and debt in the European crisis. *Psychoanalysis, Culture & Society, 18*(3), 313–324.

Therborn, G. (2007). After dialectics: Radical social theory in a post-communist world. *New Left Review, 43,* 63–117.

Thompson, G. (2008). Are we all neoliberals now? 'Responsibility' and corporations. *Soundings, 39,* 67–74.

Trust for London. (2017, October 8). *27% of Londoners in poverty.* Press notice. Retrieved from https://www.trustforlondon.org.uk/news/27-londoners-poverty/

UBS/PWC. (2017). *New value creators gain momentum: Billionaires insights 2017.* Retrieved from https://www.pwc.com/gx/en/financial-services/Billionaires%20insights/billionaires-insights-2017.pdf

Venugopal, R. (2015). Neoliberalism as concept. *Economy and Society, 44*(2), 165–187.

Wacquant, L. (2009). *Punishing the poor: The neoliberal government of social insecurity.* London: Duke University.

Walmsley, R. (2017). *World prison population list.* 11th ed. Institute of Criminal Policy Research. Retrieved from http://www.icpr.org.uk/media/41356/world_prison_population_list_11th_edition.pdf

Watkins, S. (2016). Casting off? *New Left Review, 100,* 5–33.

Neoliberalism as an art of governance: reflecting on techniques for securing life through direct social work practice

Neoliberalism als eine art und weise der Regierung: reflektieren auf die Techniken die das leben sicher machen durch direkte Sozialarbeitspraxis

Uschi Bay

ABSTRACT

Neoliberalism is a diffuse and contested term; however, as an art of government, drawing on Foucault's theorising, it posits personal responsibility as the basis of an ethical society. Neoliberalism mostly governs individuals through their freedom, where the concept of freedom presupposes a rational self that is motivated to improve and secure their life now and in the future. For those who are unable or unwilling to participate in securing a decent lifestyle within the norms of society, systematic modifications including social welfare policies that are punitive and freedom-depriving are used to attempt to modify individuals' behaviour. Direct social work practice with individuals also relies on individual autonomy as one of its central technologies guiding individuals towards choices that will improve their lives. Social work practitioners are seen to be part of an enabling network that assists individuals who are considered self-excluded due to their irresponsible choices to work on themselves to form an 'entrepreneurial self'. Social workers engage in the neoliberal art of governance through the 'conduct of conduct' of self and others in their direct practice with people. If individuals are understood as constituted through networks of power relations, then direct social work using a pastoral relationship can be a node of power where understanding of whom they are 'made to be' can enable engaging in individual and collective resistance to some of the perversions of neoliberal governance. Through pastoral care, resistance as both 'conduct of conduct' and 'counter conduct' is possible and necessary.

ABSTRAKT

Neoliberalism ist ein diffus und bestrittener Begriff, aber als art und weise der regierung, genohmen von Foucault's theroretisieren, setzt es die persoenliche verantwortung als den Grund einer ethischer Gesellschaft. Neoliberalism meistens reguliert durch die Freiheit jedem Einzelnen. Der Begriff von deiser Freiheit nimmt als selbstverständlich ein vernünftiges Selbst. Ein Selbst das motiviert ist sich zu verbessern und das sein Leben sicher machen will, heute und auch in der Zukunft. Für diejenigen wo nicht mitmachen kønnen oder die nicht bereit sind eine Anståndigkeit zu sichern innerhalb der Normen der Gesellschaft, gibt es systematische Änderungen, einschließlich von Sozialhilfe Richtlinien, die beide Bestrafung und Freiheit verwenden um individuelles Verhalten zu modifizieren. Direkte Sozialarbeitspraxis mit Individuen setzt auch auf individuelle Autonomie, eine von den zentrale Technologien, die den Einzelnen leiten zu Entscheidungen, das Ihr Leben verbessern würden. Sozialarbeiter engagieren in der neoliberal Kunst der Governance in ihrer direkte Praxis mit Menschen. Sozialarbeit benutzt pastorale Beziehungen und diese kønnen einen Knoten der Macht sein, wo das Verståndnis von wem wir 'gemacht sein sollen' erklårt wird und auch wo der individueller und kollektiver Widerstand ermøglicht würden kønnte. Widerstand zu insbesondere Perversionen von Neoliberalism sind øfter notwendig. Durch eine pastorale Beziehung konnte der Widerstand gegen beide die erwarteten verhaltungsweisen und die gegenverhaltungsweisen ermøglicht und notwendig gemacht.

Geopolitically, neoliberalism is variegated as a type of economic policy and framework for regulating labour relations and promoting 'free' markets. In the United Kingdom, United States, Australia and New Zealand there are differing historical accounts given of the rise of neoliberalism in public policy. However, even though neoliberalism is variable across different countries, recent research by Spolander et al. (2014, p. 305) indicates some common features across several EU and non-EU countries' social work contexts and practice. These features are an increasing marginalisation of service recipients and users, reductions in preventative services and a rise in managerialist supervision and management processes. Further, the framing of public service provision as competitive and as operating through market-like arrangements means that social work practice is now operating in settings that commodify and instrumentalise all engagements and tends to regard many interactions as primarily economic exchanges. Non-Government Organisations (NGOs) are also drawn into these security and regulatory strategies of governments (for an Australian example see Bay, 2008) and do not escape similar commodification and economic exchanges in framing their practices.

Neoliberalism is considered to link with capitalism in ways that further disenfranchise and marginalise those people who are already positioned at the margins of society. In social work it is common to critique neoliberalism for promoting a so-called 'free' market ideology and to resent the encroachment of a market logic into the provision of social and human services, governing policies and programme practices (Ferguson, 2007). Particularly, the inevitable creation of winners and losers that accompanies this neoliberal move, including the growing depth of poverty or on-going austerity suffered by many people, is often blamed by social work authors on the last two decades of neoliberal policies within these EU and OECD (Organisation for Economic Co-operation and Development) countries (see, for instance, Beddoe, 2014; Dominelli 1999; Healy, 2012; Mitendorf & van Ewijk, 2015). An increasing focus on the precarity of those targeted ar either not performing for society, by not contributing to it in maximally economically productive ways, or those who are considered to break the law, can signify being abandoned and possibly no longer provided for by the state. In some countries even the bare minimum of security and safety offered in the past through the welfare state are no longer guaranteed (Layton, 2010), or, as is the case in some of the neo-paternalistic and punitive policy responses to the 'failing subject' (Hyslop, 2016), they force various groups into arrangements that are intolerable. There are many examples of these kinds of policy responses impacting very negatively on marginalised groups, such as income management forced on remote Aboriginal communities in Australia (Arthur, 2015).

In this paper I will briefly outline the way that social workers have engaged with neoliberalism as context before turning to a fuller discussion of Foucault's notion of neoliberalism as an art of governance, including some of his thinking around pastoral care. Then, I will explore how neoliberal subjectivity is constituted generally, including the new relations of freedom and fear within the discourses of risk and failure. I aim to prepare the ground for discussing how to conceptualise direct social work practice to clarify the use of 'counter-conduct' (Davies, 2005) through refusing and resisting certain aspects of neoliberal subjectivity. The aim of unpacking some of the power relations in direct social work practice is to engender new ways of connecting with oneself and others that respect human vulnerability, precarious existence, connection, dependency and interdependence (Layton, 2010, p. 312; Weir, 2013).

Neoliberalism as context for social work practice

Any changes in welfare regimes or in political rationalities 'will shape the way in which social work is constituted and practiced' (Wallace & Pease, 2011, p. 133). Social work is often positioned as struggling against neoliberalism and its techniques such as managerialism in many settings (Hyslop, 2016; Bay, 2011). Resistance to neoliberalism is particularly evident in the strand of social work theorising referred to as critical social work (Baines, 2007). For instance, 'Baines's research demonstrated that social workers feel strongly impacted by numerous constraints on their work at both the macro-structural level of the policy and organizational context and the micro-interpersonal level' (Wallace & Pease, 2011, p. 133). Further, McDonald (2005) found feminist models were replaced with pathologising and individualising models of clinical case management in domestic violence services (as cited in Wallace & Pease, 2011, p. 138). This means that especially at the micro level of social work practice, in the relation to governing ourselves and governing others (a pastoral care relation), that the incursion of neoliberal rationality as an art of government needs serious attention.

Wallace and Pease (2011, p. 137) propose that some social workers, distressed by the types of changes in service delivery designs, retreated to therapeutic and clinical work to attempt to ignore these changes. My argument in this paper is that it is not possible to escape or ignore neoliberalism, both its logic and the governing practices associated with it, in direct social work. Neoliberalism cannot be escaped or ignored because the insecurity, increasing inequality and complexity of people's lives created or produced by 'precarious neoliberal capitalism' (Brunila & Valero, 2018) are expressed and experienced as our daily struggles and also form and shape our subjectivity as we adapt to these norms. The dominant effect of increasing individualism and self-responsibilisation is anxiety and over-stress (Brunila & Valero, 2018, p. 77). The frequent requests by governments and agencies for clients/service beneficiaries and social workers to account for themselves in the use of their time, their productiveness and effectiveness, to demonstrate they can cope or be resilient, is intensifying and further constitute neoliberal subjectivities. Neoliberal subjectivities require individuals to relate to themselves in an enterprising way, as self-sufficient, while totally denying the human condition of interdependence. This denial of the interdependence of people, with each other and the planet, and the disregard for the notion of needs in neoliberal political rationality, promote a relation to the self that sees 'survival as an individual responsibility'(Davies, 2005, p. 9). When social workers leave out neoliberal political rationality as the current context in responding to clients in clinical or therapeutic settings, the separation of 'the psychic and the social' are reinforced. This separation is one of the problematic contentions of neoliberal individualism (Layton, 2010, p. 317).

Further, Wallace and Pease (2011) conclude that some view social workers as ambiguous about neoliberalism and as, at times, unable to step outside it, in order to critique it. This may be partly due to the pervasiveness of neoliberal thought and the acceptance of many of its logics as common sense (Harvey, 2007). This ambivalence or ambiguousness also relates to the way vulnerability and fear are simultaneously stoked by governments and the media. It is treated as shameful to reveal any vulnerability or needs in neoliberal times (Layton, 2010, p. 311).

Davies (2005, p. 9) argues that 'vulnerability is closely tied to individual responsibility'. This vulnerability is further tied to the notion that 'workers are disposable and there is no obligation on the part of the 'social fabric' to take care of the disposed' (cited in Brunila & Valero, 2018, p. 84). Sennett (2006, p. 181) adds that indifferent institutional order breeds 'low levels of informal trust and high levels of anxiety about uselessness'. Most neoliberal subjects are engaged in activities that assure their survival particularly their economic survival. Neoliberalism as a political rationality tries to render the social domain economic and links a reduction in (welfare) state services and security systems to the increasing call for 'personal responsibility' and 'self-care" (Lemke, 2001, p. 203). Social workers are also precariously placed in relation to their own economic survival and not immune from these intensifying pressures to secure their roles and positions. Indeed, some like Rose (1999), argue that therapeutic cultures such as 'psychology and psychoanalysis helped constitute the neoliberal subject' (as cited in Clare, 2017, p. 29) through the focus on self-care and self-responsibility.

Direct social work practice aims to shape individuals and guide their behaviour and feelings, their actions and interpersonal relations as well as their self-relating through various techniques and processes. Layton (2010, p. 318) describes that in her clinical practice from a psychoanalytic perspective, neoliberal political rationality calls forth perverse defenses that mean clients/ service beneficiaries fluctuate between fantasies of 'omnipotent self-sufficiency and the cynical or apathetic sense of helplessness'. Neoliberalism as a political rationality does not recognise limits, and individuals in this context can thus oscillate between 'fantasies of having it all' and deep disappointments that leave them feeling helpless and victimised (Layton, 2010, p. 316). It is my contention that Foucault's theorising of neoliberalism as an art of governance may assist social workers in identifying and resisting concentrations of power, to struggle against powers effects even as these are embedded in pastoral and disciplinary power relations.

Neoliberalism as an art of governance

Social workers in direct practice are enmeshed in neoliberalism both as a rationality of government and as an art of government. Foucault uses the term government in a very broad sense as an activity that aims to shape and guide individuals to behave or act or comport themselves in particular ways. Modern government is understood to be exercised through 'institutions, procedures, analyses, reflections, calculations and tactics' (Foucault, 1991). It includes the relation of the self with the self, private interpersonal relations and relations concerned with the exercise of political sovereignty. In short, governmentality is concerned, according to Foucault (2008), with the way one 'conducts the conducts' of people, including how one shapes one's own conduct. Governmentality in effect indicates the interlinking between micro effects of power (including technologies of self – how we relate to ourselves) with macro strategies of power.

Neoliberalism as an art of governance focuses on technologies of security, technologies of fear and 'technologies of the self'. 'In the context of neoliberalism, fear is the basis and motive for the constitution of the responsible, reliable and rational self' (Lemke, 2014, p. 68). The enterprising self is constantly aware of economic, climatic, social and emotional risks. Fear of failure is cultivated to increase a sense of vulnerability and precarity in the individual, marginalised group and/or at the population level. This means that social workers and service users in various settings are dealing with the insecurity, fear of failure and anxiety and self-doubting this elicits in their relations to themselves and with others. As Lemke (2014, p. 69) states, technologies of fear promote an 'individual retreat to privacy' and 'coping with fear becomes a problem of individual psychology or a medical issue' rather than about social relations of mutual care and shared benefits. This retreat into individual privacy means there is an inability to see, for instance, so called mental health problems as anything other than a problem of individual psychology or as a medical issue needing medicating. Many consider their anxiety and stress to reflect a 'personal problem or deficit' rather than the outcome of increasing precarity in economic circumstances.

Neoliberalism as an art of governance focuses on individuals and technologies of the self. Social workers in direct practice are in effect supporting and steering individuals' active engagement, encouraging their hopes, inspiring their desires, stimulating their creativity, enhancing their autonomy and promoting their productivity (Foucault, 2008). Neoliberalism as an art of governance highlights the power relations in direct practice that are effected through what Foucault considers pastoral care. The direct relationship between social workers and clients/service beneficiaries within the context of neoliberalism as an art of governance also allows us to critique 'what we say and how we think', as well as 'our commitments and obligations', and to learn about 'the kinds of truths about ourselves we rely upon and reinforce in the process of doing so' (Hamann, 2009, p. 58).

Pastoral power

Foucault (1983) claims that since the beginning of the eighteenth century the modern state integrated the individual into government through pastoral power. The development of the modern welfare states, according to Foucault, must be understood as the interplay of two strategies of power encapsulated in a 'city-citizen game' that involves the self-governing capacities of free persons in a political community and a 'shepherd-flock game' concerning the needy, obedient individual. Foucault describes four unique characteristics of pastoral power:

> it seeks to deliver the individual to salvation; it is prepared to sacrifice itself for the life of the flock; it is equally concerned for the one as for the many, the part and the whole; it requires knowledge of the conscience, the inside of people's minds. (Foucault, 1983, p. 214)

Although salvation has now been replaced with norms of health, wellbeing and security in this life for most governmental interventions, it is the deviance from norms that 'attracts the attention of the 'pastor' or draws in 'mechanism of security' supposedly in order to act for the benefit of the individual or group (Mayes, 2016, p. 24). In direct social work practice this mechanism 'dovetails discipline and control with ethics and freedom' (Mayes, 2016, p. 25).

Pastoral care historically is associated with the Judeo-Christian pastor who is attributed by Foucault to be the first to seek to govern a people as distinct from a territory (Mayes, 2016, p. 25). This opens up the possibility for governing various sub populations within the same political territory say of the nation State differently, and as Foucault argued in his *Security, territory, population* (2007) lecture series that it was through state racism that specific population groups were 'separated off from the normal population for specific and unique strategies of containment and correction' (Binkley, 2016, p. 182). It is this kind of logic that reinforces the separation of population groups 'for the purposes of specialized modes of government' (Binkley, 2016, p. 182). Social workers are aware of the way marginalised groups are divided from the 'normal population' and treated differently using governmental strategies that are often punitive and oppressive.

This differential treatment and public indifference to certain groups' suffering has a psychic effect on the population as a whole. Social workers in direct practice may find that clients/ service beneficiaries are defended against the feelings of 'abandonment, helplessness, and vulnerability with the 'lie' of self-sufficiency' (Layton, 2010, p. 312). Self-sufficiency is the neoliberal norm, and many people shape their subjectivity in relation to their inner world rather than the wider world in a reaction to the lack of social solidarity evident in social, political and institutional arrangements. Paradoxically this reaction to neoliberalism opens individuals up to be even more governable through technologies of the self and learning the right way to present oneself (Brunila & Valero, 2018).

Pastoral power and political power were more or less linked to each other, according to |Foucault (1983, 2008), especially in relation to the 'conduct of conduct' in the family, medicine, psychiatry, education and employment (among others) and in reference to such life experiences as madness, illness, deaths, crime and sexuality. Foucault (1982, p, 789) refers to the 'government of children, of souls, of communities, of families, of the sick'. In modern times pastoral relations of care/government are continued through the interpersonal relationship of the 'analyst-analysand, doctor-patient, teacher-student, counselor-patient and so on' (McGuishin, 2007, p. 205). Care mediates this relationship between the pastor and each individual (McGushin, 2007, p. 201). It is out of care for oneself that 'an individual submits to the authority of the pastor in order to save himself in order to be led to his own salvation', according to McGushin (2007, p. 201). Pastoral power is thus a productive power that produces subjects. It is also a power that we exercise on ourselves as well as we let it be exercised on or over us. Clearly, social work relationships with clients in direct practice can be understood to be part of the government of individuals using care of the self as an aspect of pastoral power.

Pastoral power presumes that we have relations with 'ourselves as hidden texts' that need to be 'interpreted' by the pastor (analyst, doctor, teacher, counsellor, social worker) in order for us to be healed (Foucault, 1983). Clients can only be cared for if the pastor/social worker knows the individual client precisely and is aware of the condition of the intimate details of their life and life events. This knowledge is attained through the technique of confession, also an earlier Christian practice that morphed and changed over time and forms the basis of the caring relationship between the social worker and the client in a direct counselling relationship. Foucault (1983, pp. 201–202) discusses how

> this form of power cannot be exercised without knowing the inside of people's minds, without exploring their souls, without making them reveal their innermost secrets. It [also] implies a knowledge of the conscience and an ability to direct it.

In a sense when social workers undertake an assessment of a client or family the accumulation of detailed knowledge collected from and about the client and family feeds into the power relations evident in pastoral power. Foucault considers the confession as a 'powerful technology' that asks individuals to express their feelings and thoughts, and to discuss their deeds. The social worker in a pastoral like role uses this knowledge drawn from the client to guide and instruct the client towards taking care of their own selves through 'vigilant self-attention'. Confessional techniques focus on the articulation of the truth of the

Client's life, identity and their relationship to themselves and to others.

Thus the pastorate is an individualising power and individuals are led to take care of themselves through acknowledging the truth about themselves in front of the social worker. This articulation of the truth about oneself is considered to be highly significant in the previous religious confessional and is also reminiscent of psychodynamic understandings used in social work counselling practice. Pastoral power is often understood as a caring relation in social work where the individual or group is encouraged to 'confess' to learn the truth about themselves and to open up to the 'expert' who can 'interpret the significance and the meaning of the confession' (Mayes, 2009, p. 8). This intimate knowledge of service users' lives is considered necessary for social workers to develop assessments and to undertake counselling among other techniques in the art of mediating the needs of the 'clients and the demands of "the systems"' (Hyslop, 2016, p. 8).

It is the pastor/social worker/expert through their very being, nature, virtue, training, knowledge and spiritual life (broadly defined) who is said to know the truth of the individual and what is necessary for the individual client, family or group to produce good habits and to transform their way of thinking and living (McGushin, 2007). Self-reflexivity by social workers and their clients is important in relation to the norms, expectations and also limitations of neoliberalism. Hence, pastoral power can be exercised to reinforce neoliberal subjectivities and neoliberal governance or it can also be used to resist neoliberal governance and neoliberal subjectivities.

Reinforcing and resisting neoliberal subjectivity

There has been little empirical research into the psychic life of the neoliberal subject (Scharff, 2016, p. 107). In order to explore how to exercise pastoral power to reinforce or resist neoliberal subjectivity, I will draw on recent research that aims to explore how 'neoliberalism is lived out on a subjective level' (Scharff, 2016). Scharff focused her research on the lives of 64 female classically-trained musicians living in London and Berlin, but originally from various national backgrounds. Although this group may be particularly positioned through their vocation in neoliberal ways, the research offers some insights that are helpful in thinking about resisting and reconstituting ourselves in ways that are alternative or counter to neoliberal political subjectivity. As Allen (2011, p. 51) states this relation to ourselves is always limited and 'although deliberate self-transformation is a practice [of] freedom', such practices of 'freedom always involves strategically reworking the power relations to which we are subjected'. The following research provides a sense of how neoliberal subjectivities become normalised and the difficulties presented by the on-going vulnerabilities individuals are likely to experience without collective support. I am proposing caring relations with clients/ service beneficiaries that are mutually self-reflexive about the limitations and effects of neoliberal political rationality, arts of governance and related subjectivities.

Firstly, Scharff (2016) identified that young women musicians were doubly constituted as neoliberal subjects. It seemed that 'women are required to work on and transform' themselves in regard to 'every aspect of their conduct' to a 'greater extent than men' while presenting 'all their actions as freely chosen' (Gill & Scharff, 2011, p. 7). This implies that the work in constituting a neoliberal subjectivity as a young woman musician required a focus and determination to transform one's self into the kind of subjectivity that can be self-managing, self-sufficient, self-promoting, free of injury, to present as a freely choosing subject at all times; to show oneself able to cope with rejection and failure, as well as positioned to disavow any inequalities or structural impediments that may prevent their career success or economic survival (Scharff, 2016).

These young women further presented themselves as neoliberal subjects in that they called themselves a business (Scharff, 2016, p. 111). They related to themselves as an enterprise, as an enterprising and ambitious individual calculating their risks and gains, accountable to themselves for their successes and losses. This meant they had to take on 'personal responsibility above and beyond particular specific circumstances' (Du Gay, 1996). This indicates there was a significant shift from a 'liberal vision of people owning themselves as though *they were property* [with the logic of exchanging work for income] to a neoliberal vision of people owning themselves as though *they were a business*' (Gershon, 2011, as cited in Scharff, 2016, p. 112, my italics). This shift indicates one of the key differences between classical liberal and neoliberal subjectivities. Rather than only sell their time and skills to an employer, this new relation is far different in scope and effect. And although this vision of treating themselves as a business could be understood as potentially promoting their freedom and independence and thus as empowering, it also responsibilises and individualises each of the young women to secure their own livelihood across their career on their own. This isolation increasing their risks and vulnerability, and shifts their success solely to winning in the market place. This positioning is in line with current neoliberal subjectivities and to resist this type of neoliberal subjectivity involves relations of care with others, which can establish new modes of living together' (Mayes, 2016, p. 133).

Further, the young women's perception of time and their habits of continual self-improvement and constant activity shows us how every part of our lives and subjectivity are structured (Read, 2009, p. 34). The research participants in Scharff's study reported that their constant activity led to feelings that there is never any 'time for anything'. This sense of never having any time for anything Conlin (2014, p. 271) states, is a new sense of temporality within neoliberal subjectivity where the 'ceaseless production and consumption' 'requires 24/7 temporalities' that 'erases the division between work and non-work time', and the 'distinctions between everyday life and structured institutional environments'.

In effect, to fit the demands of a neoliberal subjectivity it is important to be activated and continually striving for self-improvement and through these processes to at least give the appearance of self-maximisation and self-optimisation. All the technologies of self (self-monitoring, planning, innovating, prioritising) produce what Gill refers to as the '"responsibilised" subject, who requires little management, but can be accorded the "autonomy" to manage herself, in a manner that is a far more effective exercise of power' (Gill, 2009, as cited in Conlin, 2014, p. 275). However, these elements of 'autonomy', maximum productivity and effectiveness in securing and managing life are not fully possessed by anyone. The fact that a neoliberal subjectivity cannot be perfectly attained because the 'inadequate subjects must always do more' is part of the seductiveness and a constant invitation to engage in technologies of the self, including those that promote self-improvement and self-care in order to perhaps address the 'almost continual feelings of insufficiency' and inadequacy that accompany this type of subjectivity (Conlin, 2014, p. 276). This feeling of lack means that neoliberal subjectivity is always opening itself up to being governable, thus making ourselves into 'someone who is eminently governable' (Foucault, 2008, p. 270).

Counter-conduct

Pastoral care relations, like those that operate in direct social work practice, may be able to encourage new relations of the self to the self and with others that work at the limits of experience and experiment (Blencowe, 2012). This in effect means devising a new ontology (a being) and epistemology (a way of knowing) the self in this time and place, counter to neoliberal norms and its arts of governance. Hence as social workers this is not so much celebrating romantic individualism or heroic mysticism as fostering 'the intrinsic creativity of everyone's impetus and capacity to constitute a difference ... in themselves, their environment and other people' (Blencowe, 2012, p. 23). This means engaging in the present moment in a way that allows for depth and expansion in ways that promote or constitute 'a politicization of present relations and the proliferation of contingency' (Blencowe, 2012, p. 24). Through pastoral power, individual clients and social workers can 'reflect on who they are and constitute themselves otherwise' as such pastoral power holds the 'promise of a self-reflexive practice of freedom to transform oneself' (McCall, 2010, pp. 581–582). 'But when it remains stuck within the confines of cognitive behavior or neurolinguistics (re)programming interventions it risks trapping us with the very neoliberal logics that are in need of critique' (Gill, 2017, p. 12)

According to Foucault (1983), bringing into the question of power relations the relationship to freedom is a permanent political task. This is particularly pertinent in relation to neoliberalism which promotes a particular relationship to freedom and security for the state, service providers and clients that is potentially perverse in some of its effects. The way in which 'these new regimes get inside us, shape our sense of self, produce particular affects and subjectivities, erode collectivity and collaboration, promote completion' (Gill, 2017, p. 14), identifies technologies of self and care of the self as an important site for counter-conduct.

Foucault's theorising suggests that pastoral power, exercised through a relationship that an individual person could establish with a social worker, can provide an avenue for subject formation in resistance to particular forms of subjectivity, such as a neoliberal subjectivity (Mayes, 2016). Neoliberal subjectivity cannot be resisted solely through refusal, rather it requires individuals to willingly participate in making daily changes, which can also generate feelings of pleasure and empowerment (Mayes, 2016). The role of the social worker as a pastoral figure is 'to help create a social environment that supports resilience to unrealistic expectations' (Beausoleil, 2009, as cited in Mayes, 2016, p. 141). '[T]hese relations may not only encourage ways to resist certain strategies and norms, but also model new ways of life that disrupt' these norms (Mayes, 2016, p. 141). This reformation of the subject is not an individual process but is achieved through relationship and collectivities (Mayes, 2016, p. 143). Through developing a critical ethos, social workers in their engagement with clients can open up new possibilities and collectively explore new modes of living together.

Some of the flavour of this kind of resistance, Conlin (2014, p. 79) suggests, would consist of an 'enthusiasm for collective decision-making, resourcefulness, informality and playfulness' as well as temporally being out of sync with neoliberalism and using outdated modes and ways of being to 're-experience the self and everyday life'. For instance, Berardi (2011 as cited in Conlin, 2014, p. 276) explored our relations to digital communicative organisation and highlighted that the continual disruption of it impacts negatively on 'our ability to cohere as subjects and to bond with each other'. Further, he argues that this continual disruption induces over-excited emotional systems that produces panic-like effects and 'competitive aggression' (as cited in Conlin, 2014, p. 276) Social workers in direct practice in many settings may wish to reconsider these effects and build on the abilities that mean we can cohere as subjects, narrate our ethics and values, and (re)bond with each other.

Social workers are not immune to neoliberal pressures and institutional violence. Social workers through analysing neoliberalism as an art of governance can develop an 'active awareness of how relations of institutional and interpersonal power shape processes of communication and under-standing' (Hyslop, 2016, p. 8). To resist neoliberal subjectivity involves relations of care with others, which can establish new modes of living together' (Mayes, 2016, p. 133). In this way 'pastoral relations can be redeployed as an ethical care of the self' (p. 134). For instance, 'Esposito points to this possi-bility in writing that the pastoral relationship can support power and increase it, but also ... resist power and oppose it' (2008, as cited in Mayes, 2016, p. 139). Hence, how social workers use pastoral power in direct practice can either support neoliberal governance and increase its intensity or enable resistance to specific tactics and goals through an attitude of critique that is 'distinct from judgment precisely because it expresses a sceptical to questioning approach to the rules and rationality that serve as the basis for judgment' (Hamann, 2009, p. 57). This critique involves exploring the modes of our practices that we accept as dominant, or normal, to show that we cannot take these neoliberal assumptions as self-evident and to continually challenge our ways of thinking.

Conclusion

Neoliberalism as an art of governance stimulates fear, anxiety and shame as mechanisms of security that focuses individuals on making 'present choices out of a concern for future consequences' (Mayes, 2016, p, 42). In this way Mayes (2016) argues that '[f]reedom and security dovetail into one another such that 'freedom is nothing else but the correlative of the deployment of apparatuses of security ... [which] cannot operate well except on condition that it is given freedom (Foucault, 2007, p. 48). Freedom in neoliberalism is arranged and limited by so called 'free choice' with the only responsible or sensible choice being the predetermined choice that promotes health and secur-ity (Mayes, 2016 p. 42). Neoliberalism in effect creates a certain type of freedom that is then duly devoured by neoliberalism. To reclaim freedom paradoxically 'does not come easily: we need to be "made free" in order to participate in the freedoms available' (Bondi, 2005, p. 512). Neoliberal sub-jectivity renders us governable through our capacities. To fully grasp these capacities and redo our freedom, requires a work upon the conditions of life and on our intrinsic creativity to constitute a difference in our selves, in our environment and with others.

Neoliberalism as a political rationality and institutional rationality disposes social workers to con-sider their actions in relation to the imposition of this new order or the *dispositif* that works at 'forcing the subject into a stance of competitive differentiation, livelihood and opportunism' (Binkley, 2011, p. 88). An analysis of neoliberalism as an art of governance assists social workers to understand the way new subjectivities are composed, operationalised and constituted in differential ways. As social workers in direct or micro practice are often positioned in a pastoral care role with clients/ service beneficiaries and service users, it is worthwhile to continually explore these power relations as a flexible and adaptable mechanism for the 'conduct of conduct' and also as a site for 'counter-conduct', to elaborate a variety of different ethical ways of being with oneself, with others and with the world.

Disclosure statement

No potential conflict of interest was reported by the author.

References

Allen, A. (2011). Foucault and the politics of our selves. *History of the Human Sciences, 24*(4), 43–59.

Arthur, D. (2015). *Income management: A quick guide.* Parliamentary Library, Parliament of Australia. Retrieved from http://apo.org.au/system/files/55973/apo-nid55973-73966.pdf

Baines, D. (2007). Anti-oppressive social work practice: Fighting for space, fighting for change in social service delivery. In D. Baines (Ed.), *Doing anti-oppressive practice: Building transformative, politicized social work* (pp. 13–42). Fernwood: Hailifax.

Bay, U. (2008). The politics of NGOs: Empowering marginal groups in a climate of micro-management and distrust. *Social Alternatives, 27*(1), 46–57.

Bay, U. (2011). Unpacking neo-liberal technologies of government in Australian Higher Education Social Work Departments. *Journal of Social Work, 11*(2), 222–235. doi:10.1177/1468017310386696

Beddoe, L. (2014). Feral families, troubled families: The spectre of the underclass in New Zealand. *New Zealand Sociology, 29*(3), 51–68.

Binkley, S. (2011). Psychological life as enterprise: Social practice and the government of neo-liberal interiority. *History of the Human Sciences, 24*(3), 83–102. doi:10.1177/0952695111412877

Binkley, S. (2016). Anti-racism beyond empathy: Transformations in the knowing and governing of racial difference. *Subjectivity, 9*(2), 181–204. doi:10.1057/sub.2016.4

Bjerg, H., & Staunaes, D. (2011). Self-management through shame. *Ephemera, 11*(2), 138–156.

Blencowe, C. (2012). *Biopolitical experience: Foucault, power and positive critique.* New York: Palgrave Macmillan.

Bondi, L. (2005). Working the spaces of neoliberal subjectivity: Psychotherapeutic technologies, professionalism and counselling. *Antipode A Radical Journal of Geography, 37*(3), 498–514. doi:10.1111/j.0066-4812.2005.00508.x

Brunila, K., & Valero, P. (2018). Anxiety and the making of research(ing) subjects in neoliberal academia. *Subjectivity, 11*, 74–89.

Clare, S. D. (2017). 'Finally, she's accepted herself!' Coming out in neoliberal times. *Social Text, 35*(2 (131)), 17–38. doi:10.1215/01642472-3820533

Conlin, P. (2014). Neoliberalism out of joint: Activists and in activists in London's social centers. *Subjectivity, 7*(3), 270–287. doi:10.1057/sub.2014.8

Davies, B. (2005). The (im)possibility of intellectual work in neoliberal regimes. *Discourse: Studies in the cultural Politics of Education, 26*(1), 1–14.

Dominelli, L. (1999). Neo-liberalism, social exclusion and welfare clients in global economy. *International Journal of Social Welfare, 8*, 14–22. doi:10.1111/1468-2397.00058

Du Gay, P. (1996). *Consumption and identity at work.* London: Sage.

Ferguson, I. (2007). *Reclaiming social work: Challenging neo-liberalism and promoting social justice.* London: SAGE.

Foucault, M. (1983). The subject and power. In H. Dreyfus & P. Rabinow (Eds.), *Michel Foucault: Beyond structuralism and hermeneutics.* Chicago, IL: University of Chicago Press.

Foucault, M. (1991). Governmentality. In G. Burchell, C. Gordon, & P. Miller (Eds.), *The Foucault effect: Studies in governmentality* (pp. 87–104). Chicago, IL: University of Chicago.

Foucault, M. (2007). *Security, territory, population.* Lectures at the College de France 1977–1978 (G. Burchell, trans.). New York, NY: Palgrave Macmillan.

Foucault, M. (2008). *The birth of biopolitics.* New York, NY: Picador.

Gill, R. (2017). Beyond individualism: The psychsocial life of the neoliberal university. In. M. Spooner (Ed.), *A critical guide to higher education & the politics of evidence: Resisting colonialism, neoliberalism, & audit culture.* Regina: University of Regina Press.

Gill, R., & Scharff, C. (2011). Introduction. In R. Gill & C. Scharff (Eds.), *New femininities: Postfeminism, neoliberalism and subjectivity* (1–17). Basingstoke: Palgrave.

Hamann, T. H. (2009). Neoliberalism. *Governmentality, and Ethics. Foucault Studies, 6*, 37–59.

Harvey, D. (2007). Neoliberalism as creative destruction. *The Annals of American Academy of Political and Social Sciences, 610*, 22–44. doi: 10.1177/0002716206296780

Healy, K. (2012). *Social work methods and skills: The essential foundations of practice.* Basingstoke: Palgrave Macmillan.

Hyslop, I. (2016). Neoliberalism and social work identity. *European Journal of Social Work.* doi:10.1080/13691457.2016.1255927

Layton, L. (2010). Irrational exuberance: Neoliberal subjectivity and the perversion of truth. *Subjectivity, 3*(3), 303–322. doi:10.1057/sub.2010.14

Lemke, T. (2001). 'The birth of bio-politics: Michel Foucault's lecture at the college de France on neo-liberal governmentality. *Economy and Society, 30*(2), 190–207.

Lemke, T. (2014). The risks of security: Liberalism, biopolitics and fear. In V. Lemm & M. Vatter (Eds.), *Foucault, biopolitics, and neoliberalism* (pp. 59–76). New York, NY: Fordham University Press.

Mayes, C. (2009). Pastoral power and the confessing subject in patient-centred communication. *Journal of Bioethical Inquiry, 6*(4), 483–493.

Mayes, C. (2016). *The biopolitics of lifestyle: Foucault, ethics and healthy choices.* New York, NY: Routledge.

Mccall, C. (2010). Edward McGushin: Foucault's askesis: An introduction to the philosophical life. *Continental Philosophy Review, 42*(4), 577–582.

McDonald, J. (2005). Neo-liberalism and the pathologising of public issues: The displacement of feminist service models in domestic violence support services. *Australian Social Work, 58*(3), 275–284.

McGushin, E. (2007). *Foucault's askesis: An introduction to the philosophical life.* Evanston, IL: Northwestern University Press.

Mitendorf, A., & van Ewijk, H. (2015) Working with social complexity in a neoliberal society: Challenges for social work in Estonia. *European Journal of Social Work, 19*(1), 78–91. doi:10.1080/13691457.2015.1025711

Read, J. (2009). A genealogy of homo-economicus: Neoliberalism and the production of subjectivity. *Foucault Studies, 6*, 25–36.

Rose, N. S. (1999). *Governing the Soul: The shaping of the private self* (2nd ed.). London: Free Association Books.

Scharff, C. (2016). The psychic life of neoliberalism: Mapping the contours of entrepreneurial subjectivity. *Theory, Culture and Society, 36*(6), 107–122. doi:10.1177/0263276415590164

Sennett, R. (2006). *The culture of the new capitalism.* New Haven: Yale University Press.

Spolander, G., Engelbrecht, L., Martin, L., Strydom, M., Pervova, I., Paivi, M., & Petri, T. (2014). The implications of neoliberalism for social work: Reflections from a six-country international research collaboration. *International Social Work, 57*(4), 301–321. doi:10.1177/0020872814524964

Wallace, J., & Pease, B. (2011). Neoliberalism and Australian social work: Accommodation or resistance. *Journal of Social Work, 11*(2), 132–142. doi:10.1177/1468017310387318

Weir, A. (2013). *Identities and freedom: Feminist theory between power and connection.* New York, NY: Oxford University Press.

Servants of a 'sinking titanic' or actors of change? Contested identities of social workers in Sweden

Passiva tjänare av 'ett sjunkande skepp' eller förändringsaktörer? Ifrågasatta identiteter hos socialarbetare i Sverige

Jessica H. Jönsson

ABSTRACT

Historically, social workers have been an integral part of a well-developed welfare state in Sweden. However, due to the neoliberal changes, which have seen the weakening of the support system for vulnerable groups and individuals, the traditional 'solidary role' of social workers has rapidly altered. This has created uncertainty and dilemmas for the identification of many social workers, who still perceive themselves as promoters of 'welfare of the people'. This article dwells, therefore, on neoliberal transformations and the changing professional identity of practitioners. The study is based on a comprehensive empirical work of interviews with social workers. The results show a growing and widespread unease with new professional roles and functions of social workers as bureaucrats within a neoliberalised organisation of public social work. Some social workers still try to find creative and new ways of working in solidarity, while others, although critical, see adjustment to the new organisational frames as a way to continue their work. It is argued that social workers are not passive actors in the process of neoliberalisation of public social work in Sweden but could actively take different stances and choose their own identifications, in order to maintain the solidary role of social workers.

ABSTRAKT

Historiskt sett har svenska socialarbetare varit en integrerad del av en välutvecklad välfärdsstat. Men på grund av de nyliberala förändringar som har inneburit en försvagning av välfärdsstaten och dess stödsystem för utsatta grupper och individer, har socialarbetares traditionella 'solidariska roll' snabbt förändrats. Detta har skapat rollkonflikter och flera dilemman för många socialarbetare som fortfarande uppfattar och identifierar sig som en profession som främjar välfärd och solidaritet. Föreliggande artikel ämnar att undersöka hur de senaste decenniernas nyliberala förändringar har påverkat socialarbetares professionella identitet i Sverige. Studien bygger på ett omfattande empiriskt material bestående av intervjuer med socialarbetare verksamma inom den kommunala sektorn. Studiens resultat visar på en växande och utbredd oro hos socialarbetare för deras nya professionella roller och funktioner som byråkrater i en nyliberaliserad organisation i offentligt socialt arbete snarare än välfärdsagenter.

Resultatet visar också att socialarbetarna reagerar på olika sätt mot sina nya nyliberala professionella roller och funktioner. En del försöker hitta kreativa och nya sätt att arbeta i solidaritet, medans andra, kritiska attityder tilltrots, ser en anpassning till nya organisatoriska ramar som ett sätt att fortsätta sitt jobb. Artikelförfattaren menar att socialarbetare inte behöver vara passiva aktörer i nyliberaliseringsprocessen av det offentliga socialt arbetet i Sverige, utan kan vara aktiva aktörer i att motverka nyliberala förändringarna inom professionen och inta solidariska arbetssätt och identiteter.

Introduction: on shaky ground

'Like a sinking Titanic'; that is how social workers describe the current state of public social services in Sweden (Sveriges Television, 4 February 2015). The similarity between the image of Titanic as an 'unsinkable ship' and the image of the Swedish welfare state as one of the world's strongest and most lasting institutions is striking. In each case, the most vulnerable groups pay the price of its failures. The image of Sweden is much stronger than the reality of its welfare state, which has undergone three decades of neoliberalisation and marketisation with substantial impact on social policy, social work education and practices (Kamali & Jönsson, 2018). Neoliberalisation as a socioeconomic doctrine believes in the ideological dominance of the necessity of a global market with the minimum control of the nation state. As Harvey (2005) puts it, neoliberalism is a theory of political economic practices that proposes that human wellbeing can best be advanced by liberating individual entrepreneurial freedom characterised by strong private property rights, free markets and free trade. The role of the state is thus to create and preserve an institutional framework appropriate to such practices. One of the consequences of neoliberalism is, according to Bourdieu (1998), the dominance of individualism and the destruction of collectivism. This leads, according to Bauman (2001), to the loss of state-centred institutions and a moral blindness attached to uncontrolled market competition.

OECD reports show that Sweden is among those countries with them highest adjustment of their societies to neoliberal transformations (OECD, 2011, 2013, 2016) (Figure 1).

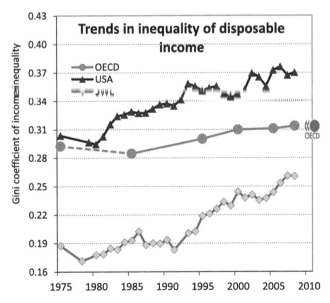

Figure 1. Trends in inequality of disposable income. Source: OECD Social Expenditures database. www.oecd.org/social/expenditure.htm.

The reconstruction of the Swedish welfare system because of the neoliberalisation of the country is challenging the established image of Sweden as a bastion of equality, equity and social cohesion.

The neoliberal reorganisation and a 'social work in crisis' in Sweden have led to a situation in which municipal authorities and social workers are not able to guarantee the rights and entitlements of people (Jönsson, 2015). The blame is often put on social workers who have the 'street-level' contact with people in need of the welfare state's interventions. This is a result of a political and media cover up of what really is happening with a welfare state in retreat from its traditional obligations. Social workers are working hard in difficult times with scarce resources to help people in need and are in a constant struggle within neoliberalised organisation and routines.

However, neoliberal changes of the Swedish welfare state have not passed without resistance. Critical voices are growing in a country where critics of the cooperation between the state and the market have traditionally not been strong. Although there have been critics against 'paternalistic features' of the welfare state during earlier periods, this critique was not against neoliberalisation of the Swedish welfare state. The critical voices of today from academics, educators and practitioners focus more explicitly on the neoliberalisation of Swedish society and the retreat of the welfare state. The Swedish state is today highly criticised for not taking its traditional responsibilities (existing even during the 1970s and 1980s) for the welfare of people. Such voices are increasingly challenging the deterioration of people's living conditions because of the rapid neoliberalisation of Swedish society. Social workers are protesting against worsening of their working conditions, managerial legal and administrative frames replacing the traditional and solidary basis of social work, limited support to people in need, individualisation and fragmentation of social work instead of holistic approaches and growing stress and burnout among social workers. Protests have been organised and carried out by critical networks among social work practitioners, students, and service users in Sweden e.g. by KAOSA, Kritiska Organiserade Socialarbetare (*Critical Organised Social Workers*), SFSA, Socialarbetare för social aktion (*Social Worker for Social Action*) and NBT, Nu bryter vi tystnaden (*Now We break the Silence*), and numerous demonstrations through social work unions and social workers organised in different parts of the country. Although there is evidence in previous literature that social workers may respond differently to transformations in their organisations, we know less about responses related specifically to the neoliberal political landscape of Swedish welfare and social work, as will be explored in this article.

The study

This study explores social workers' responses to recent decades' neoliberal transformations of the Swedish welfare state and social work. The following questions have guided the study: How has the recent political, social and organisational transformations influenced the self-image of social workers? How have such transformations influenced social workers' professional identification? How do social workers respond to neoliberal changes in and limitations to their professional activities?

Since the main objective of the study is to capture social workers' understanding of their professional roles and functions within neoliberalised frames of social work organisations, this study has a qualitative approach. The sample is composed of social workers engaged in different areas of public social work, such as child and family welfare, addiction care, economic support and social work with migrants and asylum seekers. The author have conducted interviews with 15 social workers (11 women and 4 men) during 2016–2017 in the three Swedish cities of Gothenburg, Malmö and Stockholm in which urban social problems such as marginalisation have rather dramatically increased during the last three decades of neoliberalisation of Swedish society. Three social workers have more than 20 years of experience. Eight of the social workers have between 5-10 years of experience and four of them have newly stepped into the profession with less than 5 years of experience. The 'voices from within', which are about social workers' experiences of 'being a social worker' in a neoliberal organisational landscape, have been analysed using QCA – qualitative content analysis (Graneheim & Lundman, 2004). The use of QCA aimed at interpreting variations through identifying differences and similarities in content, expressed as categories and themes at various levels of abstraction. By using this method of analysis, it was possible to identify relevant categories and themes and to provide a comprehensive understanding of its manifest and latent contents and messages in the frame of relevant critical social theoretical perspectives. Although QCA is inductive, it does not need to exclude deductive reasoning (Patton, 2002). Using theory and previous studies was useful in the process of data analysis (Berg, 2001), i.e. initial coding starts with theory and relevant research findings (Hsieh & Shannon, 2005).

The first part of the article explores the neoliberal political context of social welfare and social work in Sweden. The next part introduces the theoretical concepts of 'symbolic violence' and 'governmentality' used in the article to analyse the way social workers have been influenced by recent neoliberal transformations. The following part of the article provides illustrations of difficulties faced by social workers in their daily activities, difficulties that create ethical dilemmas and impact their professional identities and aspirations, but also evoke resistance and protests among social workers. The focus of the final part of the article is on the responsibility of social work as a profession and social workers as individuals to resist neoliberal methods and managerial techniques that reduce social workers to neoliberal administrators, which helps to reproduce inequalities and injustices in society.

Neoliberal transformation of the Swedish welfare and social work

As one of the most significant socioeconomic, political, ideological and cultural changes to the world during recent times, neoliberalism 'transmogrifies every human domain, along with human subjectivity itself, and all spheres of existence are framed and measured by economic terms and metrics, even when those spheres are not directly monetised' (Brown, 2015).

One of the major reasons behind the 'neoliberal turn' can be found in the shift in hegemonic political and economic ideology from socialism to neoliberalism, the latter privileging the private sector, which also has brought with it a 'welfare blindness', causing the general majority to be relatively uncritical of the political leaders and authorities whose traditional duties have been to provide welfare to the people (Vejlby, 2011). The weakening of political opposition to neoliberal ideology has created some kind of general 'acceptance' of neoliberal reforms as necessary for the 'wellbeing of the people'. Such a relative acceptance is important for a neoliberal *governmentality* to exist (Foucault, 1979/2008). This means a neoliberal technique of governance by which people are convinced that the superiority of the global market is the only alternative. Notwithstanding growing protests against neoliberal reforms and marketisation of the welfare state, the political message is almost the same: 'there is no alternative' to neoliberalism, in Margaret Thatcher's words. Neoliberalisation conducted by both the right wing and social democratic governments in Sweden is almost neutralised and de-politicised. As a result, the commoditisation of social welfare services as well as the adoption of private sector management philosophies and tools have 'colonised and fashioned the design, provision and implementation of social welfare policy and structures' (Spolander, Engelbrecht, & Sansfacon, 2016).

The welfare state reforms in Sweden have created a 'welfare market' in which private organisations and individuals are able to obtain considerable economic benefits from public expenditures. Many traditional political and ideological advocates of the welfare state, such as social democrats, who are now influenced by the hegemonic neoliberal ideology, are re-defining the domains of the welfare state and the role of politics and social policy in providing welfare to people.

Given that neoliberalism is about to 'make governance cheaper' and limit the scope of the government intervention of the market, it is expected that the financial burden of the welfare state should be less in a time of a neoliberal reorganisation of the welfare state. However, this is not the case in the face of evidence. Studies and statistical reports show that notwithstanding neoliberal reforms and marketisation of welfare services, the public costs of the welfare state have increased (OECD, 2016). Paradoxically, the increase of public expenditures has not been targeting people in need of such services. This is mainly due to the new profit-hunting actors in the 'welfare market', which receive a large part of social expenditures as the mediators of services (Jönsson, 2015; Jönsson & Kojan, 2017).

Such transformations have dramatically changed the way social work has traditionally been organised and practised, as well as the way social problems are defined and dealt with, including social workers professional identities (Espvall, 2018; Lauri, 2016; Tham, 2018). New techniques, such as New Public Management (NPM) and evidence-based practice (EBP), have been created to simplify and standardise responses to individuals' and families' social problems in line with this reorganisation of the welfare state (Petersén & Olsson, 2015; Ponnert & Svensson, 2016). Social workers have historically been an integral part of a well-developed welfare state in Sweden. However, the 'solidary role' of social workers has rapidly altered due to the neoliberal changes, which has weakened the social support system. This has created 'identity crises' for many social workers who still perceive themselves as promoters of 'welfare of the people'. The realm of social workers' influence on the fulfilment of their mandate for the social dimension of public life is curtailed by neoliberal constraints (|Lorenz, 2016, 2017). Social workers feel strongly impacted by numerous constraints on their work, both at the macro-structural level of policy-making and organisational context of their work and at the micro-interpersonal level (Jönsson, 2015; Lauri, 2016).

Social work in Sweden has only until recently acknowledged the limited professional possibilities for social workers to provide services, as well as the existence of serious tensions between neoliberal strategies and the professional ethics and core values of social work. As some studies have hinted, social work and social workers are increasingly detached from including and dealing with the structural and institutional aspects of social problems, with people in need of social work interventions 'becoming' responsible for their social problems (Dahlstedt & Lozic, 2017; Jönsson, 2013; Sernhede, 2018). This forces social workers to continuously negotiate the boundaries of their professional responsibilities in relation to the core values of the profession. Neoliberal imperatives and requirements create many dilemmas for social workers, who are concerned with addressing the structural conditions of social problems and with collective empowerment (Jönsson, 2018). Indeed, overemphasising the individual responsibility of people in need of social work interventions in respect to their social problems runs the risk of seeing social workers operate in the capacity of 'controller' (Cuadra Björngren & Staaf, 2014; Skjefstad, Kiik, & Sandoval, 2018) rather than as an agent of change.

Although such responses are uneven and interchangeable, they are strong signs of a profession in transition targeted by growing neoliberal political and organisational changes. The vulnerable position of social workers and the space that the neoliberal reorganisation of social work has created for those employed within public social work in Sweden creates a confusing position for social workers.

The neoliberal governance of social work

This study uses the theoretical concepts of 'symbolic violence' (Bourdieu) and 'governmentality' (Foucault) to analyse the way social workers have been influenced by recent neoliberal transformations and the changing of their professional identity. 'Governmentality', in Foucault's theoretical standpoint, corresponds well with Bourdieu's concept of 'symbolic violence' for studying the formation of power and knowledge governing society (see also Kamali, 2015). It provides a theoretical framework for analysing technologies of self as they intersect with technologies of domination. By technologies of self I mean here the combination of 'taking care of oneself' and de-politicisation of one's actions in order to protect oneself from being subjected to punishment by political and bureaucratic organisations. In the neoliberal organisation of social work, a combination of technologies of self and technologies of domination helps to reproduce inequalities. Such theoretical perspectives are necessary to explore unequal practices in society and the role of social work for promoting social justice and social change (see also Donovan, Rose, & Connolly, 2017; Garrett, 2007a, 2007b; Hewitt, 1983; Kamali, 2015; Lauri, 2016). It can be said that disciplinisation, based on power structures in society, makes the reproduction of privileged positions and structures possible. Reproduction of hierarchical positions and power structures in society is not only based on physical violence but also on the 'soft means of domination', i.e. 'symbolic violence' (Bourdieu, 1991, p. 190). Symbolic violence makes the mechanisms of domination possible, since every domination includes some degree of acceptance (Foucault, 1977, 1982). As Bourdieu (1984, 1991) puts it, human actions take place in different fields and each field has its own 'rules of games' and 'dispositions', which force individuals to adjust their actions to the field's manifest and latent rules and routines. Individuals who engage in a specific field are struggling over desirable resources and should respect and reproduce the dispositions of the field in order to guarantee obtaining privileges attached to the domination of privileged groups in society.

Neoliberalism influences more or less every field of human action and forces many to adjust themselves to neoliberal conditions. Bourdieu (1998) argued that neoliberalism involves the dominance of individualism and the destruction of collectivism. This has been one of the consequences of the increasing ideological domination of the necessity of a global market with the minimum control of the nation state. Likewise, Foucault argued that what makes states truly neoliberal is using the market to govern, distributing services and benefits according to the market logic of efficiency, competitiveness and profitability. According to Foucault (2008, p. 131), neoliberal reforms and the restructuring of society are taking place through a complex system that he calls *governmentality*. Governmentality as a process of governing over people and societies not only by 'monopoly over legitimate means of violence' but also through 'convincing' people of the necessity of governance and domination. Governmentality makes people accept the legitimacy of the system as necessary. In other words, neoliberalism is largely legitimised as the only possible system of organising economy, politics and culture. Those individuals who adjust themselves to neoliberal imperatives get rewarded and those who do not can be subjected to punishment.

Social workers in Sweden are mainly working within public organisations and institutions and are a professional group highly influenced by neoliberal governmentality. Overall, the notion of 'efficiency' underpins everyday activities in public social work arenas. This creates a situation in which social workers are left with dilemmas of their professional identity as the *helper* and not controller and agents of efficiency. Social workers are forced to react to such new working conditions in their professional practices. One such challenge is the question of identification as social workers. Traditionally, many social workers have identified themselves as solidary human beings and the workers of a 'good state' with strong welfare obligations towards people. However, in a time when the state is retreating from its traditional role as the champion of people's welfare, it is getting harder for public social workers to identify themselves as a member of a solidary profession.

Result and analysis: voices from within

In this section, social workers' experiences of working in, and responding to, the increasing neoliberal organisation of public social work is presented and analysed.

Managerial professional social workers

Overall, there is a common understanding among social workers participating in this study that recent political, social and organisational (neoliberal) reforms of the last decades have affected important aspects of social work. Such changes are expressed in the growing demand for Evidence Based Practice (EBP) , new technologies for 'simplifying' and standardising social problems and their roots, by stressing *efficiency, individual responsibility* and *standardisation* of the provision of social services. Social workers tell me about procedures akin to rationalisation and standardisation as the consequences of neoliberal reorganisation of welfare state, which in different ways have affected social work practice. 'Elena', an experienced social worker within the field of addiction care, states:

> We have standardised the way we solve complex problems by always 'choosing' the same measures, because it its cheap and does not cost much. I am indeed educated, competent and experienced enough to do professional assessments but it seems not what the organisation want me to do.

Further, the emphasis on 'efficiency' and on 'budget management skills' has led social workers away from what many social workers consider as *the heart* of social work, namely meeting the needs of people in their social realities formed by broader structural approaches in social work. Sitting behind a desk being a paper-pusher/secretary is not only extremely time consuming but also hinders social workers from meeting peoples' needs in their everyday lives, as many uttered. Interviewee 'Josephine', working with child and family care and with several years of professional experience, tells how this affects her work:

> I feel like a programmed machine. I mean, anybody could do what we are doing, there is no need for professional knowledge. This is not what I have been educated for. Everything is so standardised. I have left my jobs several times and found another, believing that it would be better somewhere else and I could work differently, but it was not the case, it is the same everywhere.

Or as another social work colleague, working in the same area with only a few years of professional experience, 'Emelie' puts it:

> I spend almost all of my time by the computer, making calls, writing documents, and so on. Following manuals, it is a hell to fill out forms and it take so much of my time and steal time from to many other things that I as a social worker should do. I would rather meet my clients face-to-face.

This technological basis for practice, represented by the 'electronic turn' in social work (Garrett, 2005), is changing the functions and mandates of social workers. Within new organisational conditions, the work is increasingly being ordered and structured by neoliberal policy makers far removed from the day-to-day encounters that social workers have with service users. The new way of standardisation of social work, which often is legitimated as making social work more effective, empties social work practice from its human qualities. Neoliberal governmentality leaves no space for social workers' autonomous evaluations of their work and consequences of their interventions. They are increasingly disciplined in new working conditions, which really do not need educated and creative social workers. Respondents to this study acknowledge that they do not have the time for comprehensive social work but take rapid and technical decisions for short-term interventions. 'We just scratch on the surface', says 'Lila', one of the interviewed social workers. She is realising that their documentation of people's social problems, and their assessments on the same, are rather simplified and watered-down:

> There is basically no time for detailed assessment writing, my colleagues have piles of papers and notes that have not been registered for many months ... We just 'sum things up', I do not think the content of the assessments make any sense to (who it concerns) our 'clients' ...

As argued here, this violates even Swedish laws, which regulate social workers' actions. Practitioners argue that in many cases they see the needs and are aware of the rights of people as well as of ethical issues in their work, but realise that they are not able to do much because of their workload and shortage of time. 'Lydia', at a child and family section, argues:

> In order to do the most urgent and short time interventions, serious and important matters and cases are ignored This leads often to the situation that we get the problems of the families back again. I don't see the point ...

There is an obvious un-ethical tendency in neoliberalised social work in Sweden. Many social workers experience that they have to accept such a strategic/rationalised documentary tendency in social work because of a top-down power structure in public organisations of social work. Not adjusting themselves to such neoliberal and managerial imperatives will not be in the individual interests of social workers, i.e. in Foucault's words 'taking care of the self'. They can be sanctioned negatively or punished, in Bourdieu's (1991) word. As 'Malin', by referring to her social work with economic support, says:

> One is always controlled. My chief is going through my documents, decisions and what I write about my clients. I have her control in my mind when writing my assessments and make decisions. I feel that my education and what I have learned is not recognised and valid here, I have simply to accept what the chief wants me to do. Otherwise, I risk my job.

Or, as 'Samuel', working with social and economic support to people in marginalised areas, says, 'accepting what the organisation and those in power – the leadership – want is emancipatory, because then you do not need to have any confrontation with them'. Such an acceptance is part of the domination, as Foucault (2008) argued. Accepting the 'rules of games' makes working easier for social workers, since the domination is not confronted with resistance and objections. Neoliberal policies and 'NPM-ethics' are characterised by stressing the importance of measurable outputs, targets and cost effectiveness in the provision of public services. However, the narratives of the social workers rather offer a critique of such and emphasise the importance of reclaiming professional ethics for social work – ethics of social justice (Banks, 2011).

Social workers act in accordance with performance-based models of NPM and private-sector-like organisational models of work based on 'tighter' management control of the labour process, ongoing intensification of work, reduction of costs, increased standardisation, reduction of waste, the use of just-in-time deliverables and close monitoring of all aspects of work (Baines, 2004). In some of the municipal public social work organisations, they have introduced 'lean thinking' (lean manufacturing or lean production) for the social services' new systems. *Lean work* highlights the general lack of funding in the social services sector, which severely reduces the capacity to provide quality social services and effectively removes the possibility for social workers to provide holistic social services.

For example, social workers' narratives suggest that the important goal of empowerment is not realised. Rather, the findings show that participatory empowerment social work is hard to achieve. Social workers describe that their expanded workloads imply that work tends to be conducted at the last minute with little or no room for assessing empowering processes. The current neoliberal model of social work needs only 'uncritical servants' who accept and work in accordance with what is defined by the leading section of the organisation as desirable social work.

The recent emphasis on 'modernisation' and 'professionalisation' in social work in Sweden has been an effort to replace critical analysis and perspectives necessary for understanding and working with social problems. An uncritical celebration of new 'theory-less' methods and manuals in social work practice has also meant a move away from traditionally strong system of preventive social work in Sweden. As social worker, 'Jenny', puts it:

> Preventive work, who has time for that? We have no time to work with long-term goals, to find real solution to people's problems. We work merely with short-term interventions, like hospital emergency centres, or like firefighters putting out fires - the most urgent actions, not more.

This also affects social workers' relations to people whom they want to help by establishing a trustful relation.

Changing the solidary role of social workers

Many social workers are aware of consequences of the neoliberal reorganisation of the Swedish public social work. Social worker 'Kathrine' means that *the system* is creating frustration, disappointment and anger among service users, which in turn leads to distrustful relations between social workers and people they intend to help within the frames of public social work organisations.

Interviewee 'Gunhild', with more than twenty years of professional experience in social work related to addiction, homelessness and prostitution, tells about how individual responsibility for welfare is built into systems of *reward and punishment* within social work interventions and how this influences the solidary role of social workers. She says:

> Those who accept the new way of the organisation of our work, which is decided over our heads, are no problems. On the contrary, they can be rewarded by being entitled to participate in new courses and short-term education that can help them up in the organisation. This is not the case for other of us, treated as 'deviants'. Who knows, we can even be forced to leave our jobs.

Referring to social work with migrants and asylum seekers, another interviewee, 'Victor', who is critical of being a controller and 'not a solidary worker' in his words, says:

> The chief has said to my colleagues that those who do not like their work and the organisation they are working in should leave, find another job. She has signalled that persons like me are not going to do any career in this organisation, and I know that she is absolutely right.

The quotes above can be understood by the theoretical perspective of symbolic violence (Bourdieu, 1984, 1991). Those who accept and adjust themselves to the NPM models of social work are rewarded and those who do not are punished in different ways.

Another social worker, 'Eva', is frustrated about the contradictory situation created for her. She sees no space for working in accordance with her education and professional intentions for helping people in need of her competency and skills. She says:

> I feel like a 'bad social worker', I am educated to help people but I can't do that. I do not have the possibilities or time to do so. I feel frustrated and incomplete. The level of social work today has fallen dramatically. I think that you cannot be the social worker you wanted to be when you choose the profession.

Another illustration of the impact of neoliberalisation on social work and its demoralising effects on the professional identity of social workers is that the influence of neoliberal ideologies and policies has seen stress placed on the 'responsibilisation' of both service users and professional social workers. This responsibilisation forces social workers to continuously negotiate the boundaries of their professional responsibilities in relation to the core values of the profession. Such neoliberal imperatives and requirements create many dilemmas for social workers. One example is the fact that policymakers define and find solutions to social problems without using social workers' professional knowledge and competency. As expressed by social worker 'Lila':

> The new forms of organising and steering social work activities show that politicians and those in leading positions do not trust our professional ability and skills. I have educated myself several years and have many years of experience in social work practice, no politicians with not enough knowledge of social work should tell me what I should do or not should do. The most important thing for them is the budget balance and economic calculations. They do not give a damn about our competency or people's social problems.

Some social workers put the blame for their problematic working situation on themselves. 'Kathrine', an experienced social worker, is reflecting back on her recent years in social work with children 'at risk' and says:

> If I had a better managerial capacity, I maybe would be able to work more effectively, and at the same time I would be able to be successful in helping clients?

This can be understood as a way to accept the dominance of neoliberal organisational domination by trying to change the focus from the problems created by the neoliberal organisational models, such as NPM, to the individual social worker's bureaucratic and managerial abilities. The acceptance and accomplishment to neoliberalism is important for the reproduction of the dominance (Foucault, 2008) and the reward (Bourdieu, 1991) from the leading section of the organisation.

The interviews with social workers grasp the contested relationships and roles within the Swedish social welfare as a system traditionally created to maintain the well-being of individuals. Social workers are forced to adjust themselves to NPM imperatives including adjustment to discontinuities and disruptions in their contacts and work with service users. As a result, service users are forced to frequently change their social workers and meet new persons. This becomes more problematic when social workers' real time for face-to-face meeting with service users is increasingly shrinking. 'Kathrine' says:

> Sometimes, my clients apologise for 'taking my time' ... even if it is me who are supposed to help them. I am here for them, it is horrible that it has gone so far ...

Such working conditions leave social workers with the choice of either adapting to such conditions or resisting them in different ways. In many ways, the difficulties for social workers are based on what has traditionally been the solidary identity of social workers. The rapid neoliberal transformations of the public social work provoke different reactions from social workers, who may adopt a variety of positions towards such changes in their daily work.

Critical stands and acts of change

The voices from the 'sinking ship' of the Swedish public social work demonstrate that the ways in which social workers have responded to such rapid changes have not been homogenous. Because of fear of punishment, many accept their 'places in the hierarchy' and the imperatives from the neoliberal organisations' leadership. They demonstrate little or no resistance at all in order to be an accepted part of the new neoliberal field of social work. Meanwhile, others have responded by adopting a more practical stance that encompasses explicit critical perspectives and activities.

However, irrespective of social workers' individual choices of alternatives and strategies towards neoliberal changes and leadership, social workers participated in this study utter severe concerns about their professional identities. All social workers mean that they have chosen the profession of social work for its solidarity content and not for a managerial control of people in need of social work interventions. They are critical of neoliberal policies and practices, which have resulted in growing rationalisation, standardisation and individualisation of social problems and social work practices in a profession, which earlier included structural and holistic perspectives in working with marginalised and vulnerable people. In outlining resistance to and struggle against such neoliberal politics, social workers are aware of the need for collective social action and organisation. Social worker, 'Malin' urges that:

> Organise yourself for change. Alone, you are not strong, there are already so many who tried to fight the situation alone and I was one of them. This is a costly way to go, you get sick and have to leave.

As a profession engaging in upholding human rights and social justice and committed to eliminate oppression, some social workers argue for the engagement of social workers in protest movements against, and resistance to, the neoliberal policies, marginalising mechanisms, welfare nationalism and racism that influence many people's life chances. They mean that many of such structural and institutional aspects of oppression are sacrificed in the process of neoliberalisation of social work practice. Some respondents provide examples of such social work action networks, e.g. social workers go together with local non-governmental organisations to support and find solutions to undocumented immigrants by taking creative and sometimes 'illegal' actions. Some social workers say that they are participating in critical networks among social work practitioners, students and service users, such as the network Social Workers for Social Action, (SFSA). As 'Walter' puts it:

> The aim of our network is to create better opportunities for social workers, We are trying to create alternative ways of working and show to social workers that another social work is possible which is not limited to just follow what the politicians want us to do and force us to just follow laws and rules. This means that we have to follow our professional ethics and knowledge in order to help people in need of our services even if it goes against laws, rules and organisational routines. It is about solidarity and compassion.

Through SFSA, social workers arrange conferences, seminars, networking days and different social activities bringing together politicians, academics, social workers and service users to critically discuss the politics of neoliberalism and to participate in the public debate to resist. In an article in *Dagens Arena* (31 January 2011) *Socialarbetare för Social Aktion* (SFSA) social work practitioners and social work students together stress the importance of informed social work educators for the development of critical knowledge in social work education, which will prepare future social workers for working in an environment in which neoliberalism creates complex social problems. Participating in critical networks helps social workers, as they put it, to 'regain the real role and function of being a social worker'. As 'Fatima', a child welfare social worker puts it:

> We have to do something, we cannot passively accept what they force us to be, passive followers of orders and documents written by those who do not know anything about our realities; administrators who are occupied with efficiency, papers, rules, laws, and end-oriented calculations. This is about human beings' lives. I participate in

SFSA because of the solidary basis of their activities, otherwise I cannot be at ease with my role as a social worker. I have chosen social work for helping people and not for having just a job.

This illustrates Michel Foucault's famous argument, i.e. 'where there is power, there is resistance' (1990).

Concluding remarks

In the current neoliberal organisational landscape and the hegemony of the political neoliberal ideology, which even have highly influenced social democratic parties and groups in Sweden, social workers seems to be in an state of uncertainty influenced by paradoxes and dilemmas of role conflicts and identification. Although some social workers are adjusting themselves to neoliberal models based on their need of having a job or accepting neoliberal reorganisation of the Swedish welfare state, many others are critical and try to resist neoliberalisation and the retreat of the welfare state.

Resistance to neoliberalisation of public social work in Sweden is a part of an active identification of many social workers to their role of solidarity with marginalised and vulnerable groups. Many consider themselves agents of helping people in need and improving unprivileged groups' living conditions, being the agents of change and not the 'servants of a sinking Titanic'. This requires taking a radical 'political stance' in social work (McKendrick & Webb, 2014), to resist the politics of neoliberalism, which reduce social workers to be neoliberal administrators and help to reproduce inequalities and injustices in society. The identity crisis of many social workers is dependent on such a situation, created by the neoliberal and managerial organisation of social work. However, social worker are not passive actors in this process but could actively take different stances and choose their own identifications. In order to maintain the solidary identity of social workers, they can find creative ways of resisting neoliberal changes and, together with movements against neoliberalism, help to hinder the sinking of the welfare ship.

Disclosure statement

No potential conflict of interest was reported by the author.

References

Baines, D. (2004). Caring for nothing: Work organizations and unwaged labour in social services. *Work, Employment and Society, 18*(2), 267–295.

Banks, S. (2011). Ethics in an age of austerity: Social work and the evolving new public management. *Journal of Social Intervention: Theory and Practice, 20*(2), 5–23.

Bauman, Z. (2001). *The individualized society*. Cambridge: Polity Press.

Berg, B. L. (2001). *Qualitative research methods for the social sciences*. Boston, MA: Allyn & Bacon.

Bourdieu, P. (1984). *Distinction: A social critique of the judgement of tastes*. New York, NY: Routledge & Kegan Paul.

Bourdieu, P. (1991). *Language and symbolic power*. Cambridge, MA: Harvard University Press.

Bourdieu, P. (1998). The essence of neoliberalism: What is neoliberalism? A programme for destroying collective structures which may impede the pure market logic. *LE MONDE diplomatique* [online]. Retrieved from http://mondediplo.com/1998/12/08bourdieu

Brown, W. (2015). *Undoing the demos: Neoliberalism's stealth revolution*. New York, NY: Zone Books.

Cuadra Björngren, C., & Staaf, A. (2014). Public Social Services' encounters with irregular migrants in Sweden: Amid values of social work and control of migration. *European Journal of Social Work, 17*(1), 88–103.

Dahlstedt, M., & Lozic, V. (2017). Managing urban unrest: Problematising juvenile delinquency in multi-ethnic Sweden. *Critical and Radical Social Work*, 5(2), 207–222.

Donovan, J., Rose, D., & Connolly, M. (2017). A crisis of identity: Social work theorising at a time of change. *British Journal of Social Work*. Advance online publication. doi:10.1093/bjsw/bcw180.

Espvall, M. (2018). Professional strategies and neoliberal challenges in Swedish social work practice. In M. Kamali & J. H. Jönsson (Eds.), *Neoliberalism, Nordic welfare states and social work: Current and future challenges* (pp. 148–158). London: Routledge.

Foucault, M. (1976/1990). *The history of sexuality, volume 1: An introduction*. New York, NY: Vintage Books.

Foucault, M. (1977). *Discipline and punish: The birth of the prison*. London: Allen Lane.

Foucault, M. (1979/2008). *The birth of biopolitics. Lectures at the Collège de France, 1978-1979*. New York, NY: Palgrave Macmillan.

Foucault, M. (1982). The subject and the power. In H. Dreyfus & P. Rabinow (Eds.), *Michel Foucault: Beyond structuralism and hermeneutics* (pp. 208–226). Brighton: Harvester.

Garrett, P. M. (2005). Social work's 'electronic turn': Notes on the deployment of information and communication technologies in social work with children and families. *Critical Social Policy*, 25(4), 529–553.

Garrett, P. M. (2007a). Making social work more Bourdieusian: Why the social professions should critically engage with the work of Pierre Bourdieu. *European Journal of Social Work*, 10(2), 225–243.

Garrett, P. M. (2007b). The relevance of Bourdieu for social work: A reflection on obstacles and omissions. *Journal of Social Work*, 7(3), 355–379.

Graneheim, U. H., & Lundman, B. (2004). Qualitative content analysis in nursing research: Concepts, procedures and measures to achieve trustworthiness. *Nurse Education Today*, 24(2), 105–112.

Harvey, D. (2005). *A brief history of neoliberalism*. Oxford: Oxford University Press.

Hewitt, M. (1983). Bio-politics and social policy: Foucault's account of welfare. *Theory, Culture and Society*, 2(1), 67–84.

Hsieh, H. F., & Shannon, S. E. (2005). Three approaches to qualitative content analysis. *Qualitative Health Research*, 15(9), 1277–1288.

Jönsson, J. H. (2013). Social work beyond cultural otherisation. *Nordic Social Work Research*, 3(2), 159–167.

Jönsson, J. H. (2014). Local reactions to global problems: Undocumented immigrants and social work. *British Journal of Social Work*, 44(1), i35–i52.

Jönsson, J. H. (2015). The contested field of social work in a retreating welfare state: The case of Sweden. *Critical and Radical Social Work*, 3(3), 357–374.

Jönsson, J. H. (2018). Välfärdsstatens försvagning, ökade sociala problem och social mobilisering [A retreating welfare state, increasing social problems and social mobilisation]. In S. Sjöberg & P. Turunen (Eds.), *Samhällsarbete – Aktörer, arenor och perspektiv* [Community work – actors, arenas and perspectives] (pp. 237–254). Lund: Studentlitteratur.

Jönsson, J. H., & Kojan, B. H. (2017). Social justice beyond neoliberal welfare nationalism: Challenges of increasing immigration to Sweden and Norway. *Critical and Radical Social Work*, 5(3), 301–317.

Kamali, M. (2015). *War, violence and social justice: Theories for social work*. London: Routledge.

Kamali, M., & Jönsson, J. H. (2018). *Neoliberalism, Nordic welfare states and social work: Current and future challenges*. London: Routledge.

Lauri, M. (2016). *Narratives of governing: Rationalization, responsibility and resistance in social work* (doctoral dissertation). Retrieved from http://umu.diva-portal.org/smash/get/diva2:923799/FULLTEXT01.pdf

Lorenz, W. (2016). Rediscovering the social question. *European Journal of Social Work*, 19(1), 4–17.

Lorenz, W. (2017). European policy developments and their impact on social work. *European Journal of Social Work*, 20(1), 17–28.

McKendrick, D., & Webb, S. (2014). Taking a political stance in social work. *Critical and Radical Social Work*, 2(3), 357–369.

OECD (2011). *Divided we stand: Why inequality keeps rising*. OECD Publishing. doi:10.1787/9789264119536-en

OECD (2013). *Increasing inequalities between 1980s to 2012*. OECD Publishing. Retrieved from http://www.oecd.org/els/soc/49499779.pdf

OECD (2016). *OECD social expenditures database*. OECD Publishing. Retrieved from http://www.oecd.org/social/expenditure.htm

Patton, M. Q. (2002). *Qualitative research and evaluation methods*. Thousand Oaks, CA: Sage.

Petersén, A. C., & Olsson, J. I. (2015). Calling evidence-based practice into question: Acknowledging phronetic knowledge in social work. *British Journal of Social Work*, 45(5), 1581–1597.

Ponnert, L., & Svensson, K. (2016). Standardisation – the end of professional discretion? *European Journal of Social Work*, 19(3-4), 586–599.

Sernhede, O. (2018). Urban marginality, social mobilisation and youth work in the shadow of neoliberalism and segregation. In M. Kamali & J. H. Jönsson (Eds.), *Neoliberalism, Nordic welfare states and social work: Current and future challenges* (pp. 238–248). London: Routledge.

Skjefstad, N. S., Kiik, R., & Sandoval, H. (2018). The role of social workers under neoliberal ideology at the Norwegian Labour and Welfare Service (NAV). In M. Kamali & J. H. Jönsson (Eds.), *Neoliberalism, Nordic welfare states and social work: Current and future challenges* (pp. 137–147). London: Routledge.

Socialarbetare för social aktion (SFSA) [Social Workers for Social Action]. (2011, januari 31). *De som inte ges utrymme finns inte!* [Those not provided space do not exist] Retrieved from http://www.dagensarena.se/opinion/socialarbetare-for-social-aktion-de-som-inte-ges-utrymme-finns-inte/

Spolander, G., Engelbrecht, L., & Sansfacon, A. P. (2016). Social work and macro-economic neoliberalism: Beyond the social justice rhetoric. *European Journal of Social Work, 19*(5), 634–649.

Tham, P. (2018). A professional role in transition: Swedish child welfare social workers' descriptions of their work 2003 and 2014. *The British Journal of Social Work,* 449–467. doi:10.1093/bjsw/bcx016

Vejlby, S. (2011). War, xenophobia, and the death agony of the Danish social democratic welfare state. *Socialism and Democracy, 25*(2), 44–57.

Human rights and social justice in social work education: a critical realist comparative study of England and Spain

Los derechos humanos y la justicia social en la formación en trabajo social: un estudio comparativo entre Inglaterra y España desde el realismo crítico

María Inés Martínez Herrero ⓘ and Helen Charnley

ABSTRACT

The history of social work as a profession and academic discipline is inextricably linked with principles of human rights (HR) and social justice (SJ). The Global Standards for social work education promote HR and SJ as unifying themes, yet there is little understanding of how these themes are embedded in social work education in specific national contexts. This article, based on empirical research in England and Spain, explores social work educators' understandings of, and strategies used in learning and teaching about, HR and SJ. Using a critical realist framework, a web survey was followed by qualitative interviews with educators in each country to identify opportunities and challenges in stimulating students' theoretical understanding of HR and SJ, and their application in practice. Findings show that prevailing neoliberal ideology has pervaded social work in both countries (more strongly in England) placing pressure on social work educators to convey narrow understandings of HR and SJ and to adopt increasingly bureaucratic and distant relationships with students. Identifying a range of factors informing educators' understandings of HR and SJ, the research identifies spaces for strengthening the focus on HR and SJ in social work education. The article argues that while university-based social work education remains a fertile site for the deconstruction of neoliberal ideology that threatens the HR and SJ foundations of social work globally, social work and social work education require the development of a distinct, alternative, HR and SJ based ideology.

RESUMEN

La historia del trabajo social como profesión y disciplina científica está estrechamente ligada con los principios de los derechos humanos (DDHH) y la justicia social (JS). Los Estándares Globales para la formación en trabajo social promueven en la actualidad que los DDHH y la JS sirvan como temas unificadores y transversales en la misma. Sin embargo, existe poco conocimiento sobre cómo éstos son incorporados en la formación en trabajo social en contextos nacionales específicos. Este artículo, basado en una investigación llevada a cabo en Inglaterra y España, explora cómo los docentes de trabajo social entienden los DDHH y la JS, así como las estrategias empleadas en su docencia relacionada con los mismos. Utilizando el realismo crítico como metodología marco, el estudio incluyó una encuesta electrónica y entrevistas cualitativas a docentes en ambos países con el objetivo de identificar oportunidades y dificultades encontradas a la hora de promover la comprensión teórica y aplicación práctica de los DDHH y la JS por parte de los alumnos. Los resultados indican que la ideología neoliberal dominante que se extiende en el trabajo social en ambos países (si bien en mayor medida en Inglaterra) da lugar a presiones a los docentes para que transmitan un contenido reduccionista en relación con los DDHH y la JS y adopten relaciones cada vez más burocráticas y distantes con los estudiantes. Sin embargo, el estudio también identifica una variedad de factores que informan la manera en que los docentes entienden estos principios, así como una serie de espacios y oportunidades para fortalecer el enfoque de los DDHH y la JS en la formación en trabajo social. El artículo argumenta que mientras que la educación universitaria continúa siendo un terreno fértil para la deconstrucción de la ideología neoliberal que amenaza globalmente los pilares de DDHH y JS del trabajo social en todo el mundo, el trabajo social y la formación en trabajo social necesitan trabajar en el desarrollo de una ideología alternativa propia, basada en los DDHH y la JS.

Introduction

Across the world people are suffering the effects of increasing inequality, the consequence of aggressive neoliberal globalisation and the rapid spread of systems and mechanisms to support and maintain its dominance. Even in countries with welfare traditions, such as England and Spain, the vast majority are experiencing reductions in their standard of living with increasing numbers experiencing poverty or extreme poverty. Human rights are being violated through the degradation of working conditions, the retreat of civil liberties on grounds of national security, austerity measures and the degradation of natural environments (Dominelli, 2012; Lundy, 2011).

Neoliberalism, as a political-economy theory, claims that the most effective and desirable way of promoting human wellbeing is removing social and political constraints to free market mechanisms, allowing their optimum operation to deliver maximum economic growth (Harvey, 2005). But these theoretical ideas are inconsistent with overwhelming evidence of increases in poverty and inequality during periods of neoliberal policy globally (Piketty, 2014), in Europe (De Vogli, 2013), and specifically in England and Spain (FOESSA, 2013; The Equality Trust, 2017).

Concepts of human rights (HR) and social justice (SJ) underpin the social work profession internationally (IFSW and IASSW, 2014) and are reflected in codes of ethics worldwide (Banks, 2006), including those of the British and Spanish national associations of social workers (BASW, 2014; CGTS, 2012). In an increasingly complex and globalised world, social problems gain an international dimension as structural inequalities are deepened by uncontrolled neoliberal market mechanisms, and the HR and SJ framework of social work gain increasing importance in countering narrow, market driven, approaches to address the needs of service users (Dominelli & Khan, 2000).

As neoliberal ideology challenges the nature of social work and social work education Lavalette (2011) has described social work as being at a crossroads. In one direction lies the reinvention and strengthening of the critical tradition towards the achievement of social justice. In the other lies the defeat of the critical tradition and further marginalisation of the profession as a force against the pernicious effects of neoliberalism in undermining HR and SJ. Higgins (2015) has recently highlighted the confrontation between 'a broad conception of social work as understood by the International Federation of Social Workers' (IFSW) and the bureaucratic approach to social work in England, aligned with a neoliberal education model focussing 'on the service user as the "problem" and disengaged from the wider socio-political context of contemporary society'

(Higgins, 2015, p. 12). This confrontation, he argues, represents a struggle for the soul of social work and presents particular dilemmas for social work educators. Human rights and social justice are central social work values, yet educators find themselves working within education systems increasingly influenced by neoliberal ideals. For social workers to feel empowered to embed HR and SJ in their practice, it is fundamental that schools of social work make HR and SJ central to social work education (Dominelli, 2004; Sewpaul & Jones, 2005).

This article draws on a doctoral study of social work education in England and Spain. Specifically, the article aims to address research findings in relation to two of the study's research questions, namely: i) what are social work educators' understandings of HR and SJ in social work education in England and Spain? and ii) what learning and teaching strategies are used in the two countries to transmit HR and SJ to social work students?

The study was set against the European socioeconomic crisis associated with unbridled capitalist mechanisms and the irresponsible behaviour of financial institutions, economic and political powers (Jordan & Drakeford, 2012; Lundy, 2011). Used to justify the imposition of austerity agendas in Europe, the crisis visibly increased suffering amongst the most vulnerable (Eurostat, 2013) presenting social workers with ever increasing challenges in fulfilling their professional roles.

The comparative focus of the study is informed by the experience of the lead author who qualified and practised as a social worker in Spain before embarking on postgraduate study in England. Despite the commitment to HR and SJ embodied in the international definition of social work and codes of social work ethics in both countries, experience of the Spanish and English contexts suggested rather different understandings and applications of these values in social work education and practice. These differences offered fertile ground to compare the responses of social work education in these culturally contrasting European countries to the impact of neoliberalism on the profession and its service users, and to identify opportunities to reclaim more emancipatory forms of social work.

The article offers an outline of the study's theoretical underpinnings, research design and methods, followed by two findings sections focussing respectively on i) educators' understandings of HR and SJ and ii) strategies used in learning and teaching about HR and SJ. Drawing on the tenets of critical realism (Bhaskar, 1979), and critical discourse analysis (Fairclough, 2010), we then discuss these findings in more detail, focussing on the oppressive ideology of neoliberalism and the factors that mediate responses to neoliberalism. Finally, using Fairclough's notion of a 'positive critique' (2010, p. 2), we argue for the development of an alternative ideology of HR and SJ-based social work (IFSW and IASSW, 2014) to counter the prevailing pressures of neoliberalism.

Theoretical underpinnings, study design and methods

Comparing social work education in the two countries required a balance between breadth and depth of understanding, leading to the adoption of a mixed methods approach within a critical realist framework (McEvoy & Richards, 2006), offering the potential for the study to 'prise open the black box' to identify opportunities to reclaim more emancipatory forms of social work (Houston, 2010). Critical realism assumes the existence of an external social reality that is not directly observable: a complex reality where social phenomena are the result of a series of generative mechanisms (Bhaskar, 1989), interacting with each other in particular contexts. From a critical perspective, theory, values and politics are inseparable from research evidence, forming 'critical contextual features' of the research process, 'intertwined with knowledge claims' (Soydan, 2010, p. 131).

Data were collected through a web-based survey of social work educators distributed to all educational institutions offering undergraduate social work qualifying courses in England and Spain. These were followed by in depth interviews with a small sample (N = 7) of social work educators from one university in each country, selected purposively for its overt commitment to HR and SJ-based social work education demonstrated through published mission statements and programme information. Acknowledging the low response rates associated with web-based surveys and challenges in generalising from interviews based on a small purposive sample as limitations of this study, these sampling strategies and methods of data collection supported the broader goals of the research in combining breadth with depth of information to identify strategies of resistance to the spread of neoliberal ideology in social work education.

The web survey, achieving responses from 41 educators in 23 English institutions and 35 educators from 13 Spanish institutions, generated qualitative information through open ended questions about educators' understandings of, and attitudes and personal commitment to, HR and SJ, as well as their strategies for learning and teaching about HR and SJ. The interviews explored these questions in greater depth. Assisted by Nvivo software (Bryman, 2016), interview transcripts and responses to open ended questions from the survey were analysed thematically and subject to elements of critical discourse analysis (Fairclough, 2003). This involved multiple readings of the data with the explicit purpose of identifying underlying discourses described by Fairclough (2003, p. 123) as 'ways of representing' aspects of the social world which are enacted in, but have greater permanence than, particular texts or speeches, being linked with deeper ideologies and social structures. A coding structure was created to bring together different expressions of the same discourse. For example, various references to the function of contemporary mainstream social work in England as a mechanism of oppressive neoliberalism were coded 'mainstream social work in England: oppressive' and considered as a single discourse.

In addressing each research question, combinations of relevant empirical research findings were interpreted in line with the principles of critical realism (Bhaskar, 1979) through a process of retroduction. This involved going back from, below, or behind, observed regularities (Blaikie & Priest, 2017) to identify the historico-political, cultural and socio-economic factors shaping understandings of HR and SJ. Involving successive cycles of deduction and induction, linking theory with empirical data, retroduction allows for differing interpretations to be drawn together to suggest causal tendencies, mechanisms that operate in subtle ways, to explain events and suggest ways of responding to them (Danermark, Ekström, Jakobsen, & Karlsson, 2002; Houston, 2010). Pursuing the example of a single discourse – 'mainstream social work in England: oppressive' – the process of retroduction revealed explicit links with the ideology of radical social work in England and with wider theoretical argument about the impact of neoliberalism on the social work profession in England. This prompted further reflection, as part of the process of retroductive thinking, about the absence of a similar discourse in data generated from social work educators in Spain. Among the possible explanations or 'potentially operating causal mechanisms' (Houston, 2010), those considered to have greater explanatory power, such as the different historical links between social work and welfare systems in each country, were explored further to offer carefully informed interpretations of the research findings. We make no claims to singular truths here. Rather we adhere to Blaikie and Priest's (2017) articulation of the process of retroduction as requiring creativity as well as deep familiarity with the contexts of the research and relevant theory to inform the development of emerging argument. In the following section we present the results of this process in identifying social work educators' understandings of HR and SJ.

Social work educators' understandings of human rights and social justice

Social work educators in England largely understood HR and SJ as separate concepts and areas of knowledge. For example:

> Many of the questions talk about 'human rights and social justice' as though these terms are inevitably lined or inextricably woven together. In fact, it is entirely possible to discuss human rights in terms of individuals' rights without any linkage to social justice. (survey 30, England)

> The notion of rights tends to individualise and I think that, although that's important there are limits to that. And I think that a collective orientation underpins notions of social justice. (interview 2, England)

As these examples indicate, human rights were understood in legal terms, focussing on first generation civil and political rights enshrined in the UK Human Rights Act 1998. The relevance of human rights for social workers' roles was understood in terms of compliance with statutory human rights and legal responsibilities towards individual service users. This narrow approach represents a techni-cal rather than a professional approach, leaving social work practice highly susceptible to party pol-itical interests illustrated starkly by the Conservative Government's recent attempts to repeal the Human Rights Act (Murray, 2017).

The British Association of Social Workers reflects similar concerns in its Human Rights Policy, which recognises and seeks to address the fact that:

> "Human rights" as they have been passed into legislation in the UK have often been given a narrower meaning than the understanding social workers have as a profession .... (BASW, 2015, p. 4)

In contrast to these narrow understandings of HR and the separate consideration given to HR and SJ found in England, social work educators in Spain understood the two concepts as being intrinsi-cally linked, including individual and collective rights. One educator explained:

> I understand that social work is closely linked with the struggle for justice, and the struggle for justice is a struggle for human rights. (interview 4, Spain)

Another explained that HR and SJ were 'closely interlinked' in teaching, 'revolving around one another' (interview 3, Spain).

For educators interviewed in Spain, the social work profession had an important and unquestion-able responsibility to defend HR and promote SJ. Human rights responsibilities were seen as being shared by government, civil society and professions, with social work having a particular responsibil-ity in line with the global definition of social work. Educators were fully aware of, and engaged with, structural, activist, preventive and developmental dimensions of SJ. This was of particular relevance as the impact of extreme austerity measures being imposed across Spain were seen as clear examples of social injustice and violations of HR. For instance, one educator referred to the relationship between HR and SJ in social work as 'extremely close' and described the triple alliance of HR, SJ and social work as 'highly powerful' (interview 1, Spain). She linked her views directly to the inter-national definition of social work:

> The IFSW's ... new definition even assimilates HR and SJ as the motivation and justification of social work. There-fore, from the very roots of our profession it is clearly being made explicit the fact that social work has as a pillar, as a foundation, and thus as a channel always to travel together with the defence of human rights and to establish norms and possible mechanisms for achieving social justice.

Another educator in Spain highlighted the importance of social work's role in promoting the struc-tural dimensions of the concepts of human rights and social justice, claiming that:

> ... that of the social worker is the par excellence professional profile concerned with denouncing, promotion, pre-vention ... with accompanying communities in the process of achieving more ability to claim their rights, to denounce living conditions that are certainly not socially just, and to promote fairer conditions ... a social worker also has capacity to have an impact on politics and on public society for the promotion of social justice and human rights .... (interview 2, Spain)

The social work educators interviewed in England also expressed strong engagement with HR and even stronger engagement with SJ, arguing the need to promote these values within the social work profession. However, their understandings of the alliance of HR and SJ in social work were closely linked with their personal and/or political values and their concerns about current and future directions in social work and social work education. One explained:

> ... from the age of about 12 I have been interested in issues of social justice and being politically oriented if you like ... And the reason I was drawn towards working in social care was because I felt it was one way of realising the notion of social justice (interview 2, England)

And another:

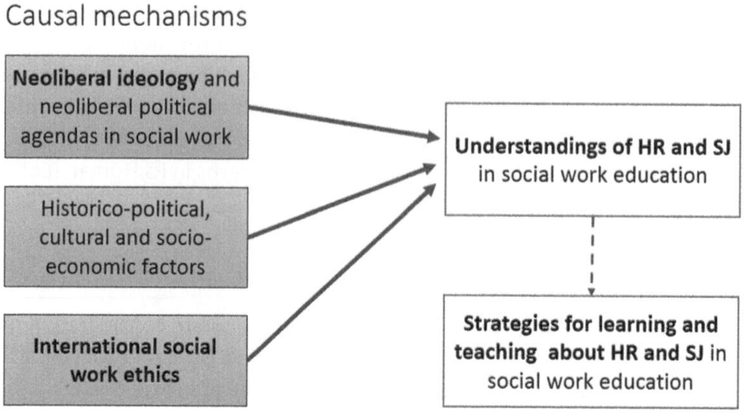

Causal mechanisms

Figure 1. Model of causal mechanisms informing social work educators' understandings of: HR and SJ and subsequent strategies for learning and teaching.

> The people that social workers work with ... get a hard time from society ... they deserve one group of professionals that will stand up and speak out for them and be alongside them, and that's my vision of what the social worker should be ... We emphasise it throughout the course, whenever we can we talk to them about the social causes of private pain .... the political nature of social workers' tasks. (interview 3, England)

Just as social work educators in Spain, those in England were concerned about the direct effects of neoliberal politics and mechanisms on the most vulnerable groups of people in society. But they also highlighted the further oppression of vulnerable groups by a welfare system and social work profession being reshaped along neoliberal lines.

> What is happening with social work ... is that it's now a system for fixing people to fit the system ... We teach students to think about human rights and social justice, [but] I wonder if that's all undone when it comes to practice. (interview 1, England)

Oppressive practice settings and the tension between students' focus on employability and social work principles were noted in survey responses as challenges for social work educators in England. For example:

> The jobs we are training students to fill now may have the label social work but in reality they are administrative agents of statutory services and if we encourage them to focus on rights and justice they will not survive that long. (survey 9, England)

These practice-based challenges did not feature in the responses of social work educators in Spain raising the interesting question of what might account for the differences.

The research findings suggested that while HR and principles of SJ were central to social work education in Spain, in England their place in social work education was highly contested. Using the process of retroduction (Blaikie & Priest, 2017) described earlier, ideological, historico-political, cultural and socio-economic factors were identified as influential in shaping different understandings of HR and SJ in social work education in England and Spain and, we argue, underpin educators' strategies for facilitating learning and teaching about HR and SJ. A model of these causal mechanisms is shown in Figure 1.

Strategies for learning and teaching about human rights and social justice

In both countries tension was evident between the ethical commitment of the social work profession to HR and SJ, and neoliberal ideology that was driving narrow models of social work education, undermining the value-base of the profession. Ideology, defined as a 'systematic body of ideas'

(Hall, 1977, p. 4) including collective beliefs, values and interests (Carey & Foster, 2013), is conceptualised in critical theory as a means of maintaining power and domination (Fairclough, 2010), setting a basis for assessing whether the use of specific discourses leads to social wrongs that require mitigation to avoid threatening human well-being. Fairclough (2010) argues that critical theory can also be used to develop 'a positive critique' to identify and analyse ways in which oppressive ideology can be resisted.

Exploring strategies used by educators to develop students' critical understandings of HR and SJ, and of the pernicious effects of, and strategies to resist, neoliberalism revealed a range of practices. These included strengthening the focus of learning and teaching about histories and theories of HR and SJ; stressing the importance of structural theory to complement theoretical understanding of social work with individuals; connecting knowledge and theoretical understanding with contemporary social work practices; and creating safe discussion spaces for the exploration of experiences and understandings of injustice. Educators' own commitment to values of HR and SJ, supporting collective action by students, raising awareness of international developments in social work, and identifying opportunities for international networking and periods of practice in international settings, were also considered effective in enabling students to develop more critical understandings of HR and SJ.

Despite these strategies for promoting greater engagement with HR and SJ, findings from the survey pointed to the predominance of a narrow neoliberal conceptualisation of social work and social work education in England posing one of the main constraints to incorporating meaningful learning and teaching about HR and SJ in the social work curriculum. Educators in Spain identified fewer challenges for teaching in these areas, referring to curriculum content and practical methods for facilitating links between theory and practice. Interview participants in both countries were openly critical of neoliberal ideology, its effects on society and the social work profession. Unsurprisingly, given their recruitment from universities and courses known for their commitment to HR and SJ, they were keen to explain how they attempted to convey through their teaching, models of social work that embody human rights and values of social justice. In both countries educators' views embodied anti-capitalist ideology, for example 'market needs are prioritised over people's needs' (England), and 'people are exploited and dehumanised' (Spain). Interview participants in both countries drew on discourses of radical social work referring to 'the public causes of private pain', and the role of social work in 'fixing people to fit a capitalist system'. It was notable, however, that educators in Spain drew heavily on ethical discourses of international social work, focussing more closely on citizenship rights and welfare state ideology.

In terms of critical realism, the ideologies of neoliberalism and international social work ethics, mediated by historico-political, cultural and socio-economic influences, were inextricably linked with social work educators' understandings of HR and SJ, which in turn informed strategies for learning and teaching about HR and SJ as illustrated in Figure 1. In the following section we discuss neoliberalism, conceptualised as an oppressive ideology, in more detail before expanding on the factors mediating responses to the threats posed to social work education and practice by neoliberalism.

The oppressive ideology of neoliberalism in social work

Numerous authors have described how government led marketisation processes have reshaped social work, diminishing its autonomy, professional scope and standards (Bamford, 2015; Dominelli, 2004, 2010; Dustin, 2007; Ferguson, 2008; Garrett, 2010; Harris, 2014; Jones, 2004). The growth of managerialism and the widespread adoption of bureaucratic models of practice have served to dilute the essence of social work as a relationship-based profession (Bamford, 2015; Munro, 2011) and policy rhetoric promising greater choice and control for service users has been used to transfer responsibility for social problems to individual service users (Barnes, 2011; Ferguson, 2007, 2012). These shifts are reflected in social work education. In England there is increasing pressure to prepare students for the workforce by maximising time in practice settings where students are socialised through exposure to statutory interventions reflecting the dominant social control elements of social work (Bamford, 2015). This minimises time available for developing deep, critical understandings of HR and SJ, fundamental concepts for the social work profession (Croisdale-Appleby, 2014; Higgins, 2015). While this situation was articulated most clearly by research participants in England, these market-oriented processes of de-professionalisation affecting social work are also found in other European countries including Spain (De la Red & Brezmes, 2009; Ioakimidis, Cruz-Santos, & Martínez-Herrero, 2014; Ponnert & Svensson, 2016).

The retreat of European welfare states and the expansion of neoliberal models of social work are explained by reference to a combination of causal factors related to global economic forces, politics and ideology (Dominelli & Khan, 2000). European governments, whether conservative or social democratic, have used the pressures of globalisation as justification to adopt and reinforce neoliberal policies associated with the retreat of welfare provision and weakening of human rights (Ferguson, 2008). This has left social work in a state of uncertainty and has seen the emergence of a 'neoliberal social work' focussing narrowly on risk management rather than broader notions of empowerment of individuals, families, groups and communities in situations where HR and SJ are threatened or denied. Social work concerns with structural causes of injustice are increasingly interpreted by governments as problematic and as evidence of the need for the reform of social work. The traditional values of social work including respect for persons, belief in individual change, and relationship-based interventions are being continuously eroded as particular social groups such as young people, those seeking asylum or migrating for economic reasons, are demonised in neoliberal societies (Ferguson, 2008). The victimisation of vulnerable groups and social work service users was highlighted by all educators interviewed in this study who were unanimous in their views about the importance of helping social work students to understand and overcome prejudices associated with negative images and ideological discourses that serve conveniently to further 'punish the poor' (Wacquant, 2009).

The philosophy, principles and values of the neoliberal market have been argued as being both antithetical to, and irreconcilable with, those of social work, rooted in notions of human dignity, human rights, social justice, universalism, democracy and citizenship (Dominelli, 2010; Eroles, 1997; Ferguson, 2008; Ife, 2008). But there are those in the social work scientific community who, however reluctantly, embrace the neoliberal view of the world and engage with the dominant social control role assigned to social work by neoliberal governments since this direction is readily perceived as the sole route to professional and scientific status within the profession (Shaw, 2003). In both England and Spain, controlling features of the profession have been evident through the history of social work although they have co-existed with more enabling practices and radical approaches designed to achieve social change. However, the new millennium, particularly in England, has seen an increasingly rapid tightening of the neoliberal grip and the establishment of a dominant neoliberal paradigm informing social work policy and practice (Higgins, 2015). In these circumstances, the development of effective forms of resistance to neoliberalism and its impact on the social work profession become ever more important, and the process of developing effective resistance requires knowledge and understanding of the contextual factors that can all too easily derail such efforts. It is to these mediating factors that we now turn.

Historico-political, cultural and socio-economic factors mediating responses to neoliberalism

Consideration of the historical links between the social work profession, western capitalist welfare states and cultural values provides a further opportunity to shed light on the greater historical and contemporary misalignment of mainstream social work with HR and SJ ideals in England compared with Spain. Social work as a profession developed to respond to the economic and social needs of people following the growth of industrialisation in the nineteenth century and rising levels of conflict between the working and ruling classes in western societies (Eroles, 1997). Responsibility for addressing the resulting social problems was first assumed by charitable organisations and gradually extended to nation states which became the main guarantors of social welfare during the twentieth century (Lundy, 2011). Thus, the growth of capitalism has been accompanied by state sponsored responses to social problems arising from the predominant economic system. The relationship between capitalism and state welfare has always been complex and highly contradictory, and their coexistence has become increasingly tense and untenable in late-stage or neoliberal global capitalism (Lundy, 2011). As Lundy (2011, p. 15) argues, 'addressing societal inequalities and social structures that contribute to such conditions is no longer part of the political agenda'.

In Spain, notwithstanding the influence of international capitalism, the relationship between capitalism, welfare and the nation state has followed a different path given the later development of a welfare state. The dictatorial Franco regime, 1939–1975, left Spain internationally isolated, lacking in democratic and welfare rights. And Spanish social work has been shaped by the process of merging the catholic charity tradition of social welfare provision with the development of a 'scientific' social work profession (Méndez-Bonito, 2005) with limited support from government. Even during the democratic era, social work in Spain has not been subject to significant government control, maintaining autonomy in its education system, its knowledge and value base. The mainly female profession has historically shown strong vocational rather than employment-oriented motivation and the profession has maintained greater resistance to market pressures in relation to recruitment (Méndez-Bonito, 2005). As one educator in Spain noted:

> There is a high level of commitment [to HR and SJ] one has and develops when making the decision to study social work.... I believe that the majority of social work students are very vocational and very eager to change the world. (interview 3, Spain)

By contrast, an educator in England suggested that:

> Students when they graduate they want to find work. They're in a position of 'do you hold on to your moral values or do you take work when you know you need work?' I think there's a real wrestle with those kinds of things. (interview 1, England)

While Spanish social work and social work education have had briefer exposure to neoliberal ideology, Spanish society, strongly influenced by Catholicism and the strength of the family as an institution, is arguably better placed to resist the values of neoliberal capitalism. While both countries have become increasingly culturally diverse and have seen sharp declines in Christian religious adherence, almost 70% of Spanish citizens continue to describe themselves as Catholic (CIS, 2015), while in 2014 only 43% of English and Welsh citizens of the UK described themselves as Anglican, Catholic or members of other Christian denominations (Sherwood, 2016).

Acceptance of neoliberal discourses among citizens and social scientists, including social workers, is more likely as societies become increasingly fragmented and plural, less secure and controllable, and where identities, values and lifestyles are reoriented to greater individualism (Dominelli & Khan, 2000). The impact of capitalist economies on individuals, legitimised through the mass media, is well documented (Bourdieu, 2005; Méndez-Fernández, Leal-Freire, Martínez-Rodríguez, & Salazar-Bernanrd, 2006) and includes the growth of individualism, consumerism, competitiveness, commodification of personal relationships, weaker social cohesion and cooperation, passivity and hedonism. Those deprived of their rights are persuaded to accept the unified discourse presented by politicians and the media, justifying inequality as the product of personal merit, legitimising the commodification of people, hindering collective action and the defence of human rights (Méndez-Fernández et al., 2006). Méndez-Bonito (2005) highlights how these traits and values are at odds with traditional Spanish social values that embrace wellbeing as relational, ambivalence towards wealth and prestige, and acceptance of help from family and social, often religious, networks. By contrast, she notes, capitalist values are more easily implanted in societies sensitive to Protestantism such as England, where individual notions of success and wellbeing, autonomy and self-determination, and a scientific approach to human problems are all held in high regard.

Spanish social work has also been more closely influenced by the radical social work tradition of Latin America sharing some common cultural elements of language and religion, and its own, relatively recent, emergence from the struggle for democratic and welfare rights. This has contributed to the profession's ongoing identity as having a role in promoting structural change and human rights, rejecting narrower neoliberal models of social work education and practice. Open rejection of neoliberalism and austerity measures is evident in the statements and discourses of Spanish social work professional associations (CGTS, 2009; Lima, 2012) and was also evident in survey responses and interviews with social work educators in Spain.

Building on this more nuanced understanding of the differences between the two countries, we turn to explore ways of challenging neoliberalism through the development of an alternative ideology built on HR and SJ, consistent with the international definition of social work.

Challenging neoliberalism through an alternative ideology of human rights and social justice-based social work: developing 'a positive critique'

This section speaks to Fairclough's (2010) argument that critical social research can contribute to struggles for better societies through a 'positive critique', analysing how capitalism's social wrongs can be mitigated and resisted. Wronka and Staub-Bernasconi (2012) claim that the commitment to human rights articulated in the international definition of social work as a profession and academic discipline (IFSW and IASSW, 2014) provides the profession with autonomy allowing for the refusal of 'illegitimate' demands from social agencies, society and service users.

Despite working in a context in which narrow neoliberal models of social work practice and education are able to flourish, interview participants in England had found ways of remaining loyal to their professional ideologies and encouraged students to do the same, employing learning and teaching practices described earlier. However, as managerialism and marketisation gain further ground in social work education, the space for this type of resistance is likely to be increasingly constrained. In Spain, mainstream social work and social work education remain more strongly aligned with the international definition of social work, supporting Carey and Foster's (2013) argument that occupations such as social work can be seen as capable of producing their own self-determining ideologies that can compete with others.

In this study, the international definition of social work, together with international and national codes of ethics, constituted a systematic body of ideas, beliefs and interests capable of producing emancipatory discourses to counter ideological expressions of neoliberalism. The tension between the ideology reflected in international social work ethics and the oppressive ideology of neoliberalism, concerned with maintaining dominant power relations, was evident in social work education in both countries, influencing educators' understandings of HR and SJ. The dynamic between these ideologies was mediated by cultural beliefs, norms and values in each country, particularly those informing notions of individualism and communitarianism and the roles and relationships between the individual, family, community, church and state (Tropman, 1986). These contextual features influenced the balance between the positive ideology of international social work ethics and the oppressive ideology of neoliberalism.

Social work educators, especially in England, continue to face attempts by those who promote, or fail to oppose, the principles of neoliberalism, destabilising the HR and SJ foundations of the profession. The ethical foundations articulated in the international definition of social work, therefore, take on an ever more important role in providing social work practitioners and educators with a legitimate framework from which to pursue the core values of social work and deconstruct neoliberalism. But the potential to realise the aspiration summed up in the expression 'another social work is possible' (Ferguson, 2009) must be accompanied by a dual note of caution. First is Carey and Foster's (2013, p. 256) warning that 'self-determining ideologies can adapt, change or even disappear over time'. And second is Foucault's (1990) assertion that while resistance and defiance are natural within discursive terrains, resistance in itself may not necessarily lead to wider change.

Conclusion

Empirical evidence from this comparative study of social work educators in England and Spain demonstrates the reach of neoliberalism into the realm of social work education where core values of respect for human rights and the pursuit of social justice lie in tension with contemporary policies shaping social work practice. Using a framework of critical realism to 'prise open the black box' (Houston, 2010), this study has sought to offer a more nuanced appreciation of social work educators' understandings of HR and SJ and their application in social work education. The broad comparison between England and Spain has sharpened the focus of understanding by using a process of retroduction, examining patterns in the empirical data in the light of their respective historico-political, cultural and socio-economic contexts. And interviews with educators overtly committed to HR and SJ-based social work have highlighted practices used to facilitate students' appreciation of the importance of HR and SJ in social work nationally and globally that can serve to inspire others in Europe.

However, the persistence of neoliberal agendas shaping social welfare policy and the delivery of public social work services means that social work practitioners and educators alike face continuing uncertainty. Challenging the status quo requires continual critical and creative thinking. Current concerns facing social work in England include political aspirations to undermine the power of the Human Rights Act and the climate of xenophobia, legitimised by policies promoting stricter immigration controls for refugees from regimes with little regard for human rights, and for European citizens whose right to free movement is under threat from Brexit. Social work education is also under attack with the introduction of fast track training programmes and apprenticeship schemes that prioritise socialisation into practice settings commonly concerned with the social control functions of social work. Government investment in these schemes, together with arrangements that incentivise the development of teaching partnerships between local government social work departments and universities, divert funds away from social work education in higher education institutions, further undermining the specialist body of knowledge and value base of the social work profession and limiting the development of critical thinking associated with higher education. In Spain, evidence of a stronger continuing commitment to the interconnected importance of HR and SJ in social work education and practice with explicit acknowledgement of the relevance of structural causes of social problems suggest that Spanish social work education is better equipped to resist the influence of neoliberalism. However, in a period marked by the consequences of continuing economic crisis and draconian austerity, and recent developments in political governance that signal the continuing power of right wing politics, the social work profession will require continuing effort to resist and challenge neoliberalism.

The study reported here suggests that the wide range of actors in the social work profession must redouble efforts, nationally and internationally, to seek strategies to counter the social injustices that are the inevitable result of neoliberalism, affecting social work service users, practitioners and educators alike. Further research is required, not only to map developments but to engage service users, practitioners and educators in action research to reclaim and sustain the values of HR and SJ in social work education and practice.

Acknowledgements

This research was supported by the UK Economic and Social Research Council. We thank two anonymous reviewers for their comments on an earlier version of the article.

Disclosure statement

No potential conflict of interest was reported by the authors.

Funding

This research was supported by the UK Economic and Social Research Council.

ORCID

María Inés Martínez Herrero (iD) http://orcid.org/0000-0002-7743-2771

References

Bamford, T. (2015). *A contemporary history of social work. Learning from the past*. Bristol: Policy Press.

Banks, S. (2006). *Ethics and values in social work* (3rd ed.). Basingstoke: Palgrave Macmillan.

Barnes, M. (2011). Abandoning care? A critical perspective on personalisation from an ethic of care. *Ethics and Social Welfare*, 5(2), 153–167.

BASW. (2014). *The code of ethics for social work: Statement of principles*. Retrieved from http://cdn.basw.co.uk/upload/basw_112315-7.pdf

BASW. (2015). *BASW human rights policy*. Kent: The British Association of Social Workers.

Bhaskar, R. (1979). *The possibility of naturalism: A philosophical critique of the contemporary human sciences*. Brighton: Harvester Press.

Bhaskar, R. (1989). *Reclaiming reality: A critical introduction to contemporary philosophy*. London: Verso.

Blaikie, N., & Priest, J. (2017). *Social research: Paradigms in action*. Cambridge: Polity Press.

Bourdieu, P. (2005). *Pensamiento y acción. 2ª edición*. Buenos Aires: Libros del Zorzal.

Bryman, A. (2016). *Social research methods*. Oxford: Oxford University Press.

Carey, M., & Foster, V. (2013). Social work, ideology, discourse and the limits of post-hegemony. *Journal of Social Work, 13*(3), 248–266.

CGTS. (2009). *Manifiesto Trabajo social ante la Crisis: Consejo General del Trabajo Social*.

CGTS. (2012). *Codigo deontologico del Trabajo Social*. Retrieved from https://www.cgtrabajosocial.es/consejo/codigo_deontologico

CIS. (2015). 3050 Barómetro de Enero 2015.

Croisdale-Appleby, D. (2014). *Re-visioning social work education. An independent review*. London: Department of Health.

Danermark, B., Ekström, M., Jakobsen, L., & Karlsson, J. C. (2002). *Explaining society. Critical realism in the social sciences*. London: Routledge.

De la Red, N., & Brezmes, M. (2009). Trabajo Social en España. In T. Fernández García & C. Alemán-Bracho (Eds.), *Introducción al trabajo social* (pp. 131–152). Madrid: Alianza.

De Vogli, R. (2013). Financial crisis, austerity, and health in Europe. *The Lancet, 382*(9890), 391, doi:10.1016/S0140-6736(13)61882-1. Retrieved from http://www.sciencedirect.com/science/article/pii/S0140673613616621

Dominelli, L. (2004). *Social work. Theory and practice for a changing profession*. Oxford: Polity.

Dominelli, L. (2010). *Social work in a globalizing world*. Cambridge: Polity Press.

Dominelli, L. (2012). *Green social work: From environmental crises to environmental justice*. Cambridge: Polity.

Dominelli, L., & Khan, P. (2000). The impact of globalization on social work in the UK. *European Journal of Social Work, 3*(2), 95–108.

Dustin, D. (2007). *The McDonaldization of social work*. Aldershot: Ashgate.

The Equality Trust. (2017). *How has inequality changed?* Development of UK Income Inequality. Retrieved from https://www.equalitytrust.org.uk/how-has-inequality-changed

Eroles, C. (1997). Derechos humanos: compromiso ético del trabajo social. In C. Eroles, N. Fóscolo, & M. C. G. d. Camín (Eds.), *Los Derechos Humanos: Compromiso ético del Trabajo Social* (pp. 15–64). Buenos Aires: Espacio Editorial.

Eurostat. (2013). *People at risk of poverty or social exclusion by age and sex*. Retrieved from http://appsso.eurostat.ec.europa.eu/nui/show.do?dataset=ilc_peps01&lang=en

Fairclough, N. (2003). *Analysing discourse: Textual analysis for social research*. London: Routledge.

Fairclough, N. (2010). *Critical discourse analysis : The critical study of language* (2nd ed.). Harlow: Longman.

Ferguson, I. (2007). Increasing user choice or privatizing risk? The antinomies of personalization. *British Journal of Social Work, 37*(3), 387–403.

Ferguson, I. (2008). *Reclaiming social work: Challenging neo-liberalism and promoting social justice*. London: Sage.

Ferguson, I. (2009). 'Another social work is possible!' Reclaiming the radical tradition. In V. Leskošek (Ed.), *Theories and methods of social work: Exploring different perspectives* (pp. 81–98). Ljubljana: University of Ljubljana, Faculty of Social Work.

Ferguson, I. (2012). Personalisation, social justice and social work: A reply to Simon Duffy. *Journal of Social Work Practice, 26*(1), 55–73.

FOESSA. (2013). *Desigualdad y Derechos Sociales. Análisis y Perspectivas 2013*. Madrid: Foessa; Cáritas.

Foucault, M. (1990). *The archeology of knowledge*. London: Routeledge.

Garrett, P. M. (2010). Examining the 'conservative revolution': Neoliberalism and social work education. *Social Work Education, 29*(4), 340–355.

Hall, S. (1977). The hinterland of science: Ideology and the 'sociology of knowledge'. In C. f. C. C. Studies (Ed.), *On ideology* (pp. 6–15). London: Hutchinson.

Harris, J. (2014). (Against) neoliberal social work. *Critical and Radical Social Work, 2*(1), 7–22.

Harvey, D. (2005). *A brief history of neoliberalism*. Oxford: Oxford University Press.

Higgins, M. (2015). The struggle for the soul of social work in England. *Social Work Education, 34*(1), 4–16.

Houston, S. (2010). Prising open the black box: Critical realism, action research and social work. *Qualitative Social Work: Research and Practice, 9*(1), 73–91.

Ife, J. (2008). *Human rights and social work: Towards rights-based practice*. New York: Cambridge University Press.

IFSW, & IASSW. (2014). *Global definition of social work*. Retrieved from http://ifsw.org/get-involved/global-definition-of-social-work/

Ioakimidis, V., Cruz-Santos, C., & Martínez-Herrero, I. (2014). Reconceptualizing social work in times of crisis: An examination of the cases of Greece, Spain and Portugal. *International Social Work, 57*(4), 285–300.

Jones, C. (2004). The neo-liberal assault: Voices from the front line of British state social work. In I. Ferguson, M. Lavalette, & B. Whitmore (Eds.), *Globalisation, global justice and social work* (pp. 97–108). London: Taylor and Francis.

Jordan, B., & Drakeford, M. (2012). *Social work and social policy under austerity*. New York: Palgrave Macmillan.

Lavalette, M. (Ed.). (2011). *Radical social work today. Social work at the crossroads*. Bristol: Policy Press.

Lima, A. I. (2012). Alliance for the defence of social services: Spanish network in defence of social rights and a public system of social services. In N. Hall (Ed.), *Social work around the world V: Building the global agenda for social work*. Nottingham: IFSW.

Lundy, C. (2011). *Social work, social justice, and human rights: A structural approach to practice*. North York: Toronto Univ Press.

McEvoy, P., & Richards, D. (2006). A critical realist rationale for using a combination of quantitative and qualitative methods. *Journal of Research in Nursing, 11*(1), 66–78.

Méndez-Bonito, P. (2005). The history of social work education in Spain: Does harmonisation make sense? *Portularia, 5*(1), 205–222.

Méndez-Fernández, A. B., Leal-Freire, B., Martínez-Rodríguez, M., & Salazar-Bernanrd, J. I. (2006). Aprehendiendo a respetar: La perspectiva de Derechos Humanos como elemento fundamental en la formación y práctica del trabajo social. *Acciones e Investigaciones Sociales, 1*, 460–487.

Munro, E. (2011). *The Munro review of child protection: Final report, a child-centred system*. London: The Stationery Office.

Murray, C. R. G. (2017). Magna Carta's tainted legacy: Historic justifications for a British bill of rights and the case against the human rights act. In F. Cowell (Ed.), *The case against the 1998 human rights act: A critical assessment*. London: Routledge.

Piketty, T. (2014). *Capital in the twenty-first century*. Cambridge, MA: Harvard University Press.

Ponnert, L., & Svensson, K. (2016). Standardisation—the end of professional discretion? *European Journal of Social Work, 19*(3-4), 586–599.

Sewpaul, V., & Jones, D. (2005). Global standards for the education and training of the social work profession. *International Journal of Social Welfare, 14*(3), 218–230.

Shaw, I. (2003). Critical commentary. Cutting edge issues in social work research. *British Journal of Social Work, 33*, 107–120.

Sherwood, H. (2016). People of no religion outnumber Christians in England and Wales—study. *The Guardian*. Retrieved from https://www.theguardian.com/world/2016/may/23/no-religion-outnumber-christians-england-wales-study

Soydan, H. (2010). Politics and values in social work research. In I. Shaw, K. Briar-Lawson, J. Orme, & R. Ruckdeschel (Eds.), *The SAGE handbook of social work research* (pp. 131–148). London: Sage.

Tropman, J. E. (1986). The "catholic ethic" vs the "protestant ethic": Catholic social service and the welfare state. *Social Thought, 12*, 13–22.

Wacquant, L. (2009). *Punishing the poor: The neoliberal government of social insecurity*. Durham: Duke University Press.

Wronka, J., & Staub-Bernasconi, S. (2012). Human rights. In K. Lyons, T. Hokenstad, M. Pawar, N. Huegler, & N. Hall (Eds.), *The SAGE handbook of international social work* (pp. 70–84). London: SAGE.

Clients and case managers as neoliberal subjects? Shaping session tasks and everyday interactions with severely mentally ill (SMI) clients

신자유주의적 주체로서의 클라이언트와 사례관리자? 정신중증질환을 경험하고 있는 클라이언트와의 상담과제와 일상적 상호작용 형성에 관한 연구

Eunjung Lee, A. Ka Tat Tsang, Marion Bogo, Marjorie Johnstone and Jessica Herschman

ABSTRACT

This article explores *how* multiple contexts – professional knowledge (e.g. case management), institutional practices (e.g. New Public Management), and mental health policies and legislations (e.g. Mental Health Act) – under neoliberal governance (re)produce ways social workers interact with their clients in moment-to-moment interactions. It is part of a larger process and outcome research project on cross-cultural social work practice in outpatient community mental health settings in an urban Canadian city. Using transcripts of audio-taped sessions between social workers and clients with severe mental illness, and inspired by critical theories of language, knowledge and power, we illustrate how neoliberal themes (re)position clients and social workers in negotiating session tasks in everyday interactions, and how these interactions shape the clients and social workers as desirable and undesirable neoliberal subjects. These detailed studies in micro-interactions can be used as practice examples in considering how social workers can be critically reflective of our own micro practice and resist the governing neoliberal ideology in the macro level.

초록

본 논문은 신자유주의적 거버넌스 하에서 전문지식(예, 사례관리), 기관실무(예, 신공공관리), 정신건강 정책과 법률(예, 정신보건법) 등과 같은 다양한 맥락들이 어떻게 사회복지사와 클라이언트의 일상적 상호작용 방식을 (재)생산하는지를 탐색한다. 이 연구는 캐나다 한 도시의 지역정신건강센터들에서 수행된 다문화 사회복지실천의 과정과 결과에 관한 전체 연구프로젝트 중 일 부분에 해당된다. 사회복지사와 정신중증질환을 경험하고 있는 클라이언트 간 상담내용을 녹음하고 이를 언어, 지식 그리고 권력에 관한 비판이론으로 분석하였다. 이를 통해 신자유주의적 테마들이 어떻게 사회복지사와 클라이언트와의 일상적 상호작용 속에서 상담과제를 설정하는지, 그리고 이러한 상호작용들 속에서 어떻게 그들이 바람직한 혹은 바람직하지 않은 신자유주의의 주체로 결정되는지를 규명한다. 이러한 일상 언어의 미시적 상호작용에 관한 연구는 사회복지사가 자신의 실무에 영향을 미치는 신자유주의적

이데올로기를 어떻게 비판적으로 성찰하고 변화시키고자 노력할 수 있는지를 보여주는 실천사례로 활용될 수 있을 것이다.

Introduction

Literatures on the effective 'standard of care' for the severely mentally ill (SMI) support the claim that case management (CM) services are the most beneficial in community mental health contexts (Greene et al., 2006; Ziguras & Stuart, 2000). Earlier models of Case Management (CM) trace their roots to the social liberation movements of the 1960s and 1970s, which resulted in an increased awareness of the oppression and discrimination faced by persons living with SMI. Before this time, mental health services were largely limited to institutional care and hospitalised settings (Martin, Peter, & Kapp, 2003). The new, rights-based discourses promoted a socio-political movement towards a community mental health model, which was supported by the advent of psychotropic drugs. Subsequently, a financial imperative for health care costs was downloaded onto lower levels of government (i.e. federal-to-state/provincial-to-municipal). This context positions CM models as an alternative liberal treatment plan to costly institutional health settings; at the same time, however, case managers became responsible for reducing programme costs, increasing pro-ductivity and maintaining higher caseloads, medical adherence and symptom management of clients (Vourlekis & Ell, 2007; Williams, Forster, McCarthy, & Hargreaves, 1994). Due to these increasing roles of case managers, CM services have been critiqued for 'managing cases' rather than 'providing care' to clients and 'disempowering' clients rather than achieving the proposed goal of 'empowering' them (Dustin, 2007; Meeks, 2001; Spitzmueller, 2014). Instead of criticising individual case managers, we attest that these mishaps can be attributed to neoliberal ideology and practice, which govern and shape case managers' tasks and interactions with clients. While focusing on self-sufficiency, effective-ness and efficacy, social workers are consumed by 'services that count and are measurable' with endless record-keeping and tracking. Meanwhile, although unintended, social workers are managed and co-opted into costing the importance of the alliance instead of learning about the 'person' of the client and his/her needs (Dominelli, 2010; Dustin, 2007; Sewpaul & Hölsher, 2004).

We echo this critical scholarship and furthermore aim to illustrate *how* this unintended practice occurs when providing CM services. Our research focus is on unveiling manifestations of how the macro systems and underlying ideology (i.e. neoliberalism) impact on our micro interactions (i.e. turn-by-turn communi-cation) and consequently position the client and social worker in certain identities (i.e. neoliberal subject making). Using selected excerpts from actual interactions between clients with SMI and social workers, we illustrate this neoliberal subject-making process: *how* social workers' own subject formation under neoliberal governance (e.g. thrift, on self-efficiency and accountability,) influences their interactions with clients, and meanwhile, though unintended, positions clients as lesser neoliberal subjects.

To locate the structural context for social service delivery in Ontario, Canada where our data are drawn from, we first briefly review Canadian mental health policy and the pervasive practice of case management. Second, we introduce our theoretical framework – critical theories of neoliberalism and social work (Dustin, 2007; Moffatt, 1999; Rose, 1999) along with several critical Foucauldian concepts (Foucault, 1983, 1980, 1976). Then, using critical discourse analysis (Fairclough, 2013), we examine the actual interactions between the clients with SMI and their case managers. We close with a discussion of the implications of, and training issues for, social workers in serving clients with SMI in community mental health practice.

Case management and mental health policy and practice in Canada

In Canada, the federal government sets the standard for the national health policy, but each provin-cial government is responsible for the delivery and regulation of service in health policy administration. In Ontario, case management, especially intensive case management models such as Assertive Community Treatment (ACT), along with community-based crisis response systems, have become the dominant practice in mental health treatment. The ACT programme is a multidisciplinary team treatment approach for people with SMI, consisting of a psychiatrist, a psychiatric nurse, a social worker, a rehabilitation counselor and a peer support worker. Its principles include community-based services toward community integration, highly individualised assertive and proactive primary services on a 24/7 basis, emphasis on vocational services toward employment, substance abuse services, family support and education, psychoeducational service, and attention to health care needs (Ontario ACT Association, 2018). Social workers in the team provide much of the psychosocial services to clients. Among various services (e.g. housing and transportation support, medication monitoring, supportive counseling, etc.), securing financial stability becomes central, and social workers support clients in their application for the income assistance programme, the *Ontario Disability Support Programme (ODSP)* offered under the *Ontario Ministry of Community and Social Services* (Gewurtz, Cott, Rush, & Kirsh, 2012).

Critical scholars in Canadian mental health policy note that the standards set by *the Ministry of Health* in each province are closely aligned with the New Public Management approach in a neoliberal welfare state (Gourlay, 1998; Goering, Wasylenki, & Durbin, 2000). They argue that, despite the explicit task-oriented approaches that guide case managers, the prescribed service requirements (e.g. focus on employment and individual/family responsibilities) appear to structure (and even limit) the case managers' daily tasks and (inter)actions with clients and their families. Meanwhile, government cutbacks on social spending, the redistribution of funding through large over-seeing organisations, and their 'fee-for-service' billing practices (e.g. numerous case notes and transactional units measuring client/worker interaction) have become the 'practice standard', negatively impacting and changing the face of case management and community mental health practice (Spitzmueller, 2014). Greene and his colleagues (2006) also critique that, despite varied perspectives on CM practice, the main objective has been one that has continued to 'focus on keeping consumers stabilised in the community' and to encourage consumers to 'accept the limitations their illness created, encouraging them to manage their illness and to lower their expectations for future achievement and growth' (p. 340).

The idea of mentally ill people as dangerous, sick and/or incompetent, who need to be managed, controlled and contained from/by so-called healthy people, has been a driving force in Canadian mental health (Goering et al., 2000; Magnus & Shera, 2012). The *Mental Health Act* (MHA) in Ontario sets out the criteria for voluntary, informal and involuntary admissions to psychiatric facilities and the MHA amendment in 2000 established *Community Treatment Orders* for the management of psychiatric outpatients, a legislation that over-rode patient consent to treatment (Ontario Hospital Association, 2016). Although this *Act* applies to people whose capacities are compromised severely and globally, and the empirical studies clearly note that people with SMI are less violent compared to their counterparts (Stuart, 2003), this pervasive rhetoric may impact discourses of how mentally ill people are constructed in society – in the minds of social workers as well as in the minds of clients themselves. Thus, the pervasive discourse of mentally ill people as *dangerous* and/or *incompetent*, in conjunction with the emphasis on *managing care* through intensive case management services under neoliberal policy and practice, may work as *reference points* governing social workers' (inter)-actions in working with SMI people, spurring questions such as: Is he/she able to handle his/her daily care? Does he/she have the capacity to understand financial management to be self-sufficient?

Constructing neoliberal subjects in the community mental health practice

The idea of 'many realities' is intrinsic to social construction theory and acts to broaden social workers' understanding of the many realities/complexities embedded in clients' experiences-in-contexts. It cautions social workers against the danger of 'claiming to know' and understand the clients' everyday experiences without being carefully reflexive of underlying socio-cultural-political values and norms

(Krause, 2002). What critical scholars in language, discourse and power contribute is a further broadening of our focus into the 'gaze of the observer' and its impacts on the observed (Foucault, 1976). Social workers' own multiple realities (based on their own individual and professional socio-cultural-political values and knowledges) influence their (inter)actions in constructing many realities of the client-in-context. We concur with Foucault (1983) who explores the ways in which power relations privilege the production and dissemination of certain forms of knowledge over others. He refers to the means by which this occurs as *'apparatuses of control'* (Foucault, 1980, p. 102). When conflicted and contested knowledge/discourses co-exist, he argues, disciplinary power enables actors in institutions to privilege selected knowledge against and/or over others using apparatuses of control, and thus claim privileged knowledge as the objective fact, truth, reality and norm. He further articulates how the *'apparatuses of control of others'* (e.g. governing ideology, surveillance, setting expectations, explanation, persuasion and questioning the position/capacity of others) also produces the *'apparatuses of control of self'* (e.g. self-surveillance and self-policing) (Foucault, 1983, p. 212). Thus, a process of positioning/claiming as a dominant subject is part of a process of constructing a subordinate subject.

We situate the 'gaze of the observer' re-contextualised and re-scaled in multiple layers within the current pervasive neoliberal ideology: we wonder how case managers are constructed and disciplined by the governing ideology and policy directives; how clients are treated and managed by their case managers in everyday discursive practice; and how this might contribute to the ways clients view themselves. The British critical social work scholar Dustin (2007) argues that the neoliberal values of small government, individualisation, privatisation, commodification and cost-efficiency are now the governing principles of public management – this is called New Public Management (NPM). State-funded services have been deinstitutionalised, fostering individual responsibility, self-sufficiency and volunteerism, transforming clients to consumers and increasing the monitoring, assessment and regulation of both service providers and organisations. This change has been inculcated in our minds as apparatuses of control of others/self and moves from the *'is'* (e.g. a funding cut *is* the fact) to the *'ought to'* (e.g. we *ought* to make our services efficient), in order to ensure the survival of our profession and prove its legitimacy, instead of challenging policy decisions around the 'is' (e.g. *why is* there a funding cut?) (Fairclough, 2013). Meanwhile, the salience of the client's values and meanings of their own experiences, the professional foundation of striving for social justice (not efficiency/effectiveness) and the social work practice principles based on the relationship between client and social worker have been moved from the centre to the periphery (Dominelli, 2010; Dustin, 2007).

Neoliberal subject making: The ideology of neoliberalism and its dominant social values contribute to the ways clients and social workers are constructed within our society and in turn influence the ways they perceive themselves (Dustin, 2007; Rose, 1999). A neoliberal subject (e.g. client) who is independent, self-reliant, self-sufficient and self-responsible is valued and desirable while dependency, inter-dependency and incompetence is undesirable; thus, this 'less desirable neoliberal subject' needs to be managed. A neoliberal subject (e.g. social worker), who is productive, cost-efficient and accountable in keeping endless records of the close surveillance and managing of cases, is considered the best practice in the New Public Management paradigm (Dustin, 2007; Rose, 1999). Under the close regulation and organisational standards in NPM, spending time to support clients with SMI for their house transfer or listening to their stories do not count; yet, filling out a form for income assistance or a housing application *do* as effective services. Doing so may *pre-empt* other exchanges between clients and social workers and *objectifies* clients. Rather than making meaning of their own experiences and knowledge, clients become re-constructed as service consumers; instead of building connections with clients for care, social workers come to operate as technocrats and/or managers. Dustin (2007) argues that the increase of 'managerial surveillance of social work activities' (p. 37) reduces the scope of social work tasks and results in the 'de-skilling' of social workers (p. 42). Subsequently, *managing cases* to produce cost-efficient, accountable services replaces *providing care* through the professional use of self in the therapeutic relationship. Social workers in the neoliberal state endlessly negotiate their professional identities (Dominelli, 2010; Dustin, 2007; Moffatt, 1999; Sewpaul & Hölsher, 2004). Quoting Donald Schön's appeal for professionalism marked by 'reflection-in-action' rather than 'technical rationality' (1983), Dustin (2007) heightens our awareness of the danger of managing cases as technical rationality and awakens us to explore ways of fostering our reflection-in-action. In this article, as a part of this reflection-in action, we illustrate how the neoliberal agenda permeates social work practice and governs the micro-interactions with clients.

Method

The data used in the present study come from a naturalistic process-outcome study of clinical social work encounters conducted at a Canadian university (PI: the second author). The project underwent an ethics review and was approved by the affiliated institutes. The original study collected both quantitative data (i.e. several outcome and alliance measures at pre- and post-treatment, and follow-up) and qualitative data (i.e. after-session interviews and audio-recorded therapy sessions ranging from 2 to 22 sessions per dyad) to explore how differential treatment outcomes can be understood by in-session treatment processes. (For details of the original research and findings, see Lee et al., 2018; Tsang, Bogo, & Lee, 2011). Table 1 summarises the participants in the original study who were recruited through professional networks using snowball sampling in various community outpatient clinics.

The second and third authors read all transcripts of the 15 therapy dyads and identified two cases where the clients have a history of psychosis (i.e. a diagnosis of schizophrenia). The first, fourth and last authors and the research team members consisting of seven graduate students independently read the full transcripts of two cases (in total 21 sessions) and identified segments reflecting CM services (e.g. disability application, medication management, housing application, financial management, etc.). We met and compared our selected segments, discussed discrepancies and chose mutually agreed upon segments. Then, the first author conducted a critical discourse analysis of the final selection of segments (details to follow) and the authors jointly reviewed the analysis. The first author kept a log of reflections on the analysis process.

In Case A,[1] the client, Lan, is a single, second generation Vietnamese immigrant to Canada, currently in her forties, living in a house with her older sister and her family. The social worker, Mike, was born and raised in Canada, self-identified as of British descent Caucasian, with a Master's Degree in Social Work (MSW) and over 15 years of post-graduate practice experience in the community mental health field. They met weekly for 32 sessions in total and the initial three sessions were taped and fully transcribed verbatim.[2] In Case B, Kuai is a single, second generation Japanese Canadian in his forties, living in the basement of his parents' home. The social worker, Tim, self identifies as white, in his forties, with a MSW and over 10 years of post-graduate clinical experience in community mental health settings. They met for 19 sessions which were taped and fully transcribed verbatim, mostly for individual sessions and at times, with other service providers and the client's parents. The verbal texts in these transcripts served as the data for the current paper. Considering the

Table 1. Demographic information of the participants.

	Clients	Social Workers
Gender	15 (2 male and 13 female)	12 (2 male and 10 female)
Age	3 adolescents, 6 in the twenties, 2 in the thirties, 3 in the forties, and 1 in her fifties.	Late 30's to 60's
Ethnic/racial groups by self-identification	9 as white, 2 as Asian, and 4 as African with various ethnic and religious backgrounds	11 white with various ethnic and religious backgrounds and 1 Asian Canadian
Others		At least 10 years of post-graduate clinical experience

space limits, among various session tasks of CM in both cases, we chose segments around the *Ontario Disability Support Programme (ODSP)*, which was one of the prominent CM services discussed in both cases: in the selected excerpt from Case 1, the social worker helps the client to complete an ODSP financial assistance application form, and in Case 2, the conversation centres on the client's spending and saving habits and the risks of being cut off from ODSP. Securing income toward financial self-sufficiency and independent community living is an important task for a case manager in community mental health services. However, what we would like to emphasise here is *how* this is established and discursively performed in constructing the client's very own needs, and how it impacts upon the client's identity.

A framework of analysis

A primary focus of the *critical discourse analysis* (CDA) is on 'the effect of power relations and inequalities in producing social wrongs' (Fairclough, 2013, p. 8). Among varied CDA scholars, we are inspired by Fairclough's work (2013) because his main analyses and its broad objectives are to develop ways of analysing languages that address and represent the workings of contemporary capitalist societies, especially 'the 'neo-liberal' version of capitalism' (p. 1). According to him, social reality is relationally and dialectically textualised in both *social structures* and *social events/elements* (i.e. texts, utterance) and mediated by *social practice* (i.e. 'orders of discourse' as ways of acting/representing/being). Variations and differences in social structure are not random but socially organised in relatively stable and pervasive dimensions of social practice and selectively actualised in social events/elements.

What CDA analysts do is '*not* analysis of discourse "in itself" … but analysis of dialectical *relations between* discourse and other objects, elements, or moments as well as analysis of the 'internal relations' of discourse' (p. 4). Therefore, his textual analysis pays attention to the mediating link between 'linguistic analysis' and 'social analysis' (Fairclough, 2013). Linguistic analysis pays attention to micro details of language – how ways of being, (inter)acting and representing in a text is 'realised in its semantic, lexico-grammatical, and phonological features' (p. 291) in turn-taking, while social analysis pays attention to macro context of language – how this linguistic analysis is situated within contextual and governing social structures. This 'mixed' approach to the discursive text analysis will be used to understand how the governing neoliberal agenda is reified by clients and case managers in their interaction. Initially in each excerpt we will analyse utterances between the clients and social workers especially semantic, lexico-grammatical choices and topic changes (i.e. linguistic analysis); and then by contextualising them we will consider how these utterances work to enact/interact between the clients and social workers, to represent their power and authority or lack thereof, and to elaborate their being (identity) within Canadian mental health policies and case management approaches governed by a neoliberal agenda (i.e. social analysis).

Findings

Constructing the client's needs

In Session 3, Lan and Mike discuss completing a self-report section on the ODSP application form that requires details of how her illness results in difficulties with daily activities. In Line 37 of this session, Mike reads from the form: 'tell us what impact your physical and mental illness has on your daily ability. You may choose to provide details about the following: your own personal care, such as bathing, dressing, etc.; work activities; hobbies; activities in your community; emotional problems. And do you have someone to help you if you need it, and wanted help from your family, or social supports; and your general help'. Subsequently Lan notes her feeling of depression (Line 38) and the difficulties associated with depending on her family for support (Line 40) due to the family's own issues (Line 42) including her sister's health concern with an impending operation (Line 44). As Mike reads the disability form in Line 37, this item asks 'You may *choose* to provide details about the following'. Despite the fact that Lan already *chose* and clearly told him that she wanted to address her depression and difficulties of relying on family support, Mike (in the subsequent turn Line 45) changes the topic to personal care (Excerpt 1).

Excerpt 1. Source: Session 3.[a]

45.	Mike	Do you want to talk about anything about your personal care in terms of your bathing, is it any difficulty for you or there's any demands for bathing?
46.	Lan	I like to, sometimes if I don't go out, I'll take a bath, but what, where, own personal care?
47.	Mike	Such as bathing, dressing. Some people
48.	Lan	Take a bath every day, like that?
49.	Mike	Yah, some people spend a lot of extra time in bathing, or some people have, they get pretty occupied with bathing, sometimes that can be part of their illness, they wash too much, so many times,
50.	Lan	Yah, because my sister Lia it was me that used the water in the house, but I usually take a bath every day, I use a lot of water, I like to wash.
51.	Mike	So is it more than once a day or is it once a day?
52.	Lan	Just once a day,
53.	Mike	Okay, and is it for, how long does it usually take to bathe?
54.	Lan	Around thirty minutes, not too long, that's okay,
55.	Mike	Yah, mmm ... the reason I'm asking is because I was talking on the phone with your sister and she mentioned that this might be an area that you have some difficulty in, that's all, I'm just asking.
56.	Lan	If I'm, you know, if I ...
57.	Mike	Like with washing,
58.	Lan	If I wash a lot?
59.	Mike	Yah.
60.	Lan	Yah, I use water a lot,
61.	Mike	Okay. The reason I'm asking is because if they think it might help to go in here,
62.	Lan	It might help?
63.	Mike	Yes, if you're trying to explain some of your difficulties, it might help to go in that.
64.	Lan	I have no problem.
65.	Mike	To perform
66.	Lan	Oh, if I need help to take a bath, to take a shower like that?
67.	Mike	No, not help, but if, if you tend to spend more time bathing than other people do, maybe that's something they should know, trying to explain it,
68.	Lan	Okay, I spend more time.
69.	Mike	Okay, do you know roughly how much it would be, like is it a half hour a day?
70.	Lan	More than an hour,
71.	Mike	More than an hour, okay,
72.	Lan	Okay, because sometimes I wash my face
73.	Mike	Is it two hours? Or
74.	Lan	And I brush my teeth, and I wash my face, yah, it takes approximately two hours a day

[a]In all excerpts, numeric numbers indicate speaking turns in each session. A bracket [ ] indicates the transcribers' or authors' notes.

Linguistic analysis: Mike abruptly changes the topic to bathing by explicitly inviting her to talk about 'personal care in terms of your bathing' (Line 45). Lan tries to answer to Mike's question, yet soon appears to 'notice' the abrupt topic change, which does not align with previous turns in the conversation and tries to locate the personal care topic on the disability form (' ... what, where, own personal care?' in Line 46). Then, Mike appears to read from the form: 'Such as bathing, dressing'; Lan checks back in with her understanding of the topic: 'Take a bath every day, like that?' (Line 48); and follows Mike's confirmation 'Yah'. Meanwhile, her experiences of depression and difficulties getting family support are *pre-empted* from the conversation.

In Line 49, Mike continues with his previous inquiry from Line 45 on Lan's personal care, bathing, but with more *explanation*. In Line 50 Lan hints at difficulties around different views on her bathing between her and her sister ('I use a lot of water') but maintains her position ('I like to wash'). From Lines 51 to 54, the organisation of turns is mainly a Question-Answer format where Mike inquires, even interrogates ('more than once a day or is it once a day?' 'How long?') and Lan answers, still firmly noting 'not too long' and voicing her opinion clearly 'that's okay' (Line 54).

Then, Mike discloses his having had contact with Lan's sister who considered bathing as 'the area that you have some difficulty' (Line 55), which overrides Lan's own voice ('that's okay' in the previous turn, in Line 54). She appears momentarily disoriented about the topic focus: 'If I'm, you know, if I ... '

(Line 56). Mike notes 'Like with washing' (Line 57) and Lan is *questioning* for clarification 'If I wash a lot?' (Line 58), and soon *clarifies* her point 'I use water a lot' (Line 60), which she already claimed as her view in Line 50. This interaction of questioning and resisting signifies dis-alignment between the client and worker (Stivers, 2008). This pattern is repeated again. Mike explains (Line 61), Lan requests clarification (Line 62), Mike further elaborates (Line 63), and Lan asserts that 'I have no problem' (Line 64). Lines 64 and 66 show a dis-alignment where Lan 'interrupts' Mike. In Line 67 Mike attempts to re-align with Lan by making a further 'explanation' to Lan: he seeks to make a compelling case for her disability application by illustrating difficulties in her daily activities ('something they should know'). Lan then not only acknowledges and aligns with Mike on the topic of bathing but also affiliates with his stance by affirming 'Okay I spend more time' (Line 68). In subsequent turns, she then adjusts her answers drastically from 'Around thirty minutes, not too long' (Line 54) to 'more than an hour' (Line 70) to 'approximately two hours a day' (Line 74). Subsequently, Mike no longer explains, but accepts Lan's answers (e.g. *'Okay'* in Line 69, 'More than an hour, *okay'* in Line 71) and even pools her answers (e.g. 'Is it two hours?' in Line 73, to which Lan answers 'approximately two hours a day' in Line 74), which are now deemed as the valid truth.

Social analysis: Initially Lan says bathing is something she enjoys ('I like to wash'). Then, by each turn as described above, her enjoyable activity is recruited into a 'problematic' act that brings conflict with her sister who sees it as 'the area that you have some difficulty'. There appear to be power struggles between Lan and Mike enacted in this excerpt – how Lan's utterances are discursively managed and disciplined by Mike. Initially Lan actively resists: 'not too long, that's okay' (Line 54), 'If I wash a lot?' (Line 58), (but according to my sister!) 'I use water a lot' (Lines 50, 60), and finally 'I have no problem' (Line 64). However, Mike consistently recruits Lan's compliance through repeated *explanations* such as, 'the reason I am asking is because ... ' (Lines 55 & 61) and 'trying to explain ... ' (Lines 63 & 67). Mike also uses *questions* (Lines 51, 53, & 73) as 'persuasion' tactics. Juhila and Abrams (2011) note that, subtle forms of persuasion (e.g. explanation) in interactional situations are used not only to encourage and construct clients into certain identities but can also be used as 'ways to reduce clients' interactional resistance' (287). Subsequently, Lan reduces her active resistance and adjusts her answers about bathing time, even dramatically, to fit in with Mike's authoritative utterances. Her own enjoyable experience thus becomes the object of discipline and close scrutiny by the professional gaze, and further serves as an 'indicator' of her illness by both the professional (social worker) and the institution (the disability form).

This discursive interaction also appears to construct the client's need and identity (a way of being). For example, Mike appears to construct what 'mentally ill type behaviour' (Smith, 1978, p. 37) is – 'that can be part of their illness, they wash too much, so many times' (Line 49). In her work on *'K is mentally ill'*, Smith notes that 'it is the teller of the tale's privilege both to define the rule or situation and to describe the behavior' (p. 39). As the teller of the tale in the mental health field, Mike's authoritative utterance seems to make a rule/claim of what constitutes 'mentally ill type behaviour' – bathing too much – thus constructing Lan's identity/ways of being as *Lan is mentally ill* (Smith, 1978). With the task of securing income in this session, the client's own choice of topic (i.e. depression and difficulties of getting family support) is silenced, and her initiative of exploring them becomes hermeneutically void in the dialogue. Instead, the institutional practice in this excerpt is centred on completing the disability form with compelling examples of 'mentally ill type behaviours' (Smith, 1978).

We acknowledge that a task-oriented work (e.g. financial support with disability checks, medication monitoring, etc.) is critical in supporting clients with severe mental health challenges in community mental health practice (Greene et al., 2006). Nonetheless, it should be noted that there is no talk from Lan that indicates she was asking for 'financial support' or any help in completing ODSP in the previous turns of this excerpt, or in this session (Session 3) and even in Sessions 1 and 2. Lan could have indicated during the intake that getting financial support was one of her expectations for the service, and yet Mike did not bring up this point before changing the topic here. How, then, was Lan's *need* for financial support *constructed* at this very moment by abruptly changing the topic in Line 45?

As a case manager in a community mental health setting, Mike may have 'professional knowledge' of the client's financial struggles and 'expertise' on how to help them. However, in this interaction, his professional knowledge and institutional agenda are privileged to the point where he *skips* consulting the client about her knowledge of what she needs for herself and *omits* even asking her: e.g. 'I wonder if you have any financial struggles that you may need some support with?' We argue that the power from professional knowledge/expertise (e.g. we know what they need given our CM knowledge), in combination with institutional demands and close surveillance that are legitimatised by the bureaucratic service management (e.g. what services count as effective), may cause a social worker to become unwittingly trapped into claiming and reifying institutional knowledge and power, and overriding (and potentially degrading) the client's experience, knowledge and power, while re-positioning the client as a 'mentally ill person'.

Constructing the client's identity

In the next excerpt, Tim, Kosi, and his father discuss how to secure Kosi's disability check from ODSP so that he can be self-sufficient. In the past, Kosi saved the ODSP funds he received, thus jeopardising his ODSP eligibility due to his accumulated assets. Previously he had a record of not completing the ODSP form and had not had any income assistance from ODSP (Excerpt 2).

Excerpt 2. Session 2.

71	Kosi	And I went without money for about a year,
72	Father	Yeah
73	Kosi	And I didn't need any money
74	Tim	Was it because he couldn't get to the office?
75	Father	We got him there, but he wouldn't answer the questions that he thought ...
76	Kosi	But I didn't want anything, I didn't, I was sick for a while, so I was thinking of getting better, and I didn't want to take government money at the time, because that was like in 6 or 7 years ago. But I mean I refused the money at first because I didn't need it, I had food and [........]. I was sick, I didn't get better, and now I don't know what's going to happen with my health, like I can continue with what's happening,
77	Tim	Well hopefully we'll get as much money as you're entitled to, until you're able to do.

Linguistic analysis: Initially, Kosi verbalises his desire to *not* take government money repeatedly, in Lines 71, 73, and 76, using multiple *I*-statements (i.e. 'I went without money', 'I didn't need any money', 'I didn't want anything, I didn't', 'I didn't want to take government money', 'I refused the money', and 'because I didn't need it'). Upon Kosi's explicit statements, Tim first addresses this issue with the father in Line 74, instead of asking Kosi directly, although it is Kosi who spoke in the previous turn. Then, it is revealing to see the lexical choices of the father: 'We got him there, but he wouldn't answer ...' making the division between we (him and his wife) and he (Kosi). Then, Kosi elaborates with a lengthy self-disclosure in Line 76: there appears to be a struggle between resistance ('I *didn't* want anything, ... I *was* thinking of getting better') and compliance ('*now I don't* know ... what's *going to happen* with my health') which is manifested in the contrast of Kosi's use of *tense*: in the past, Kosi appeared hopeful and strived to be self-sufficient and independent whereas in the present (and even future), he appears insecure and maybe even hopeless. Instead of exploring this struggle, Tim again deploys the contrast of the lexicon, we versus he/you in Line 77 ('*we'll* get as much money as *you*'re entitled to, *until you're able to* do').

Social analysis: Here, there has been little exploration of how Kosi constructs the meaning of receiving a disability pension from the government. Repeatedly he asserted not needing the disability pension using multiple *I*-statements. We interpret this discursive pattern as representing his position as a neoliberal subject (a way of being), valuing his own free will with no financial reliance/dependence. And yet his own assertion to be a neoliberal subject is dismissed by both Tim and his father discursively as described above. Why does Tim not ask him directly? Not only is Kosi's talk (and his presence) dismissed here, but also his identity appears implied. We wonder if Tim considers Kosi's identity as being incompetent (to comprehend the need of the financial support thus being sick and abnormal) to the point that there seems no reason to directly ask him why he does not need money. This conversational gesture seems to set out discursively the next turns in their interactions; for example, in Line 74, it appears that the father refers to 'we' as himself and his wife (Kosi's mother) but at the same time it appears as setting out a division between normal and abnormal, as if *we as normal people* would know the need of financial security by obtaining money and *he as an ill person* who is incompetent to comprehend it and did not answer the questions despite the fact that 'we got him there.' Then, in Line 76: on the one hand, Kosi resists the discourse of 'he = sick and not self-sufficient' versus 'we = normal and logical,' using multiple *I*-statements to legitimise his reason for not needing ODSP money; and on the other hand, he negotiates with the gaze of others (the view of 'we') and describes himself as being ill and incompetent ('I was sick for a while' & 'I was sick, I didn't get better, and now I don't know'). Instead of inviting Kosi to explore other *counter-discourses* to construct the meanings around his experiences (e.g. What it was like for him to go without money, why he did not need money and thus refused it, or any of his cultural values that positioned him against receiving the government money), Tim changes the topic to his disability check in Line 77. Here, Tim again deploys 'we = normal/healthy' versus 'you = ill and incompetent' ('*we*'ll get as much money as *you*'re entitled to, *until you're able to* do').

Fairclough (2013) describes this type of split as the *fallacy of division* by deploying the pronouns of we versus other. This division then seems to discursively and dialectically set out a movement here from the 'is' (i.e. what Kosi wants/does not want) to the 'ought to' of the case manager's/institutional task (i.e. economic self-efficiency) (Fairclough, 2013). This discursive pattern legitimises and rationalises the neoliberal task of securing financial independence while the client's needs/aspects of the services and the other tasks of the social worker (e.g. listening to and joining the client in making meaning of the client's experiences) disappear. Meanwhile, Kosi is positioned as a lesser neoliberal subject, which is in essence *hybrid within* the neoliberal subject-making discourse (i.e. producing and consolidating the division between who is up to the expectation of the neoliberal agenda and who is not) (Dustin, 2007).

From this session and onward, this task becomes dominant as shown in the next excerpt. Session 12 starts with a discussion around Kosi saving his money (Excerpt 3).

Excerpt 3. Session 12.

21	Tim	So do you have any idea what you might do with the money when it comes, she's saying [Kosi's ODSP worker] if you put it in the bank it'll just be a matter of time that you'll go over that again, [inaudible]
22	Kosi	I don't know, it's either that or try and find a part-time job, cause if I do that it's around similar money anyway, it's about the same amount.
23	Tim	It's the same amount when you're living at home.
24	Kosi	Right
25	Tim	But if you moved out you might not get as much from a part-time job as you would from ODSP, if you were living in an apartment, cause then they give as much as nine hundred
26	Kosi	That's how I started, cause I was in my own place and they just sent it to me, I didn't apply, before that they put me on I think it was welfare, and then they changed it to disability.
27	Tim	Well I'm not trying to tell you how to spend it, I just want to make sure that you really understand that these are options that are available to you when this money keeps on coming on you're not sure what to do with it, it's sort of growing in your bank account.
28	Kosi	Ya that's the problem cause I'm not too sure.
29	Tim	Is there anything that you would like to do with that money?
30	Kosi	Not really, I'd like to save up some money for the future just in case something goes wrong, that's another reason why I want to take a part-time job, if I could find part-time work, because then I could save more, there's no limit if I'm on my own right?
31	Tim	There's still a limit of how much assets you can accumulate.
32	Kosi	No within, if I stay suspended from that and then I'm on my own, that's what I was thinking about, only reason for getting the part-time work because then I can save as much as I want without worrying about it, assuming I could find work.
33	Tim	Well there'd also be some implications for if you go off, how many years you know, like if you go off and let's say it's two or three years that you're not receiving this income, it might make it very difficult to apply again, so if you're thinking of getting a part-time job, it may be a wonderful thing to get a part-time job, but please speak to your worker before you do that, ask her how easy or difficult it would be to apply after a year, two years, four years, five years, cause I think they have a rule that if someone is off it for a while it may be very difficult to apply again.

Linguistic analysis: In Line 21, Tim anticipates that Kosi will save the money when he resumes receiving ODSP and explores how Kosi can come up with strategies to prevent this. This anticipation is on target since Kosi replies in Line 22 that he would do the same or keep trying to find a part-time job. Instead of inviting Kosi to explore his ideas, Tim continues to 'explain' the situation as if Kosi does not get it and finally notes 'Well I'm not trying to tell you how to spend it, I just want to make sure that you really understand … ' (Line 27). Kosi then complies with Tim's authoritative utterance and even doubt of what he wants ('Ya that's the problem cause I'm not too sure … ') in Line 28. This discursive pattern of Kosi's assertion for what he wants/plans followed by Tim's explanation repeats in Lines 30–33.

Social analysis: Instead of exploring how Kosi likes to manage his money and its meanings in his life, and what a part-time job may signify to him, the discursive patterns in Lines 23–26 position Tim as 'logical' with rational explanation and Kosi as 'illogical and incompetent to comprehend the situation'. Here, Tim repeatedly *explains* why Kosi risks losing his income, what is involved in re-applying and in what ways he can lower his savings to maintain his ODSP eligibility. Explanation as a persuasion tactic (i.e. apparatus of power/control of others) is also telling in Tim's lexical choice in Line 27: 'I' as the one with authority 'want to make sure' that 'you' as someone who cannot comprehend/ 'really understand'. This self-evident authority and truth-claim again moves the 'is' (what Kosi does not understand) to the 'ought to' (what the case manager/institution should do), thus discursively embodying the task of CM.

In Lines 29–30, the same pattern of Lines 21–22 is replicated, only this time, Kosi elaborates to further position himself as a neoliberal subject who can 'save some' for a rainy day while actively looking for employment. Again in Line 31, Tim 'explains' the limits of the assets Kosi can eligibly accumulate. Discursively and dialectically, the ways they interact seem like a clash of different discourses/meanings around *what safety is for Kosi*: Kosi's utterances suggest that he would feel secure if he saves money and finds a part-time job whereas Tim seems to view safety for Kosi as following his authoritative utterances, which are logical and normal – i.e. spending the money to comply with the qualification requirements for ODSP/income.

Although Kosi actively resists this authoritative utterance in Line 32, Tim provides more explanation in Line 33. Here, similar to Line 77 in Excerpt 2, Tim considers not only the current state of safety/normalcy but also forecasts into the future – 'if you go off, how many years you know, like if you go off and let's say it's two or three years' and 'after a year, two years, four years, five years' as if being unable to ensure safety is a given characteristic of a client with a history of SMI. Invoking the competent other ('please speak to your worker') versus Kosi, the fallacy of division occurs again and the client is infantilised (i.e. 'not competent' to comprehend it so better ask the 'competent and normal' other). Through this discursive pattern, as Martin and his colleagues (2003) critique of CM, Kosi was constructed as a 'passive recipient of professional services … [and] judged to be childlike, and, like children, incapable of judging what was good for them' (p. 212). Consequently, these discursive ways of interacting and representing position Kosi as a less competent (neoliberal) subject now and in the future (Greene et al. 2006).

Discussion

Across the three excerpts presented, the linguistic analysis shows the following common patterns: the client's story was initially dismissed and not explored → the social worker chose the topic/focus of session tasks → the client resists in both implicit and explicit ways → the social worker deploys explanations and invoke authoritative voices while managing the client's resistance → after several cycles of resistance and management, the client complies with the social worker's initial tasks. The common themes in social analysis across the excerpts include: while dismissing the clients' voices and even their presence and invoking the difference between us and them, clients are positioned as being mentally ill, incompetent, illogical and lesser neoliberal subjects whereas the social workers with the authoritative and logical voices position themselves as the *knowers* of what the clients need and at times could even foresee the clients' future.

We acknowledge that our analysis is not the only possible interpretation of the data and there might be various ways of understanding the complex micro-interactions between clients and case managers in the selected excerpts. Thus, we encourage readers to actively engage in their own analysis and make use of this rich data. We also acknowledge that detailed non-verbal behaviours (e.g. sighs, tone and intonations of utterances, and body language) were not available in the original transcripts, compromising our ability to analyse even more minute details of the interaction.

Our critical analysis of the selected interactions was not intended to diminish any particular social worker, but rather to increase our collective understanding of how their (inter)actions with clients are constructed and performed within contexts, especially a governing neoliberal ideology. We aim to hold 'a stance of critical solidarity' between practitioners and researchers (Hall & White, 2005, p. 387), to find ways to counter-(inter)act and resist the neoliberal power and oppression that govern our everyday practice in serving clients with SMI in the community. Therefore, we attempted to interpret interactions in our data as reflexive social workers would do in their own practice. We find that reflexively examining the moment-to-moment interactions in actual sessions is one useful way to illustrate how the neoliberal agenda is absorbed into social workers' everyday practice.

We underline our concern in the current pervasive discourse around 'subjects' under neoliberalism: 'being normal' = 'being able to manage financial security.' Within this dominance, having hope ('I was thinking of getting better' and 'saving some for later') – a potential dream for obtaining a job and being independent, and one's own identity in pursuing one's mental health *with* mental illness, like 'normal' people – appear to be pre-empted in conversation. Their existence as a full human being is narrowed to that of a less competent neoliberal subject. The professional identity of social workers becomes that of an authoritative neoliberal agent, explicitly and implicitly invoking neoliberal values with their clients. Meanwhile their own professional identity as the 'carer' is significantly compromised.

We hope that the detailed illustration of moment-to-moment interactions between clients and social workers around CM tasks will assist social workers in critically reflecting upon their own practice and may provide detailed *ways of resisting* the overwhelming neoliberal impact and dominance on our everyday practice. Instead of taking the institutional tasks in serving the clients with SMI for granted, we first propose *questioning the 'is'* and closely explore the *movement from the is to the ought to* in our practice: why are we talking about Lan's bathing? How come her enjoyable bathing is questioned here? Why did Kosi refuse the government money? Next, we propose that social workers wonder what is *pre-empted* from the dialogue with clients with SMI. While we are consumed by current dominant discourses around being effective in service delivery and fostering client self-sufficiency, social workers need to pay attention to *what has not been talked about* and what has been *rendered peripheral*. What would Lan's most pressing concerns around her history of mental illness be? What is it like for her as a person who does not have her own place? What future plans might Kosi have once he accumulates enough savings to be independent and hold a part-time job? Lastly, we suggest paying attention to details of discursive communicative patterns such as lexical choices and repetitions that both we and clients use to convey each other's goals and tasks for sessions, and being conscious of using professional power through persuasive tactics (e.g. explanations and pooling certain answers). Why is Lan repeating that she enjoys bathing? And why might Kosi be using multiple I-statements to convey his position? Paying attention to these details in social work interactions would make social workers vigilant to clients' response/resistance, which often reveals pathways towards re-defining and re-constructing meaning in life beyond the (less valued) neoliberal subject, and case management beyond technical service provision.

Notes

1. All identifying details are disguised and pseudonyms are used to protect the privacy and confidentiality of the participants.
2. Audio files were destroyed after complete transcription. Unfortunately, no notations were used in the transcripts in the original study. Thus, we analysed only verbal texts of interlocutors in the transcripts.

Acknowledgments

The authors wish to acknowledge the research assistance from Sara Abura, Sophia Lam, Norangie Carballo-Garcia, Danielle Pearson, Tristan Gerrie, Diana Salih, and Bradyn Ko.

Disclosure statement

No potential conflict of interest was reported by the authors.

Funding

This project is funded from the Social Sciences and Humanities Research Council of Canada, Standard Research Grant (PI: Tsang).

References

Dominelli, L. (2010). Globalization, contemporary challenges and social work practice. *International Social Work, 53*(5), 599–612.

Dustin, D. (2007). *The McDonaldization of social work*. New York: Routledge.

Fairclough, N. (2013). *Critical discourse analysis. The critical study of language* (2nd ed.). New York: Routledge.

Foucault, M. (1979). *Discipline and punish*. New York: Pantheon.

Foucault, M. (1980). *Power/knowledge: Selected interviews and other writings, 1972–1977 (1st American ed.)*. New York: Pantheon.

Foucault, M. (1983). The subject and power. In H. Dreyfus, & P. Rabinow (Eds.), *Michel Foucault: Beyond structuralism and hermeneutics* (2nd ed., pp. 208–228). Chicago: University of Chicago Press.

Gewurtz, R. E., Cott, C., Rush, B., & Kirsh, B. (2012). The shift to rapid job placement for people living with mental illness: An analysis of consequences. *Psychiatric Rehabilitation Journal, 35*, 428–434.

Goering, P., Wasylenki, D., & Durbin, J. (2000). Canada's mental health system. *International Journal of Law and Psychiatry, Special Issue: Mental health policy 2000: An international review, 23*(3/4), 345–359.

Gourlay, D. (1998). *A fiscal and legislative governance map of the Canadian health and mental health systems*. Ottawa: Mental Health Promotion Unit, Health Canada.

Greene, G. J., Kondrat, D. C., Lee, M. Y., Clement, J., Siebert, H., Mentzer, R. A., & Pinnell, S. R. (2006). A solution-focused approach to case management and recovery with consumers who have a severe mental disability. *Families in Society, 87*(3), 339–350.

Hall, C., & White, S. (2005). Looking inside professional practice: Discourse, narrative and ethnographic approaches to social work and counselling. *Qualitative Social Work: Research and Practice, 4*(4), 379–390.

Juhila, K., & Abrams, L. (2011). Constructing identities in social work settings. *Qualitative Social Work, 10*, 277–292.

Krause, I. B. (2002). *Culture and system in family therapy*. London: Karnac.

Lee, E., Tsang, A. K. T., Bogo, M., Wilson, G., Johnstone, M., & Herschman, J. (2018). Joining revisited in family therapy: Cross-cultural encounters between a therapist and an immigrant family. *Journal of Family Therapy, 40*, 148–179.

Magnus, M., & Shera, W. (2012). Beyond community treatment orders: Empowering clients to achieve community integration. *International Journal of Mental Health, 41*(4), 62–81.

Martin, J. S., Peter, C. G., & Kapp, S. A. (2003). Consumer satisfaction with children's mental health services. *Child and Adolescent Social Work Journal, 20*(3), 211–226.

Meeks, J. B. (2001). A social work case management experience in a managed care setting: The need for effective communication. *Home Health Care Management and Practice, 13*(6), 444–451.

Moffatt, K. (1999). Surveillance and government of the welfare recipient. In A. Chambon, L. Epstein, & A. Irving (Eds.), *Reading Foucault for social work* (pp. 219–245). New York, NY: Columbia University Press.

Ontario ACT Association. (2018). *Ontario Program of Standards for ACT Teams*. Ontario, Canada.

Ontario Hospital Association. (2016). *A practical guide to mental health and the law in Ontario*. Retrieved from: https://www.oha.com/Legislative%20and%20Legal%20Issues%20Documents1/A%20Practical%20Guide%20to%20Mental%20Health%20and%20the%20Law%20in%20Ontario%20(2012)%20(PUBLICATIONS).pdf

Rose, N. (1999). *Powers of freedom: Reframing political thought*. Cambridge: Cambridge University Press.

Schön, D. A. (1983). *The reflective practitioner: How professionals think in action*. New York: Basic Books.

Sewpaul, V., & Hölsher, D. (2004). *Social work in times of neoliberalism: A postmodern discourse*. Pretoria: Van Schaik Publishers.

Smith, D. (1978). 'K is mentally ill' The anatomy of a factual account [Special issue: Language and practical reasoning]. *Sociology, 12*(1), 23–53.

Spitzmueller, M. C. (2014). Shifting practices of recovery under community meatal health reform: A street-level organizational ethnography. *Qualitative Social Work: Research and Practice, 13*(1), 26–48.

Stivers, T. (2008). Stance, alignment, and affiliation during storytelling: When nodding is a token of affiliation. *Research on Language and Social Interaction, 41*(1), 31–57.

Stuart, H. (2003). Violence and mental illness: Overview. *World Psychiatry, 2*(2), 121–124.

Tsang, A. K. T., Bogo, M., & Lee, E. (2011). Engagement in cross-cultural clinical practice: Narrative analysis of first sessions. *Clinical Social Work Journal, 39*(1), 79–90.

Vourlekis, B., & Ell, K. (2007). Best practice case management for improved medical adherence. *Social Work in Health Care, 44*(3), 161–177.

Williams, M. L., Forster, P., McCarthy, G. D., & Hargreaves, W. A. (1994). Managing case management: What makes It work? *Psychosocial Rehabilitation Journal, 18*(1), 49–59.

Ziguras, S. J., & Stuart, G. W. (2000). A meta-analysis of the effectiveness of mental health case management over 20 years. *Psychiatric Services, 51*(11), 1410–1421.

'NEET' to work? – substance use disorder and youth unemployment in Norwegian public documents

'NEET' i arbeid? Rusproblemer og ungdomsarbeidsledighet i norske offentlige dokumenter

Anne Juberg and Nina Schiøll Skjefstad

ABSTRACT

The aim of this paper is to provide insight into the degree to which and how relevant Norwegian policy documents conceptualise the chances for inclusion in working life among young adults (18–30) who are not in employment, education and training (NEET) and who have exhibited problems with alcohol or other drugs. We analysed a sample of policy documents inspired by Foucault and Fairclough`s methodology and discussed the results in light of prevailing policy trends within contemporary welfare states and results from relevant research. We found three predominant discourses that tend to govern public opinion in the area: *The Medicalisation Discourse, The Stigma Discourse* and *The Social Investment Discourse*. All three can be related to the neoliberal tendency of individualising and medicalising social problems. There seems to be little evidence in epidemiology and other research that substance abuse represents any direct reason for the NEET status among young people. Neither is there any clear evidence that problems with alcohol and drugs among young adults will, in the long run, unambiguously reduce their working capacity. Thus, the identified discourses may contribute to the creation of myths about the NEET population in question.

SAMMENDRAG

Målet med denne artikkelen er å bidra til innsikt i hvordan jobbsjansene til unge voksne (18–30 år) som verken er i arbeid, utdanning eller arbeidstrening (NEET: Not in Employment, Education or Training) og som har fremvist problemer med alkohol eller andre rusmidler, blir beskrevet og begrepsfestet i norske offentlige dokumenter. Inspirert av Foucault`s og Fairclough`s metodologi har vi analysert et utvalg av disse dokumentene. I artikkelen diskuterer vi resultatene i lys av rådende trender innenfor dagens velferdsstater og resultater fra relevant forskning. Vi fant tre fremtredende diskurser som synes å styre offentlig opinion på det beskrevne området: *Medikaliseringsdiskursen, stigmadiskursen og sosial investeringsdiskursen.* Alle tre diskurser kan relateres til den nyliberale tendensen til å individualisere og medikalisere sosiale problemer. Det synes imidlertid å være begrenset forskningsbelegg innenfor epidemiologisk og annen forskning for at rusproblematikk representerer noen direkte årsak til NEET – status blant ungdom. Det foreligger heller ikke klart belegg for at problemer med alkohol og andre rusmidler i det lange løp vil redusere arbeidskapasiteten deres. De diskursene vi identifiserte kan likevel bidra til å skape myter omkring den gruppen av ungdom som står utenfor arbeidsliv, utdanning og arbeidstrening og som samtidig har rusproblemer.

Introduction

In the Anglophone countries, there has been a shift from *welfare* with focus on people's rights, to *workfare* with focus on people's responsibilities (Johansson & Møller, 2009). This shift in focus is underpinned by the contemporary tendency that work permeates all sides of contemporary society and makes most people view working life participation as the only path to well-being (Garrett, 2014). The mantra is 'make work pay'. A problem social workers may encounter in relation to this is that the labour market does not include everybody.

In 1991, the Norwegian Government adopted the term 'workfarè (St.meld. nr. 39 (1991–1992)). The principle of workfare was later passed on to the Norwegian Labour and Welfare Administration (NAV) that was established in 2005. One of the major goals of NAV was to get more people employed and active and to reduce the use of benefits (NOU, 2004:13). Work is, by the Norwegian government as by many other countries, now considered the key to active citizenship in society (St.meld. nr. 39 (1991–1992)). The central stance in workfare policy is to view unemployment and poverty as matters of individual responsibility and not as lack of work opportunities (Dahl, 2003; Marthinsen & Skjefstad, 2011). Workfare is thus closely related to neoliberalism, which according to Schwartzmantel (2005) is an economic policy not simply designed to cut government spending. Its aim is also to pursue free-trade policies and to free market forces from government regulations. A neoliberalist labour market requires flexible, self-governed, healthy and well-educated individuals (Giddens, 2004), which in return requires a focus in social work towards measures like 'personalisation', 'self-directed support', 'rehabilitation' and 'reactivation' (Madsen, Judd, & & Boeckh, 2015, s. 339).

For young people who often are described as NEET – Not in Education, Employment or Training (Yates & Payne, 2006) – and who have additional problems, like Substance Use Disorder (SUD) (APA – American Psychiatrist Association, 2013), the above-mentioned working life requirements may seem unattainable in the first place. Neoliberal societies take exception to people who do not control their intake of alcohol or other drugs and shape negative myths about them (O `Malley & Valverde, 2004). Besides, former studies suggest that Norwegian policy documents, political speeches, media presentations etc., depict people with mental health problems or SUD as individuals who *stay far away from work* (Frøyland, 2015). The same tendency is present in other European countries (Madsen et al., 2015).

Thus, at the same time as Norwegian labour policy still embraces participation in the work force as a general principle also for disabled people or people with temporarily reduced working capacity (Meld. St. 30 (2011–2012), there are some mechanisms that work against these principles, at least when it comes to certain groups. A fresh report from OECD (2018) points to how the Norwegian NEET population distinctly deviates from the general youth population by representing lower basic skills, higher prevalence of mental health problems, lower degrees of life satisfaction and lower job seeking activity. According to the same source, the gap between NEETs and same- age peers who are not NEET is significantly higher than in other European countries. This may represent a special challenge for Norwegian social workers with regard to attempts at including this population into working life. Social workers tend currently to be involved in both labour market inclusion and exclusion through demands on them to promote and make ontology judgments about clients with regard to working readiness (Johansson & Møller, 2009).

This article aims at studying predominating discourses in public documents about the inclusion and exclusion in the Norwegian labour market of young people (18–30) who use alcohol or other substances in problematic ways. This category corresponds with one or more criteria in the DSM-V category of Substance Use Disorder (SUD) (APA, 2013). We find the topic interesting for social work in the neoliberal era as it may enhance consciousness around how the workfare state indirectly governs social policy and thus social work practice by controlling discourses on working life participation. We assume an inherent connection between policy documents, research articles, social workers' attitudes and actions, and young unemployed problem substance users' self-image, interpretations and definitions of situations and problems. Social workers may contribute to the disqualification of young people who are potentially capable of contributing in the workforce. By concluding so, we do not mean that social workers execute their tasks without employing discretion, even though some argue that social workers no longer have discretion because of the increase in control of procedures, budgets and surveillance (Evans, 2016). According to Evans, there is evidence that social workers, despite this increase, execute discretion to a considerable extent.

We will discuss the following research questions:

- Which discourses related to young NEETs with SUD (18–30) could we identify in our material of political documents?
- To what extent do these discourses implicate that NEETs with SUD 'stay far away from work'?
- How do these findings fit with relevant research?

We will now present the method and our way of analysing our data, before we discuss the findings.

Method

Texts from the seven most central Norwegian governmental policy documents on workfare and substance rehabilitation, dating from 1991 to 2016, shape the basis for our textual analysis[1]. The texts are thus strategically chosen. We will show examples of how the texts reflect assumptions on the young substance users` ontology. A limited, but strategic qualitative sample like ours may provide a glimpse into more basic systems of thought (Engebretsen & Heggen, 2012).

The analysis has been inspired by Foucault (2002, 1999) and Fairclough (2001). The concept of discourse has been a key term in our analysis. Foucault's concept of discourse refers to an institutional way of thinking. His emphasis is on a connection between the forces in society and the way in which they materialise in institutions, in the language and in the individual's conceptions of self (Foucault, 2002). The governmental policy documents in our sample may be viewed as texts that reproduce and reinforce their power by being commented on and quoted over and over again in line with *the principle of commentary* (Foucault, 1999). They can be viewed as a 'place' where determination of meaning occurs (Kleppe, Engebretsen, & Heggen, 2012), and hence suitable for analysing discourses of NEET substance abusers' possibility for inclusion in the job market.

Subjectivation is an important concept in Foucault's understanding of power, where the starting point is that a subject is not something you are or have, but something that is created and assigned by discourse. By shaping the discourse, the state offers service users certain positions of subject and excludes others. In this way, the state governs in an indirect manner; the governing takes place by governing the governing of the self. This is what Foucault calls Governmentality (2002). Therefore, when exploring our research issues, it seems important to reveal the discourses that will partly determine the group´s possibilities in the job market.

Like Foucault, 'discourse' in the works of Fairclough (2001) is oriented towards how language (and semiosis) is dialectically linked to social relations as well as to ideology. His primary emphasis is on processes of social change. His critical discourse analysis (CDA) involves a close look at textual structures.

Discourse, according to both authors, contributes to the social actor's self-image, interpretations and definitions of situations and problems. Thus, relations of dominance are produced, re-produced and transformed in discourse. According to this, we can assume an inherent connection between policy documents, research articles, social workers' attitudes and actions, and young unemployed substance users' self-image, interpretations and definitions of situations and problems. According to Fairclough (2001) political documents are often characterised by a rhetorical, one-way kind of communication. Moreover, analysis of texts can be organised under four different concepts: 'words', which deals mainly with individual words or metaphors, 'clauses' which deals with words combined into clauses and sentences, 'clauses combinations', which deals with how clauses and sentences are linked together, and finally, 'whole- text language organisations', which deals with largescale organisational properties of texts. In this study, we have been interested in the words, concepts and understandings that occupy hegemonic positions in the policy documents. It has, for instance, been suggested that shifts in terminology (e.g. 'workfare' instead of 'welfare') along with the shifting configuration of the welfare state, reflect this kind of dynamic. The use of terms is not accidental, rather they are expressions of conscious ideology even when the terms themselves may seem self-evident and natural (Garrett, 2015). Since the small terms are equally important as clauses and structures of words, we tried to focus on all four concepts described by Fairclough when we did our analysis.

Discussion of tendencies in the material

When analysing the texts, three discourses emerged as the most predominant. (1) *The Medicalisation Discourse*, (2) *The Stigma Discourse* and (3) *The Social Investment Discourse*. In the subsequent section, we will first present the discourses we identified one by one before we discuss each of them in the light of relevant research.

The medicalisation discourse

Clarke and Shim (2010) define medicalisation discourse as the tendency to include an increasing number of life domains into the realm of medicine and redefine the phenomena that belong to such domains. Redefinition or reconceptualisation of vital life spheres in this way is a part of the neoliberal paradigm (Schwartzmantel, 2005). A study among young, unemployed people, for instance, concludes that attention towards their real or potential mental health disorders often camouflage social problems (Ose & Jensen, 2017). The term 'disorder' when occurring in workfare policy documents and practice is an example of a 'word' (cfr. Fairclough) that by means of the 'clause' *far away from work* designates statuses for which the Norwegian Labour and Welfare Administration (NAV) does not have to take any responsibility (see Frøyland, 2015). However, 'Substance Use Disorder', as expressed in DSM-V (American Psychiatrist Association, 2013), is a highly heterogeneous concept, spanning from mild to severe statuses. SUD does not necessarily implicate incapacity to work (Corrigan & McCracken, 2005). Authors that address more general inclusion in the job market in Norway (Myklebun, 2013) also note within group heterogeneity.

The medicalisation discourse is also apparent in the Norwegian government's proposal from 2006 for new measures related to the new administrative model for labour and welfare (St. meld. no. 9 (2006–2007)). Interestingly, the title of the proposal, which is one of the most important policy documents in this field, is 'Work, Welfare and Inclusion'. In the first phrase of the report, it is even underscored that: 'Norway is a society of opportunities' (p. 13).

However, the content of this report with regard both to NEETs in general and NEETs with additional substance problems is not that of inclusion. Rather, the report conceptualises them as having so-called work-hurdles, defined as physiological or physical problems, social behavioural problems or problems with alcohol or drugs. In addition, lack of education, lack of work experience, lack of employment and lack of social skills are among the 'defects' that the cited proposal mentions. Moreover, the proposal with more specific regard to people with alcohol or other drug problems states that they often lose their jobs. By its focus on dysfunction, the above-cited proposal establishes a linkage between problems with alcohol and other drugs and instability and non-employability.

The central stance in workfare policy is to view unemployment and poverty as matters of individual responsibility (Marthinsen & Skjefstad, 2011). Even though the proposal (St. meld. no. 9 (2006–2007)) suggests that the reasons for the changes in the work market are structural, in terms of downsizing of industrial workplaces etc., its obvious basis is workfare ideology, which tends to focus more on individual failure than lack of jobs. As a consequence, the report merely delineates individual solutions to young peoplès problems about getting a job. For instance, the proposal states that the above-mentioned hurdles must be '… overcome or compensated before they can get a job' (p. 33). Moreover, the report states that individuals with substance use problems, more so than people without such problems, may have greater difficulties with getting motivated for those measures that could lead to employment.

So-called labour market disengagement among young people is generally poorly understood in relevant research (Goldman-Mellor et al., 2016; Ose & Jensen, 2017). According to Ose and Jensen, definition of the disengagement relies on the eye of the beholder. Interviewing social workers, the authors identified three main barriers to education or employment: client motivation, the sense of lack of achievement/defeat and unrealistic expectations about working life. Interviewing the young people themselves, the same study revealed quite other barriers, spanning from general health problems to low self-esteem. Most often, substance use among NEETs is described as a part of a greater individual problem syndrome, like criminal history, poorer social functioning, greater disability and economic difficulties (Chen, 2011). Some studies also report that NEETs in general tend to have fewer skills in performing teamwork, decision-making and communication than non-NEETs (Goldman-Mellor et al., 2016). According to some, individual variations in work aspirations may be owed to variation in economic conditions (Carcillo, Fernández, Königs, & Minea, 2015; Newton & Buzzeo, 2015). Yet some conclude that the aspirations of the young and unemployed mirror the aspirations of the wider society (Barry, 2005). A Norwegian longitudinal study ($N = 481$) on people having undergone long-term substance treatment (Lauritzen, Ravndal, & Larsson, 2012) showed that as much as one third of this clinical cohort had ordinary, paid work 10 years after discharge from treatment, whereas the portion of health-related benefits had also increased. The scientific basis for a full-fledged medicalisation discourse on the link between SUD and employability is ambiguous at best.

The above-reported increase in use of health-related benefits in the clinical cohort, however, needs to be commented on, as health concepts tend to invite to the shaping of 'clauses' or 'clauses combinations' that establish new structures to serve a neoliberal ideology. The rationale behind the increasing tendency to put people on disability pension for a mental disorder in Norway as well as in other OECD countries (OECD, 2012 in Mykletun, 2013) remains partly obscured.

Much of the Norwegian literature that addresses the link between SUD and inclusion in the labour market refers to the relatively broad category of co-occurrent substance disorder and psychiatric statuses (Bjaarstad, Irane, Hatling, & Reinertsen, 2014; Frøyland, 2015), as if all people with SUD belong to this category. The impression that NEETs with SUD stay 'far away from work' because of their double burden (see Frøyland, 2015) and accordingly are not worth public investment is thus reinforced.

Indeed, comorbidity between substance misuse and psychiatric disorders like depressions and anxiety – so-called dual diagnosis – is common (Lai, Cleary, Sitharthan, & Hunt, 2015). Yet, several well-documented facts related to co-occurrent mental health and substance use disorders seem to be under-communicated. For instance, the concept 'dual diagnosis' for co-existing mental health and SUD covers up the fact that such co-existence relies on quite incompatible etiology models and that the term encompasses groups that are relatively well-functioning (Guest & Holland, 2011). Although Guest & Holland's concern is not lack of access to the job market, but rather limitations in access to adequate treatment facilities, their warnings are against 'words' in policy documents with gloss-over effects.

Research on the relationship between SUD and NEET for statistical association (MacDonald & Pudney, 2000; Richardson, DeBeck, Feng, Kerr, & Wood, 2014), etiology (Henkel, 2011) and compounding factors in the linkage (Fergusson, Horwood, & Woodward, 2001; Hammer & Hyggen, 2010; Lee et al., 2015) is inconclusive. The lack of unitary research results about the role of substances in a NEET career may be owing to the fact that studies differ considerably with regard to both scope, age span (with 12 and 34 years as extremes) and type of study. There seems, therefore, to be no solid evidence on dysfunctionality in NEETs that could exclude them from the labour market on the group level. The reason to 'medicalise' them is therefore vague.

The stigma discourse

Stigma is by Goffman (1963) described as a visible spot or a social category that is not acknowledged in society and is apt to reduce a person`s reputation. The stigma discourse and the medicalisation discourse are interrelated in many respects. A medical diagnosis, though, may yield acknowledgement and strengthen certain rights for patient groups and individual patients (Clarke & Shim, 2010). Stigma, however, by being socially rather than scientifically constructed, is in the neoliberal era more likely to be underpinned by a moralising kind of framework in which the clients who are immediately prepared to sell their labour are favoured (Garrett, 2014).

Negative expectancies towards substance misusers prevail among employers (Baldwin, Marcus, & De Simone, 2010) and even among professionals in professional services aimed at assisting people with such problems to a decent life and social citizenship (Askheim, 2009). We found a striking example of stigma in terms of non-evidenced, moral justification in a so-called 'Report to the Storting'.[2] Instead of discussing how NAV and related services can help people with alcohol or other drug problems, the report states that these people are not able to make use of relevant services:

> In addition to dropping out of work life because of problems with alcohol and drugs, it is also difficult to get these people back to into the job market. A lot points to the fact that people with alcohol or drugs problems, to a considerable extent, are not able to make use of the ordinary set of measures provided through the Labour and Welfare Administration. (St.mld. no. 9 (2006–2007) p. 51)

Even managers of NAV agencies and some employees in NAV share the view expressed in the excerpt (Fossestøl, Breit, & Borg, 2016). Based on a study on the role of social work in the NAV offices, these researchers conclude that many NAV employees regard people with alcohol or other drug problems as 'miles away from work' and that helping them is beyond NAV's mandate. 'Substances' in this context have thus the function of 'words' in order to justify attitudes with a moral, not scientific basis, and alludes that problem substance users are not worthy of attention.

The neoliberal tendency of stigmatising substance use problems or disorders was addressed in the introduction of this article (O`Malley & Valverde, 2004). An example that those authors provide is how the addict is portrayed as being driven by a chemical dependency that is conceived of as 'beastliness'

In relevant literature, we find that merely being a NEET also has negative connotations verging on stigma. Through the lenses of Fairclough`s discursive analysis we may, for instance, observe certain uses of dichotomy, 'clauses' or 'clauses combinations' that constitute stigma discourse. Skjefstad (2015) identified the tendency to use the underlying dichotomy of active/passive in public documents about groups that are not immediately embraced by workfare policy. This dichotomisation portrays NEETs as passive individuals, with the lack of capability or will to be active and engaged. This also implicates that they are lazy and not motivated, and thus morally inferior. In contrast, some policy documents conclude that NEETs are 'committed to work *but* vulnerable'. Here vulnerability represents a certain stigma.

The dichotomy of active/passive is also at play in other countries in Europe (Johansson & Møller, 2009). The tendency to use the active/passive dichotomy tends to derive from the neoliberal emphasis on austerity. Since citizens in late modern societies are responsible for their own self-development, they have only themselves to blame for any problems that arise from their actions or inaction (Andersen, 2003).

Several titles of the scientific papers concerning NEETs may also reflect stigma related to the NEET category or constitute stigma by using the NEETs concept in rhetorical ways. Examples of such titles are 'Preventing young people from becoming a NEET statistic', 'Once a NEET always a NEET?', 'Not a Very NEET solution (about Early School Leavers)'. In Japan, the government, by means of a strategically effective wordplay, has constructed a 'NEET problem' and used it in political campaigns in order to scare young people from becoming NEET (Toivonen, 2011).

For such reasons, some tend to renounce on the entire NEET construct because it defines young people by what they are not (Yates & Payne, 2006). NEETs tend to share many characteristics with mainstream youths (Toivonen, 2011). The strategies that NEET employ to improve their situation are often silenced (Hammer, 2007). Some also point to the evidence that even the most disadvantaged NEETs can benefit from a variety of targeted interventions (Carcillo et al., 2015). An unambiguous focus on what NEETs are not could thus function as one of those 'words', 'clauses', 'clauses combinations' etc (crf. Fairclough, 2001). that may govern mindsets in a workfare climate.

Interestingly, the NEET concept was from the beginning meant to be a substitute for more value-laden concepts[3] (Beck, 2015). Over the course of time, however, the concept, according to Beck, has gained a significance of precariousness. In the above examples, we could observe how the vocabulary *'not'* shapes an unfavourable contrast to the terms 'employment', 'education' and 'training' all of which are labour promoting. Together the terms shape a 'clause' in the Faircloughian sense.

The social investment discourse

Social investment can be defined as strengthening peoples' current and future capacities (Leibetseder, 2018). Recovery is especially important in this discourse. 'Social investment' is above all associated with the OECD (2010) agenda to promote activity instead of dependency on benefit. It represents a 'culture of inclusion' (Hemerijck, 2013). Although having a pronounced neoliberal fundament, the trend according to Hemerijck implies a certain willingness to view public investment as productive. The ideological underpinnings of the strategy are, like the ideological underpinnings of workfare, that only active and full participation in the job market ensures citizenship and realisation of adult life (Harris, Owen, & Gould, 2012). The social investment framework is also related to the concept of 'human capital'. The human capital approach is based on the belief that there is a link between productivity of people in market situations and investments in education, skills, knowledge, habits, social and personality attributes, etc (Becker, 1964/1993).

In line with both workfare and social investment principles, in 2007, the Norwegian Government launched a strategy plan for people with psychiatric problems (Ministry of Work and Inclusion and Ministry of Health and Care (2007–2012)). This strategy also includes people with alcohol or drug related problems. It mentions workplaces and managers as necessary partners in the undertaking of the strategy. The notion that the responsibility for inclusion in the workforce lies with both the user, the welfare organisations and the employers is continued in a governmental report that specifically addresses substance policy (Meld. St. 30 (2011–2012). Economic incentives are involved, in terms of extra money from NAV to employ people with special needs. The report states that:

> People with substance use problems are in danger of dropping out or are excluded from the workplace. Many are recipients of benefits. As a part of government efforts to combat poverty, targeted measures are being taken towards specific groups such as people in the medical assistance rehab program LAR. Many participants in LAR have complex problems and history of long-tern use of opiates which makes re-entry to society difficult and demanding. Evaluation of targeted measures indicates that investing in a long-term perspective gives results. (Meld.St. 30 (2011–2012) p. 82) our translation)

Although there is a focus on recovery and inclusion in the document, there is an underlying assumption that everybody must contribute to society, regardless of their problems. As stated in this policy document: 'The government builds its policy on the idea that assets must be created before they can be shared' (Meld. St. 33 (2015–2016), p. 5). In line with the principles of workfare, it is therefore necessary to create flexible workers who are willing to take risks to fill the jobs demanded by the Norwegian labour market today (Skjefstad, 2015). Thus, despite growing individualisation, late modern society is more regulated that ever, and this is a subtle form of power (Meyer, 2003). This can be related to what Foucault calls *governmentality*. People are 'tricked' into believing they want to be this flexible person, at almost any cost. Yet, the focus in our text material is not merely on the job seeker's flexibility. In the excerpt below authorities, by employing vocabulary 'words' like 'openness' and 'flexibility' about the labour market, communicate that the labour market has an accommodative, welcoming character. At the same time the motives behind social investment, namely to lower public costs in the long run (Hemerijck, 2013) and to create assets before sharing, are not directly undercommunicated.

> A well-functioning labour market, where it is better to work than receive benefits, is important for achieving a high employment rate and including people in the workplace. An open and flexible labour market provides multiple opportunities for one to try out the workplace. (Meld.St. 33 (2015–2016), p. 5)

Much of the research literature we refer to in the three sections of the paper, namely the section on medicalisation discourse, the stigma discourse and even the social investment discourse, do not unambiguously support the accommodation principles that the report seems to convey. When use of the 'word' 'flexibility' remains undefined' it also remains unclear which labour market policy lies behind it. 'Flexible citizenship' can be synonymous with a precarious existence (Turner, 2016). Do the 'clauses' in the report represent a policy that shapes a precariat of young, unexperienced workers who are likely to resign to what they get? Indeed, the above-cited report states that young people on the fringes of the labour market, in order to be included, should have primacy over others when it comes to testing their working potential. Adequate assistance measures will be offered and guarantee systems simplified 'in order to achieve a clearer and less ambiguous priority of young people'. (Meld. St. 33 (2015–2016), p. 19). All the same, Norway is subject to the same global neoliberal currents in economy as other countries. Some suggest, yet based on relatively scarce research results, that a policy of greater flexibility in the workplace in regard to working hours and job protection may be beneficial for so-called new entrants (youth, immigrants and women). This may, however, occur at the cost of the relative low-level wage inequality and economic security in Scandinavian countries for those already in the job market (Kahn, 2012).

Examples of assistance apt to enhance the profitability of young NEETs with additional problems are models inspired by Recovery (Anthony, 1993) or Supported Employment (Latimer et al., 2006). These are also in use in Norway (Bjaarstad et al., 2014). Certainly, these are models that view work as more curative than harmful even in cases of illness (Waddel & Burton, 2006 in Mykletun, 2013). They allow paid work while treatment is still going on, if the people in question govern the pace of the process at the same time as they get advice from an inter-professional team (Bjaarstad et al, 2014). Both regular and maintenance substance treatment seem to have acknowledged this need to 'recover while you work' (Blankertz et al., 2004) and report positive results (Everly et al, 2011; Silverman, Svikis, Robles, Stitzer, & Bigelow, 2001). 'Place & train' programmes (Corrigan & McCracken, 2005) and the 'Therapeutic Workplace' (Silverman et al., 2001) are other examples of models that base themselves on Recovery principles. Such models, which imply ordinary, paid work are particularly promising with regard to symptom reduction and improved social inclusion (Borg, Karlsson, & Stenhammer, 2013).

In the documents we scrutinised, however, an 'unsurmountable' dichotomy was shaped between the terms 'citizen' and 'service user'. For instance, traces of this dichotomy could be found in the previously mentioned report on welfare policy (St.mld. no. 9 (2006–2007)) and in a report on disabled peoplès participation in society (NOU, 2001: 22). The term user in the above-mentioned dichotomy connotes something negative. One is a passive recipient of welfare services. Because this position is not recognised, it leads to stigmatisation and shame. The term citizen, on the other hand, has positive connotations in the sense that one is active and has control over one's own life. This position is recognised and provides affiliation to society and creates an identity that is appreciated. Again, we

encounter the active/passive dichotomy. The displacement that social investment discourse designates from so-called passivity to active measures is based on a logic of control and discipline of
the so-called passive user (Skjefstad, 2015; Johansson & Møller, 2009).

How feasible is a social investment strategy, though? The effort made to get marginalised people
into regular jobs seldom produces outcomes that lead to self-sustainability as the success rate never
exceeds 25% (Marthinsen & Skjefstad, 2011). Many providers of social investment measures feel that
young NEETs are fooled by this. Despite investment in strategies that aim at enhancing agency and
self-confidence, access to relevant workplaces for these young people is far from adequate (Beck,
2015). Based on this information, the workfare emphasis on 'aspiration' seems paradoxical
(Spohrer, 2011). In research on disability hurdles for access to the labour market, the imbalance
between discourse on activity and individual responsibility for participation and the lack of necessary
support is underscored (Harris et al., 2012). These authors describe how social exclusion often
becomes the result.

Final reflections

The specific aim of this paper was to explore discourses that are prevalent in central Norwegian policy
documents relevant to understanding the position of youths and young adults (18–30 years) who are
unemployed, not in education or in vocational training, and who in addition exhibit problematic substance use. The texts appear rhetorical and based on certain ontological assumptions about the
clients. In the policy documents, we found three predominant discourses, all of which, by means
of rhetorical 'techniques', represent a grip on both the defined target group and authorities: *The Medicalisation Discourse, The Stigma Discourse* and *The Social Investment Discourse*. The first and the
second discourses imply that the young people in question are put into categories that connote pathology or reinforces stigma, though without any solid scientific evidence. They are portrayed as individuals who 'stay far away from work'.

This may seem paradoxical, as the documents in their headlines, and partly in their content, underscore how inclusion in the labour market is what grants access to welfare and well-being. Although
our material suggests that work is good for people, and the documents seem apt to shape an ambi-
ence of inclusion, there are some apparent contradictions that overrule this. We view these tendencies, in connection with governmentality tendencies, which have been described by Rose,
O'Malley, and Valverde (2006), as the way in which neoliberal societies govern people in ways that
individualise and naturalise topics of social inequality and leaves responsibility to the individual.
As Foucault (2002) has shown us, institutional practices have characteristic ways of shaping the individual's minds, what he calls *Governmentality*. This is a way of implementing the individualisation
characteristic of the neoliberal ideology and discourse.

All three of the discourses we found in the government documents may be related to the development of neoliberal society and the tendency to individualise people's problems and to establish
certain beliefs. By and large, the research literature we scrutinised supports the idea that the problems said to be associated with NEET may contribute to the creation of myths about the NEET population. But the picture is ambiguous, at least at first sight. There is a will, in line with social investment
ideology, to include various groups of NEETs into the job market since Norwegian authorities regard
this as the primary solution for eradicating poverty and for becoming 'the most inclusive society in
the world' (St.meld. no. 9 (2006–2007)). All the same, the social investment has proved to rest on
ontology assumptions that in practice fail to include NEETs in society. The impression that NEETs
with SUD stay 'far away from work' (see Frøyland, 2015) and accordingly are not worth public investment, is thus reinforced.

Social work and social policy are closely related as social work practice is in many ways a reflection
of the policy. Norwegian legislation, as an effect of the obligations in the Human Rights Declaration,
demands that citizens should have rights of participation and inclusion. This is also stated in the IFSW
and IASSW definitions of social work (IFSW, 2012). Young people with additional problems are often

denied those rights, opportunities, skills and responsibilities that could have granted them citizenship. Further research should therefore look more concretely at the present issues in a rights' perspective.

Notes

1. The translations of the documents are made by the authors.
2. 'Storting': The Norwegian parliament.
3. 'Status 0' is mentioned by the author (Beck) as the former designation in a British context

Disclosure statement

No potential conflict of interest was reported by the authors.

References

Andersen, NÅ. (2003). *Borgerens kontraktliggørelse.* København: Reitzel.

American Psychiatric Association. (2013). *Diagnostic and statistical manual of mental disorders.* 5th ed. Arlington, VA: American Psychiatric Publishing. doi:10.1176/appi.books.9780890425596.744053

Anthony, W. A. (1993). Recovery from mental illness: The guiding vision of the mental health service system in the 1990s. *Psychosocial Rehabilitation Journal, 16*(4), 11–23. doi:10.1037/h0095655

Askheim, O. P. (2009). Brukermedvirkning – kun for verdige trengende? Om brukermedvirkning på rusfeltet. *Tidsskrift for psykisk helsearbeid, 1,* 52–59.

Baldwin, M. L., Marcus, S. C., & De Simone, J. (2010). Job loss discrimination and former substance use disorders. *Drug and Alcohol Dependence, 110*(1–2), 1–7. doi:10.1016/j.drugalcdep.2010.01.018

Barry, M. (2005). *Youth policy and social inclusion: Critical debates with young people.* London: Routledge.

Beck, V. (2015). Learning providers' work with NEET young people. *Journal of Vocational Education & Training, 67*(4), 482–496.

Becker, G. (1964/1993). *Human capital: A theoretical and empirical analysis, with special reference to education.* London: University of Chicago Press.

Bjaarstad, S., Trane, K., Hatling, T., & Reinertsen, S. (2014). Nye trender innen arbeid og psykisk helse - sett i sammenheng med recovery. *Tidsskrift for psykisk helsearbeid, 11*(3), 232–240.

Blankertz, L., Magura, S., Staines, G. L., Madison, E. M., Spinelli, M., Horowitz, E., & Young, R. (2004). A New work placement model for unemployed methadone maintenance patients. *Substance Use & Misuse, 39*(13-14), 2239–2260.

Borg, M., Karlsson, B., & Stenhammer, A. (2013). *Recoveryorienterte praksiser. En systematisk kunnskapssammenstilling -rapport nr.4/2013.* Oslo: Nasjonalt kompetansesenter for psykisk helsearbeid.

Carcillo, S., Fernández, R., Königs, S., & Minea, A. (2015). *Neet youth in the aftermath of the crisis: Challenges and policies.* OECD. doi:10.1787/5js6363503f6-en

Chen, Y.-W. (2011). Once a NEET always a NEET? Experiences of employment and unemployment among youth in a job-training programmer in Taiwan. *International Journal of Social Welfare, 20*(1), 33–42.

Clarke, A. E., & Shim, J. (2010). Medicalization and biomedicalization revisited: Technoscience and transformations of health, illness and American medicine A blueprint for the 21th century. In B. Pescosolido, J. Martin, J. McLeod, & A. Rogers (Eds.), *Handbooks of sociology and social research* (pp. 173–199). New York: Springer.

Corrigan, P. W., & McCracken, S. G. (2005). Place first, then train: An alternative to the medical model of psychiatric rehabilitation. *Social Work, 50*(1), 31–39.

Dahl, E. (2003). Does 'workfare' work? The Norwegian experience. *International Journal of Social Welfare, 12*(4), 274–288.

Engebretsen, E., & Heggen, K. (2012). Tilsynskunnskap. In E. Engebretsen, & K. Heggen (Eds.), *Makt på nye måter* (pp. 59–69). Oslo: Universitetsforlaget.

Evans, T. (2016). Street-level bureaucracy, management and the corrupted world of service. *European Journal of Social Work, 19*(5), 602–615. doi:10.1080/13691457.2015.1084274

Everly, J. J., DeFazio, A., Koffarnus, M. N., Leoutsakos, J.-M. S., Donlin, W. D., Aklin, W. M., & Silverman, K. (2011). Employment-based reinforcement of adherence to depot naltrexone in unemployed opioid-dependent adults: A randomized controlled trial. *Addiction, 106*(7), 1309–1318. doi:10.1111/j.1360-0443.2011.03400.x

Fairclough, N. (2001). The discourse of new labour: Critical discourse analysis. In Wetherell, Taylor, & Yates (Eds.), *Discourse as data: A guide for analysis* (pp. 229–266). Milton Hall: The Open University.

Fergusson, D., Horwood, L., & Woodward, L. (2001). Unemployment and psychosocial adjustment in young adults: causation or selection? *Social Science and Medicine, 53,* 305–320.

Fossestøl, K., Breit, E. & Borg, E. (2016). *Betingelser for sosialt arbeid.* AFI rapport 2016:02.

Foucault, M. (2002). *Forelesninger om regjering og styringskunst.* Oslo: Cappelens Akademisk Forlag.

Foucault, M. (1999). *Diskursens orden: Tiltredelsesforelesning holdt ved college de France 2. Desember 1970.* Oslo: Spartacus.

Frøyland, K. (2015). Å stå langt frå arbeid' – refleksjonar og førestillingar om kven som kan jobbe. *Tidsskrift for psykisk helsearbeid, 12*(4), 307–316.

Garrett, P. M. (2015). Words matter: Deconstructing 'welfare dependency' in the UK. *Critical and Radical Social Work.* doi:10.1332/204986015X14382412317270

Garrett, P. M. (2014). Confronting the 'work society': New conceptual tools for social work. *British Journal of Social Work, 44* (7), 1682–1699.

Giddens, A. (2004). *Modernity and self-identity. Self and society in the late modern Age.* Cambridge: Polity Press.

Goldman-Mellor, S., Caspi, A., Arseneault, L., Ajala, N., Ambler, A., Danese, A., & Moffitt, T. E. (2016). Committed to work but vulnerable: Self-perceptions and mental health in NEET 18-year olds from a contemporary British cohort. *Journal of Child Psychology and Psychiatry, 57*(2), 196–203.

Goffman, E. (1963). *Stigma.* London: Penguin.

Guest, C., & Holland, M. (2011). Co-existing mental health and substance use and alcohol difficulties - why do we persist with the term 'dual diagnosis' within mental health services? *Advances in Dual Diagnosis, 4*(4), 162–172. doi:10.1108/17570971111197175

Harris, S. P., Owen, R. & Gould, R. (2012). Parity of participation in liberal welfare states: Human rights, neoliberalism, disability and employment. *Disability & Society, 27*(6), 823–836. doi:10.1080/09687599.2012.679022

Hammer, T. (2007). Labour market integration of unemployed youth from a life course perspective: The case of Norway. *International Journal of Social Welfare, 16*(3), 249–257.

Hammer, T., & Hyggen, C. (2010). Lost in transition? Substance abuse and risk of labour market exclusion from youth to adulthood. *Norsk epidemiologi, 20*(1), 93–100. doi:10.5324/nje.v20i1.1299

Hemerijck, A. (2013). *Changing welfare states.* Oxford: University Press.

Henkel, D. (2011). Unemployment and substance Use: A review of the literature (1990-2010). *Current Drug Abuse Reviews, 4*(1), 4–27.

International Federation of Social Work. (2012). Statement of Ethical Principles.' http://ifsw.org/policies/statement-of-ethical-principles/.

Johansson, H. & Møller, I. H. (2009). Vad menar vi med aktivering? In H. Johansson & I. H. Møller (eds.) *Aktivering – arbetsmarknadspolitik och socialt arbete i förändring* (pp. 9–29). Malmø: Liber

Madsen, A., M., Judd, D., & Boeckh, J. (2015). Chicken or egg? Global economic crisis or ideological retrenchment from welfare in three European countries. *Critical and Radical Social Work, 3*(3), 339–355. doi:10.1332/204986015X14392797857418

Kahn, L. M. (2012). Labor market policy: A comparative view on the costs and benefits of labor market flexibility. *Journal of Policy Analysis and Management, 31*(1), 94–110. doi:10.1002/pam.20602

Kleppe, L., Engebretsen, E., & Heggen, K. (2012). Asylmottak og innsnevring av ansvar. In E. Engebretsen, & K. Heggen (Eds.), *Makt på nye måter* (pp. 92–100). Oslo: Universitetsforlaget.

Lai, H. M. X., M. Cleary, T. Sitharthan, & G. E. Hunt (2015). Prevalence of comorbid substance use, anxiety and mood disorders in epidemiological surveys, 1990–2014: A systematic review and meta-analysis. *Drug and Alcohol Dependence, 154*(1), 1–13. doi:10.1016/j.drugalcdep.2015.05.031

Latimer, E. A., Lecomte, T., Becker, D. R., Drake, R. E., Duclos, I., Piat, M., & Xie, H. (2006). Generalisability of the individual placement and support model of supported employment: Results of a Canadian randomised controlled trial. *British Journal of Psychiatry, 189*(1), 65–73. doi:10.1192/bjp.bp.105.012641

Lauritzen, G., Ravndal, E., & Larsson, J. (2012). *Gjennom 10 år : En oppfølgingsstudie av narkotikabrukere i behandling- SIRUS-rapport nr. 6/2012.* Oslo: Statens institutt for rusmiddelforskning.

Lee, J., Hill, K., Hartigan, L., Boden, J., Guttmannova, K., Kosterman, R., & Catalano, R. (2015). Unemployment and substance use problems among young adults: Does childhood low socioeconomic status exacerbate the effect? *Social Science & Medicine, 143,* 36–44. doi:10.1016/j.socscimed.2015.08.016

Leibetseder, B. (2018). Social investment and social welfare: International and critical perspectives. *Journal of Social Policy, 47*(4), 850–852. doi:10.1017/S0047279418000405

MacDonald, Z., & Pudney, S. (2000). Illicit drug use, unemployment, and occupational attainment. *Journal of Health Economics, 19*(6), 1089–1115. doi:10.1016/S0167-6296(00)00056-4

Marthinsen, E., & Skjefstad, N. (2011). Recognition as a virtue in social work practice. *European Journal of Social Work, 14*(2), 195–212.

Meyer, S. (2003). *Imperiet kaller: et essay om maktens anatomi.* Oslo: Spartacus.

Ministry of Work and Inclusion and Ministry of Health and Care. (2007–2012). Strategiplan for arbeid og psykisk helse 2007-2012.

Meld. St. 30. (2011–2012). (2011). *Se meg! — alkohol – narkotika – doping.* Report to the Storting. Retrieved from https://www.regjeringen.no/no/dokumenter/meld-st-30-20112012/id686014/25.10.2017.

Meld. St. 33. (2015–2016). NAV i en ny tid – for arbeid og aktivitet. Ministry of Labour and Social Affairs.

Mykletun, A. (2013). Young people, disability pension and mental illness. In T. Olsen, & J. Tägtström (Eds.), *For that which grows: Mental health, disability pensions and youth in the Nordic countries* (pp. 41–49). Stockholm: Nordic Centre for Social and Welfare Issues.

Newton, B., & Buzzeo, J. (2015). Overcoming poverty and increasing young people's participation. *Criminal Justice Matters, 99*(1), 10–11.

NOU 2004:13. En ny arbeids- og velferdsforvaltning. Sosialdepartementet.

NOU 2001:22. Fra bruker til borger. Sosial- og helsedepartementet.

OECD (2018), *Investing in youth: Norway.* Paris: Investing in Youth, OECD Publishing. doi:10.1787/9789264283671-en

OECD (2010). 'Sickness, Disability and Work: Breaking the Barriers - A Synthesis of Findings across OECD Countries.' Published on November 24, 2010. Retrieved from http://www.oecd.org/publications/sickness-disability-and-work-breaking-the-barriers-9789264088856-en.htm. Downloaded 5.5.2016

Ose, S. O., & Jensen, C. (2017). Youth outside the labour force — Perceived barriers by service providers and service users: A mixed method approach. *Children and Youth Services Review, 81,* 148–156.

O`Malley, P., & Valverde, M. (2004). Pleasure, freedom and drugs: The uses of 'pleasure' in liberal governance of drug and alcohol. *Consumption Sociology, 38*(1), 25–42. doi:10.1177/0038038504039359

Richardson, L., DeBeck, K., Feng, C., Kerr, T., & Wood, E. (2014). Employment and risk of injection drug use initiation among street involved youth in Canadian setting. *Preventive Medicine, 66,* 56–59. doi:10.1016/j.ypmed.2014.05.022

Rose, N., O'Malley, P., & Valverde, M. (2006). Governmentality. *Annual Review of Law and Social Science, 2,* 83–104. doi:10.1146/annurev.laws&social sciences.2.081805.105900

Schwartzmantel, J. (2005). Challenging neoliberal hegemony. *Contemporary Politics, 11,* 85–98.

Silverman, K., Svikis, D., Robles, E., Stitzer, M. L., & Bigelow, G. E. (2001). A reinforcement-based therapeutic workplace for the treatment of drug abuse: Six-month abstinence outcomes. *Experimental and Clinical Psychopharmacology, 9*(1), 14–23. doi:10.1037/1064-1297.9.1.14

Skjefstad, N. S. (2015). *Sosialt arbeid i overgangen til NAV – utfordringer for en anerkjennende praksis* (PhD), Norwegian University of Technology and Science Trondheim, Norway (2015:227).

Spohrer, K. (2011). Deconstructing 'aspiration': UK policy debates and European policy trends. *European Educational Research Journal, 10*(1), 5–163.

Stortingsmld nr 9 (2006–2007). *Arbeid, velferd og inkludering.* Oslo: Arbeids-og inkluderingsdepartementet.

Stortingsmld nr 39 (1991–1992). *Attføring og arbeid for yrkeshemmede. Sykepenger og uførepensjon.* Oslo: Arbeids-og inkluderingsdepartementet.

Turner, B. S. (2016). We are all denizens now: On the erosion of citizenship. *Citizenship Studies, 20*(6-7), 679–692.

Toivonen, T. (2011). `Don't let your child become a NEET!' The strategic foundations of a Japanese youth scare. *Japan Forum, 23*(3), 407–429.

Yates, S., & Payne, M. (2006). Not so NEET? A critique of the Use of 'NEET' in setting targets for interventions with young people. *Journal of Youth Studies, 9*(3), 329–344.

Responsibilisation, social work and inclusive social security in Finland

Vastuullistaminen, sosiaalityö ja osallistava sosiaaliturva Suomessa

Suvi Raitakari, Kirsi Juhila and Jenni-Mari Räsänen

ABSTRACT

In this article responsibilisation in social work is studied by analysing two Finnish state-level policy documents (called final report and research report) which concern a current activation initiative called inclusive social security (ISS). It is asked how social workers and clients are constructed as responsible subjects in these documents. Responsibilisation refers to the advanced liberal mode of governmentality, which aims to strengthen citizens' abilities to self-governance through various techniques that include the intertwined elements of surveillance and empowerment. It is demonstrated that the policy documents construct the social workers' and the clients' responsibilities partly in different ways. The final report leads activation to be based on shared responsibility and social work to be more community-based, whereas the research report strengthens more individual-based responsibility of clients and social workers. For the clients, the interpretation of ISS based on shared responsibility would probably be less stigmatising and paternalistic than the one based on individual responsibilities, i.e. approaching long-term unemployed citizens as being personally 'at risk' and thus a justified target group of individualised techniques for activation. For social workers and clients, future activation appears to be a wide mix of different techniques, moral expectations and possible ways of being a responsible subject.

TIIVISTELMÄ

Artikkelissa tarkastellaan vastuullistamista suhteessa sosiaalityöhön analysoimalla kahta valtiollisen tason poliittista dokumenttia (teksteissä loppuraportti ja tutkimusraportti). Dokumentit käsittelevät ajankohtaista, kansalaisten aktivointiin pyrkivää poliittista aloitetta eli osallistavaa sosiaaliturvaa. Artikkelissa eritellään sitä, miten sosiaalityöntekijät ja asiakkaat rakennetaan dokumenteissa vastuullisiksi toimijoiksi. Vastuullistamisella viitataan uusliberalistiseen hallinnan tapaan, jonka tavoitteena on vahvistaa kansalaisten kykyä omatoimisuuteen ja 'itsehallintaan' käyttämällä erilaisia tekniikoita, joissa yhdistetään kontrollin ja voimaannuttamisen elementtejä. Sosiaalityöntekijöitä ja asiakkaita vastuullistetaan dokumenteissa osin eri tavoin. Loppuraportissa aktivointi määrittyy yhteiskunnalliseen, sosiaaliseen vastuuseen perustuvana toimintana, jolloin myös sosiaalityö näyttäytyy ennen kaikkia yhteisöllisenä työnä. Tutkimusraportissa osallistava sosiaaliturva taas tulkitaan enemmän sekä sosiaalityöntekijän että asiakkaan henkilökohtaisiin vastuisiin perustuvaksi, jolloin korostuu näkemys pitkäaikaistyöttömistä 'riskissä olevina' ja siten yksilöön kohdistuvien, sosiaalityöntekijän kanssa neuvoteltavien ja toteutettavien aktivointitoimenpiteiden kohteina. Asiakkaiden näkökulmasta sosiaaliseen vastuuseen perustuva tulkinta osallistavasta sosiaaliturvasta olisi oletettavasti vähemmän stigmatisoiva ja paternalistinen kuin yksilön vastuullisuutta korostava lähestymistapa. Asiakkaalle ja sosiaalityöntekijälle aktivointi näyttäytyy tulevaisuudessa kuitenkin sekoituksena erilaisia tekniikoita, moraalisia odotuksia ja mahdollisuuksia toimia vastuullisena subjektina.

Introduction

'On whose responsibility?' has been one of the core questions during the last three decades in discussions concerning the future of the welfare state. *Responsibilisation* is a concept that has increasingly been used and developed in these discussions. The origin of the concept can be found in the governmentality literature that draws especially on Rose and Miller's writings (e.g. Miller & Rose, 2008; Rose, 1990, 2000) and, through them, in Foucault's writings (e.g. 1988, 1991). Foucault approaches governmentality as 'techniques and procedures for directing human behavior' (Rose, O'Malley, & Valverde, 2006, p.1). Responsibilisation in turn refers to the advanced liberal mode of governmentality, which aims to produce active citizenship by strengthening citizens' abilities to self-governance through various techniques that include intertwined elements of surveillance and empowerment.

The concept of responsibilisation has been applied in various settings such as when creating an 'active welfare state' where entitlements to benefits are conditioned upon the adoption of certain kinds of behaviour (Barnett, 2003) and when analysing the relationship between the political construction of the 'active citizen' and the experiences of food bank users and volunteers (Garthwait, 2017). Responsibilisation has also been approached as an interactive accomplishment of professionals and clients at the margins of the welfare service (Juhila, Raitakari, & Hall, 2017a).

In this article we study responsibilisation in social work by analysing the Finnish state-level policy documents concerning a current activation initiative called *inclusive social security* (from now on ISS), which is targeted especially at long-term unemployed citizens. For the time being ISS in Finland is without a valid, specific law. However, the first pilot projects were launched in 2014 and recent ones have begun in 2018. ISS is not just specific to Finland. It has been introduced in many western welfare states as a promising technology in the battle against long-term unemployment and social exclusion and as one solution for sustainability in societies that are facing challenges in regard to austerity and increasing expenses due to an aging population and low workforce rates. ISS is also presented as an alternative to traditional activation policies that are said to be inadequate for employing citizens who are at risk of social exclusion and for preventing externality from working life (Hiilamo et al., 2017). ISS is a political initiative that strengthens the conditionality and reciprocity of services and brings together public employment services and social services (including social work).

The ISS policy documents examined in this article mark out the future prospects of social work by (re)defining both clients' and social workers' responsibilities in the context of activation. Notably, the documents are based on the idea of active citizenship, which means that those citizens who are seen to be 'passive' and at risk of social exclusion become the targets of particular guidance and surveillance steered by the Government and carried out by social workers. We analyse the responsibilisation in ISS documents from the point of view of social work and ask *how social workers and clients are constructed as responsible subjects in them.*

The article is structured as follows. We begin by creating a theoretical framework based on the concept of responsibilisation and in particularly on responsibility projects that shed light on the role of social work in responsibilisation. Then we describe the relations between activation policies and responsibilisation, after which we present the data and their analysis. Following this we present the findings of our analysis and then conclude by summarising and reflecting critically on the different ways of constructing social workers and clients as responsible subjects in the documents.

Responsibility projects and social work

According to O'Malley (2009), the concept of responsibilisation as developed in the governmentality literature refers to:

> The process whereby subjects are rendered individually responsible for a task which previously would have been the duty of another – usually a state agency – or would not have been recognized as a responsibility at all. The process is strongly associated with neoliberal political discourses, where it takes on the implication that the subject being responsibilized has avoided this duty or the responsibility has been taken away from them in the welfare state era and managed by an expert or government agency. (p. 276)

A mode of governmentality that is based on responsibilisation resonates with the premises of active citizenship (e.g. Ilcan, 2009; Juhila et al., 2017a; Newman & Tonkens, 2011), which emphasise taking responsibility for oneself and others instead of being dependent on welfare state and its safety nets. All citizens are subjects (and objects) of responsibilisation (Liebenberg, Ungar, & Ikeda, 2015).We are expected to govern our own lives according to the expectations of the 'normal' and 'good' life. There are, for example, governmental instructions on what constitutes a healthy diet as well as various experts such as counsellors who help to make wise choices for attaining a better life in complex situations. The aim of this kind of responsibilisation may be to empower citizens to become strong actors in the fragmented and plural western societies. Lemke (2001, p. 201) argues that social risks (such as illness, unemployment and poverty) have been transformed into problems of personalised self-care. Citizens' responsibilisation is thus linked to the retreat, 'irresponsibilisation', of the public governance and to the shifting of responsibilities to individuals and communities (Cradock, 2007, p. 162; Liebenberg et al., 2015; Peeters, 2017).

Responsibilisation is also accomplished in a more focused way by the control, guidance and support conducted by different welfare professionals, including social workers. This kind of respon-sibilisation is targeted at citizens who are categorised as unable to make responsible life choices or unwilling to meet the requirements of active citizenship. They are often defined as being at risk of social exclusion. There is a growing tendency to develop various institutional and professional enabling programmes that seek to strengthen the responsibilities of 'citizens at risk' in their own lives. These programmes can be named as *responsibility projects* (Ilcan, 2009, pp. 220–221; Juhila, Rai-takari, & Hansen Löfstrand, 2017b, pp. 19–22). In these projects welfare professionals work in close contact with clients and try to promote the expected changes in clients' lives, thinking and behaviour patterns by using various techniques such as education, encouragement, interviews, assessments, agreements and plans. The focused responsibilisation is targeted at people who are often categorised for example as long-term unemployed citizens, (former) prisoners and people with mental health, substance abuse or housing problems (Kemshall, 2002; Muncie, 2006, pp. 780–781; Pollack, 2010; Teghtsoonian, 2009, p. 29). When the responsibility projects emphasise individual conduct they move the focus away from structural exclusion and social explanations of individual adversities (see Ferguson, 2007, pp. 395–397; Scoular & O'Neill, 2007, pp. 770–771). They also easily divide citi-zens into polarised categories, such as 'independent' and 'dependent' or 'compliant' and 'incompli-ant' (e.g. Lantz & Marston, 2012; Liebenberg et al., 2015).

Applying specific techniques of responsibilisation for those categorised as 'risky citizens' has a long history in western societies. However, in advanced liberal responsibility projects welfare pro-fessionals are increasingly seen as being personally responsible for recognising risks and transform-ing 'risky citizens' into more self-governed and active citizens (Pollack, 2010). The clients, for their part, have a responsibility to strengthen their independence and capabilities to make better risk assessments and life choices as well as to become more active and integrated members of society. In this sense welfare professionals and clients are mutually dependent, as clients have to help workers to help themselves (Juhila et al., 2017b, p. 26; Matarese, 2009). Mutual dependency between welfare professionals and clients is maintained by the Government's steering practices such as performance auditing, which emphasises professionals' responsibility to effectively promote clients' activation and participation in the society. However, welfare professionals can achieve these expected results only if clients are able and willing to act towards the aims of being responsible, active and participating sub-jects. The participants have an option to resist the expectations of the responsibility projects, such as the ISS, but this puts them at risk of being labelled as 'bad clients' and 'bad social workers'.

Extending sphere of activation and responsibilisation

Many European countries increased the use of active labour market policies in the 1990s, yet signifi-cant variations are found across different countries. As Heidenreich and Graziano state (2014, p 1): '[...] the notion of activation has been used extensively in order to characterise new types of employ-ment policies'. Common to these policies is that they oblige the unemployed citizen to participate in various programmes and measurements – responsibility projects – that are meant to promote activity, participation, 'workability' and 'work readiness' in return for unemployment benefits and social security. Finland has also a long history of active labour market policies (Karjalainen & Saikku, 2011; Keskitalo, 2008; Sama et al., 2017, pp. 3–4).

Activation policies comprise conflicting objectives, expectations and techniques. Hence it is no wonder that a wide range of justifications have been expressed for and against these policies. These range from the authoritative enforcement and 'no work, no pay' and 'carrot and stick' view-points to the viewpoints of how well-organised activation programmes reduce social exclusion and increase the probability of returning to the labour market. Accordingly, there are 'softer' and 'harder' interpretations of activation (Keskitalo & Karjalainen, 2013, pp. 11–12; Sama et al., 2017, p. 4). The 'harder' interpretation emphasises the use of coercive measures to increase workforce invol-vement, whereas the 'softer' one emphasises making investments to decrease social exclusion and promote social inclusion. Despite these differences, activation policies are in general assumed to give rise to savings in public expenditures and bring about positive outcomes in regard to citizens' living conditions, health, self-esteem, well-being as well as to their integration into society (Breidahl & Clement, 2010; Inclusive social security, 2015, pp. 40–42).

In the 1980s and 1990s activation was targeted at those citizens with no serious problems besides unemployment. Since then the ideas of activation have extended to the sphere of social and welfare policies and practices (Heidenreich & Graziano, 2014, p. 1; Hultqvist & Nørup, 2017; Karjalainen & Saikku, 2011). For that reason employment, social and welfare policies have increasingly been inter-twined and focused on activating various social groups such as the long-term unemployed, women, younger and older people, migrants, young mothers, the unskilled and the disabled (Heidenreich & Graziano, 2014; Lantz & Marston, 2012). Due to these developments, the obligations and terms of getting services and benefits have tightened: the relationship between rights and responsibilities for unemployed citizens and other social groups has been redefined (Breidahl & Clement, 2010). The demand of active, responsible citizenship has been extended to concern also the most excluded citizens that need social support and benefits but who often have the least resources to reach the requirements of the activation policies (Keskitalo & Karjalainen, 2013).

Activation policies as a whole can be seen to imply and realise responsibilisation targeted to 'risky citizens' in various responsibility projects. The policies direct the citizens to be active and responsible by both investing in them and forcing them to adopt the 'right' course of action towards labour market involvement and inclusion in society. Activation policies emphasise strict regulations and indi-vidualised follow-up procedures, reciprocity, rewards, sanctions and agreements as techniques to affect unemployed citizens' conduct. Welfare professionals and especially social workers are commonly the ones responsible for putting these activation policies into practice in face-to face encounters with clients.

Analysing the state-level policy documents

ISS is briefly mentioned in the Finnish Government Programme, 2015 and in the Government Action Plan, 2017–2019 as one of the Government's key projects (Finland, a land of solutions, 2015; Finland, a land of solutions, 2017; see also Europe 2020 Strategy, 2016, pp. 20, 32). More thorough descriptions of these recent ideas of ISS can be found in two state-level policy documents. At the time there are no other detailed documents available. So these two documents serve as our empirical material for ana-lysing the connections between social work, responsibilisation and the political initiative of ISS. The two documents are as follows: (1) *Inclusive social security: Final report of the task force* (published by the Ministry of Social Affairs and Health in 2015) and (2) *Four models for inclusive social security in Finland* (printed in a series of publications concerning the Government's analysis, assessment and research activities, Hiilamo et al., 2017).

The origin of the *Inclusive social security: Final report of the task force* (from this on final report) goes back to 2013 when the National Institute for Health and Welfare set up an expert group commis-sioned by Minister Paula Risikko to think about ways to include more incentives in the current Finnish social security system and to make it more activating. As a result Antti Parpo, a member of the group, presented preliminary ideas of ISS, which led to setting up a ministry-led task force to develop the ideas further. The task force launched pilot projects in six regions and wrote a final report. The final report includes 55 pages and is available only in the Finnish language. It starts with a description of the present state of the national unemployment services and social security benefits and continues by depicting the pilot projects and conclusions drawn from them. The last part of the report is based on previous research findings that address the (economical) effectiveness of activation. The final report describes ISS as a new initiative of activation policy in Finland.

Following the work of the task group that produced the final report in March 2015, the Prime Min-ister's office awarded University of Helsinki, Department of Social Sciences the task of evaluating and proposing specific models for ISS in Finland. A research group published in Finnish a research report called *Four models for inclusive social security in Finland* (from now on called the research report) (Hiilamo et al., 2017), which includes as an attachment a literature review in English called *Inclusive social security – ideas and models in Finland, The Netherlands, Denmark and Germany* (Sama et al., 2017). The research report includes 33 pages, and the attachment of 36 pages. The research report presents the current employment services and benefits in Finland, applications of ISS in other European countries and previous research on the effectiveness of activation policies. It com-prises a chapter 'Inclusive social security model in Finland – Participant income' that is (at this moment) the most detailed description of the ideas of ISS in the Finnish context and is thus a key piece of text for this article.

When analysing the realities and relations constructed in the documents we lean on the concept of responsibilisation as developed in the governmentality literature. We pay specific attention on how social workers and clients are constructed as responsible subjects in the policy documents. The chal-lenge within advanced liberal governance is 'to find means by which individuals may be made responsible through their individual choices for themselves and those to whom they owe allegiance' (Miller & Rose, 2008, p. 214; see also Hansen Löfstrand & Juhila, 2012). Accordingly, the analysis has been focused on such pieces of texts in the documents that include notions of the distribution of responsibilities and the use of specific techniques to regulate social workers' and clients' conduct in the context of ISS.

We conducted the analysis by reading the policy documents carefully and picking out all the sen-tences and sections dealing with the responsibilities of different stakeholders, especially social workers and clients in the context of ISS. The documents include a lot of discussion for instance about current service systems, unemployment benefits and international activation models that are not relevant material for the analysis. Hence, the text material to be studied in detail turned out to be quite definite. In the next two sections we present and analyse such pieces from the documents that are relevant in regard to our theoretical framework and the research question.

Towards inclusive social security and active citizenship by means of sharing responsibilities

This section is based on a final report *Inclusive social security: Final report of the task force* (2015). It makes visible critical questions that are to be solved when implementing ISS and how ISS comprises a mix of governing techniques. The first question is whether or not the objective of labour market integration is expected to be the first priority and aim for those unemployed citizens suffering from severe social or health problems. The question illustrates the tricky interconnectedness of employment, social and welfare policies. However, as seen from the piece of text below, in spite of the anticipated and recognised difficulties in labour market integration the objective itself is not to be abandoned, but whenever it is possible the target groups of ISS should be supported and directed step by step by using low-threshold strategies to reach the ultimate goal of activation. Although the text does not address any actual actor, it still clearly constructs a 'good' and 'responsible' worker that leads the client forwards:

> The aim of inclusive social security is to make the first step of participation as easy as possible. The target group consists of people outside the labour force, whose primary goal is not necessarily to find a job due to serious social and/or health reasons. However, the participant is always, when possible, supported in his/her progress towards a working life and the job market. (Inclusive social security, 2015, p. 46)

The second question is located between 'soft' and 'hard' activation policies, between 'carrot' and 'stick' approaches. This question is present in the final report in reflecting the pilots' ability to balance the voluntariness and conditionality of ISS. These aspects of ISS are not defined as being mutually excluded. On the contrary, they are both seen to fit the ISS as crucial elements that are in line with the advanced liberal way of governing. Voluntariness is realised for instance in the possibility for long-term unemployed citizens to choose where and how they want to participate. Participation is also encouraged with small incentive 'carrots', such as bus tickets and free lunches that can be seen as techniques to guide an individual's decision making in a desired direction. Nevertheless, sanctioning 'sticks' (e.g. reducing the amount of employment benefit) are simultaneously part of ISS, when a person refuses to carry out activities agreed in the individual activation plan. Thus, sanctions can be pivotal techniques for carrying out activation plans. The long-term unemployed client is constructed as one needing resources and opportunities in order to be able to make such responsible choices that serve their inclusion:

> The experiences of the workers and participants in the pilots highlighted the fact that voluntariness is not unequivocally the opposite of obligatoriness. Despite being obligatory, rehabilitative work activity can be carried out as a voluntary activity by enabling people to choose where and when they participate, and by not employing sanctions. These principles were followed in the pilots. However, sanctions are always possible if a person opts out of activities agreed on in the activation plan. (…) Participation is voluntary and declining or terminating participation will not affect a person's social security. Possible incentives for participation include offering meals, bus tickets or transportation. (…) The work force sees that unemployed persons must be offered opportunities to contemplate and make choices for their own well-being and to promote their inclusion. (Inclusive social security, 2015, pp. 30, 46, 50)

The third crucial question dealt with thoroughly in the final report is whose responsibility it is to organise inclusive activities and participation possibilities for the long-term unemployed citizens. It is stated clearly that municipalities have the main responsibility to organise and coordinate ISS activities in close collaboration with non-governmental organisations (Inclusive social work, 2015, p. 46). The important lesson to learn from the pilots is that not only should the social welfare sector be responsible for organising the options and places for participation, but other municipal sectors and different non-governmental actors also should be. This kind of a mixed activation model including multiple actors is defined as cost effective and adequate. It is based on the idea of shared responsibilities; not only social workers and clients are made responsible but ultimately the whole community:

> Inclusive social security is a misleading term since it possibly implies that organising activities that promote inclusion is the sole responsibility of social services. In this sense as well, the pilots demonstrated the limitations of rehabilitative work activity. They included many activities more suited to be run by adult education centres or culture and sports services. This would enable the containment and smart allocation of expenses. (…) Activities could include guided group activity, open group activity, courses, meeting places, recreational spaces etc. Offering such activities requires the municipalities to allocate human resources or to obtain those resources in the third sector because the participants need support, guidance and counselling. (Inclusive social security, 2015, pp. 30, 46)

To conclude, our interpretation is that the final report represents more a 'soft' than a 'hard' interpretation of activation by emphasising the following aspects of ISS: prevention of social exclusion, importance of social support, voluntariness, sufficient level of public investments and the importance of low-threshold opportunities for participation for everyone. Nevertheless, the final report also constructs long-term unemployed citizens as a focus of step-by-step responsibilisation and as a responsible subject. A true and stable labour market position and active citizenship is presented as an ideal aim, although it is admitted that reaching this aim often takes time and includes various phases. But not just long-term unemployed citizens but also municipalities and various non-governmental actors are allocated to have responsibilities, for example to arrange meaningful places for participation with reasonable costs. Hence, long-term unemployed citizens are not seen as solely, personally responsible for 'breaking' into working life and communities. The core message of the final report is that active citizens can be created by means of sharing responsibilities: ISS is about transforming society to be active, supportive and inclusive.

Despite the idea of shared responsibility welfare professionals do not play a large part in the final report and, on the whole, responsibilities are not distributed specifically to particular professions. The term social worker is mentioned only three times and social work is not mentioned at all. All three mentions are in the description of the current context of public employment and social services, not in the visioning of ISS. Hence, social workers are not direct targets of responsibilisation in this policy document. That is mostly due to the fact that the final report does not make any concrete proposal for an realization of ISS in Finland. However, the final report recommends many practices whose enforcement seems to necessitate that social workers and other professionals who support long-term unemployed citizens should take the first steps in promoting participation, through advising clients when making choices concerning where and how to fulfil the participation obligations of ISS, making agreements and activation plans with the clients or by assessing the justification of sanctions in such cases where these obligations are declined.

Participation income as an example of a targeted responsibility project

In the other policy document, *Four models for inclusive social security in Finland*, a key term in planning the ISS model is participation income (PI) that was originally used in the Finnish discussions by Kanninen (2014). Atkinson (1996) had previously used the same concept to introduce such a basic income model that obligates the citizen to engage in socially beneficial activities in order to be entitled to the benefit (see also Sama et al., 2017). This kind of conditionality is also the basic idea of PI introduced in the research report. At the macro-level PI strives to extend what is understood as 'work' in Western societies (Hiilamo, 2014). Hence, the research report suggests a wide variety of activities that can be accepted as entitled to PI, such as voluntary work, rehabilitative work and studying in various institutions. In limited cases also informal child or elderly care may be considered as acceptable activities. From the point of view of responsibilisation it is essential, as De Wispelaere and Stirton (2007, p. 526) stress, to ask: ' […] how (and by whom) the precise scope of participation is to be determined' and '[…] how compliance is to be enforced'.

According to the research report PI would be targeted at long-term unemployed citizens that are in a difficult labour market situation and at young unemployed citizens that are at risk of social exclusion (Hiilamo et al., 2017, p. 10). PI can thus be characterised as a targeted responsibility project. The target group is estimated to be about 90,000 citizens in Finland (Hiilamo et al., 2017, pp. 18–19). What is notable is that social work is addressed as a key profession for putting PI into practice – to support, assess and monitor the aforementioned target groups' participation endeavours in society and communities. Social workers are thus positioned as responsible subjects for translating PI to concrete activation instruments. The research report offers objectives and techniques for making this translation, which we examine in the following.

First, PI is described as a 'new service and social benefit package' and as an 'instrument' to be implemented in social work for activation and empowerment (Hiilamo et al., 2017, pp. 18, 20). PI is understood as a social service distinct from the employment services, though it serves also the aims of employment policies. This 'package' is said to include particular responsibilities, tasks and activities for social workers to conduct, such as giving instructions, making agreements and assessing the clients' progress, all of which can be recognised as familiar techniques used in responsibility projects. Social workers are expected to help, encourage and motivate clients to achieve their goals concerning suitable participation and simultaneously to oversee and control their activation endeavours. All this should be based on trust and shared agreements between social workers and clients and allow solutions that fit clients' personal paths towards active citizenship. So, the combination of 'soft' and 'hard' measures in directing the citizens defined as socially excluded or as being at risk of social exclusion is in the core of targeted responsibilisation:

> The services associated with participation income would be administered by social services and would be separate from employment services. Social workers in municipalities and later in regions (from the beginning of 2019) would employ participation income as an instrument of activation and empowerment. The service package associated with participation income would comprise guidance, instructions, agreements about participatory activities and the monitoring of participation (see more in the Sanctions section). The social worker's job would be to help, support and encourage the clients to choose an activity that best suits them and support the clients in achieving their goals. Social workers would monitor participation. The monitoring should not be too controlling, rather it should be based on trust that the participants will honour the agreements made. (Hiilamo et al., 2017, pp. 20–21)

Second, within the service package a service plan is the most important technique for implementing PI. Making plans includes an idea of progress towards expected and desired aims, in this case towards more participating and active citizenship. The research report directs social workers and clients to make the service plan in collaboration. The plans should individualise and define the activities in which the long-term unemployed citizens agree to take part in return for PI benefit. Both social workers and clients should assess the realisation of the plans on a regular basis. In practice, plan making and assessment would include regular negotiations between the long term unemployed citizens and social workers. These practices make long-term unemployed citizens accountable and responsible for their life choices and the possible problems that may arise from these. In turn, social workers from their part are responsible for asking questions and making inquires and assessments related to progress in reaching (workforce) participation objectives. Social workers and clients are thus constructed as being mutually dependent on each other in fulfilling the expectations and duties of ISS:

> A service plan would be created for each client's participatory activity. In the beginning, the plan would outline the client's goals, activity and contextual factors. The social worker and the client would do the first evaluation while drafting the service plan. The second evaluation would be carried out when reviewing the results (for example after 6 months). In the second evaluation, the client would be asked to what extent they feel they have reached their goals, what kind of participatory income-related activities they have participated in and which factors have supported or obstructed their participation. Through the evaluation of individual cases, it is possible to monitor changes in the client's situation and identify factors that have prompted possible positive or negative changes. Each time when creating a service plan, other available employment-promoting services would be discussed (for example work try-outs and pay subsidy). (Hiilamo et al., 2017, p. 21)

Third, the power to make consequential assessments of a demanded amount of participation would be delegated to social workers in PI. This means that they would be given discretion and responsibility to define and evaluate what is approved in each individual case as a sufficient and beneficial amount of participation and activity. Social workers would decide when the criteria for being an 'active enough citizen' for receiving PI are obtained and thus they are constructed as decision-makers and 'gatekeepers':

> The intensity of participation required for participation income (how many hours a day, how many days a week) would be determined by the social worker. (Hiilamo et al., 2017, p. 20)

Forth, in addition to having the power to assess the intensiveness of each client's participation, social workers would be in a position to decide on a sanction embedded in PI; namely on transferring such clients who refuse to participate in any kind of activities from the active to 'passive level' of PI (meaning also a lower level of benefit). Although these transitions should be based on negotiations and agreements between social workers and clients, social workers have the ultimate power in using the financial sanctioning measure: they are the ones drawing the line between the active and passive level and putting plausible sanctions into force. For long-term unemployed citizens the choice of non-participation is made unpleasant and consequential and there are limits to clients' choice and will. It is recognised in the research report that sanctions are easily targeted at the most disadvantaged citizens – and this results in an ethical problem. In line with the fundamental ethical premises of social work, it is stated that citizens getting sanctions require also support. Hence, the report addresses a common dilemma in social work: the responsibility to protect and care as well as monitor and set boundaries to unwanted behaviour:

> If a client belonging to the target group will decline to participate in any type of activity or cooperation after discussions, they may receive a passive-level participation income, which would be an amount equal to basic social assistance. The client and the social worker agree that the client will opt out of participatory activities and that the participatory income will remain on a passive level. (…) The client will receive a passive-level participation income until they express they intend to participate and make an agreement of their participation with a social worker. (…) Some of those who decline participation activities are in the most vulnerable positions, and they may suffer from coping problems, substance abuse and mental health issues. They require special support. (Hiilamo et al., 2017, pp. 22)

In sum, our interpretation is that PI has many characteristics of a responsibility project and advanced liberal governance. It is targeted at citizens 'at risk', in this case at long-term unemployed people. Its implementation requires close contacts between social workers and clients. It is an individualistic solution to long-term unemployment and social exclusion that focuses on citizens' obligations and commitments, on strengthening their know-how, activity-level and 'entrepreneurship'. PI also comprises, as responsibility projects do, mechanisms for rewarding and sanctioning and for empowering and punishing in guiding citizens towards 'good' and 'normal life'. Accordingly, It implies clear moral standards for preferred behaviour in advanced liberal societies. A passive level of PI makes this moral aspect very clear. As Rose (2000, p. 335) writes: 'those who refuse to become responsible, to govern themselves ethically, have also refused the offer to become members of our moral community. Hence, for them, harsh measures are entirely appropriate.'

Furthermore, PI is based on mutual dependency between clients and social workers: it is only through their co-operation that PI is accomplished as outlined in the report. PI makes long-term unemployment citizens responsible for their own conduct and choices in regard to various participation options. But it also makes social workers responsible for directing clients towards the right kind of conduct and reasonable choices by using service plans, assessments and the possibility of financial sanctioning. It can be claimed that a successful social worker is able to keep as many clients as possible at the active level of PI and on a progressive path that ideally ends in labour market inclusion. This kind of success demands clients who accept and are able to follow the regulations of PI. The research report does not give a direct answer to the tricky question of what happens to those citizens who resist or are unable to follow the guidelines and rationales of PI.

Conclusions

In this article we have studied responsibilisation and social work in the context of activation policies by focusing on two state-level policy documents that outline the Finnish initiative of inclusive social security (ISS). We found that the policy documents construct the social worker and the client as responsible subjects partly in different ways.

In the document *Inclusive social security: Final report of the task force* (2015) ISS is more about strengthening voluntary participation that in the long-term and step-by-step should lead a person into working life. The governance of the long-term unemployed citizens is based on offering low-threshold opportunities for participation as well as small incentives that can be seen as techniques for guiding responsible decision making and actions according to desired ends. Nevertheless, sanctioning is simultaneously present, although not very openly explicated. The responsibilities are managed in various ways in the report. The long-term unemployed client is constructed as one needing recourses and opportunities in order to be able to make responsible decisions that facilitate integration. The client's responsibility is to make accepted choices, co-operate and utilise support according to given terms. Above all, the final report stresses what we call a shared responsibility as a means to create active citizenship – not only long-term unemployed citizens but also municipalities as well as various (non-)governmental actors are defined as responsible in implementing ISS. As Karjalainen and Saikku (2011, p. 233) stress, the idea of shared responsibility and inter-agency co-operation has gradually developed, nowadays being one of the prerequisites of the Finnish activation policies.

The other document *Four models for inclusive social security in* Finland (2017) introduces one specific model of ISS, the participation income (PI) that reminds in many ways of the responsibility projects described in the governmentality literature. According to the research report, social workers are to employ PI as an instrument in activating and empowering long-term unemployed clients. The instrument includes several techniques, such as service plans, the assessment of a suitable participation level for each client and the right to decide on sanctions in those cases where clients refuse or are not able to take part in participation activities. However, it is also stated that social workers should accomplish these responsibilities in close collaboration with clients, for instance by making decisions in a client-centred and negotiable way. Accordingly, in order to produce the good 'responsibilisation results' expected by the Government social workers need to empower responsible subjects who are willing to struggle and make an effort to fulfil the criteria related to active citizenship.

It is difficult to forecast which one of the above mentioned orientations of ISS and ways to manage responsibilities will attain a stronger position in the current activation policies in Finland. Hence, it is also uncertain what future changes will take place in social work. The final report leads social work to be more community-based, whereas by focusing on PI the research report strengthens individual based social work. From the point of view of the clients the interpretation of ISS based on shared responsibilities would probably be less stigmatising and paternalistic than the one based on individual responsibilities, i.e. approaching long-term unemployed citizens as being personally 'at risk' and thus a justified target group of individualised techniques for activation.

In addition, in the very recent activation pilot projects (Activation model for unemployment security, 2018; The basic income experiment 2018; Osallistavan sosiaaliturvan kokeilu, 2018) launched after publishing the studied policy documents, various community and individual-based orientations as well as 'soft' and 'hard' activation techniques are discussed and developed. For social workers and clients this makes future activation a wide mix of different techniques, moral expectations, rules and possible ways of being a responsible subject.

To conclude, social workers' roles and responsibilities in ISS can be manifold and are highly dependent on the future directions of governmental policies of activation that are at the moment very much in a state of flux. For social work it makes a difference as to what is seen as preferable techniques and rationales for activation: what actually activates and empowers citizens? What is seen as sufficiently active responsible subject? What does being a responsible subject require from the individual and the community? Only the future will ascertain how social workers' and clients' responsibilities constructed in the state-level documents will be translated, applied and resisted at the grassroots level: what ISS will turn out to be as the everyday experience of social workers and client.

Disclosure statement

No potential conflict of interest was reported by the authors.

References

Activation model for unemployment security. (2018). Retrieved from http://stm.fi/en/unemployment/activation-model-for-unemployment-security

Atkinson, A. B. (1996). The case for participation income. *Political Quarterly, 67*(1), 67–70.

Barnett, N. (2003). Local government, new labour and 'active welfare': A case of 'self responsibilisation'?. *Public Policy and Administration, 18*(3), 25–38.

Dahl, K. N., & Clement, S. L. (2010). Does active labour market policy have an impact on social marginalization?. *Social Policy and Administration, 44*(7), 845–864.

Cradock, G. (2007). The responsibility dance: Creating neoliberal children. *Childhood (Copenhagen, Denmark), 14*(2), 153–172.

De Wispelaere, J., & Stirton, L. (2007). The public administration case against participation income. *Social Service Review, 81* (3), 523–549.

Europe 2020 Strategy, Finland's National Reform Programme. (2016). Ministry of Finance publications 11c/2016. Helsinki, FI: Ministry of Finance, Economics Department. Retrieved from http://urn.fi/URN:ISBN:978-952-251-763-0

Ferguson, I. (2007). Increasing user choice or privatizing risk? The antinomies of personalization. *British Journal of Social Work, 37*(3), 387–403.

Finland, a land of solutions. Strategic programme of Prime Minister Juha Sipilä's government. (2015). Government publications 12/2015. Retrieved from http://valtioneuvosto.fi/en/sipila/government-programme

Finland, a land of solutions. Mid-term review. Government action plan 2017–2019. (2017). Government publications 7/2017. Retrieved from http://valtioneuvosto.fi/en/implementation-of-the-government-programme

Foucault, M. (1988). Technologies of the self. In L. H. Martin, H. Gutman & P. H. Hutton (Eds), *Technologies of the self: A seminar with Michel Foucault* (pp. 16–49). London, UK: Tavistock.

Foucault, M. (1991). Governmentality. In G. Burchell, C. Gordon & P. Miller (Eds), *The Foucault effect: Studies in governmental rationality* (pp. 87–104). London, UK: Harvester Wheatsheaf.

Garthwait, K. (2017). 'I feel I'm giving something back to society': Constructing the 'active citizen' and responsibilising foodbank use. *Social Policy and Society, 16*, 283–292.

Hansen Löfstrand, C., & Juhila, K. (2012). The discourse of consumer choice in the pathways housing first model. *European Journal of Homelessness, 6*(2), 47–68.

Heidenreich, M., & Graziano, P. R. (2014). Lost in activation? The governance of activation policies in Europe. *International journal of social welfare*, Supplement *23*, 1–5.

Hiilamo, H. (2014). Voisiko osallistava sosiaaliturva lisätä osallisuutta? [could inclusive social security increase societal inclusiveness?]. *Yhteiskuntapolitiikka, 79*(1), 82–86.

Hiilamo, H., Komp, K., Moisio, P., Sama, T. B., Lauronen, J-P., Karimo, A., Mäntyneva, P., Parpo, A., & Aaltonen, H. (2017). Neljä osallistavan sosiaaliturvan mallia [four models for inclusive social security in Finland]. Publications of the Government's Analysis, Assessment and Research Activities 18/2017. Retrieved from http://urn.fi/URN:ISBN:978-952-287-351-4

Hultqvist, S., & Nørup, I. (2017). Consequences of activation policy targeting young adults with health-related problems in Sweden and Denmark. *Journal of Poverty & Social Justice, 25*(2), 147–161.

Ilcan, S. (2009). Privatizing responsibility: Public sector reform under neoliberal government. *Canadian Review of Sociology, 46*(3), 207–234.

Inclusive social security: Final report of the task force. Osallistava sosiaaliturva. Työryhmänloppuraportti. (2015). Helsinki, FI: The Ministry of Health and Social Affairs. Retrieved from http://urn.fi/URN:ISBN:978-952-00-3581-5

Juhila, K., Raitakari, S., & Hall, C. (Eds.) (2017a). *Responsibilisation at the margins of welfare services*. London, UK: Routledge.

Juhila, K., Raitakari, S. & Hansen Löfstrand, C. (2017b). Responsibilisation in governmentality literature. In K. Juhila, S. Raitakari & C. Hall (Eds.) *Responsibilisation at the margins of welfare services* (pp.11–34). London, UK: Routledge.

Kanninen, O. (2014, April). *Osallisuustulo kestävän hyvinvoinnin yhteiskunnassa* [Participation income in a society of sustainable welfare]. Sitra's seminar, Panel introduction. Retrieved from http://www.slideshare.net/SitraFund/osallisuustulokestavanhyvinvoinninyhteiskunnassa20140131ohtokanninen

Keskitalo, E., & Karjalainen, V. (2013). Mitä on aktivointi ja aktivointipolitiikka? [What is activation and activation politics]. In V. Karjalainen, & E. Keskitalo (Eds.) *Kaikki työuralle! Työttömien aktiivipolitiikkaa Suomessa [Activation policies of unemployed in Finland]*. Helsinki, Finland: The National Institute for Health and Welfare. Retrieved from http://urn.fi/URN:ISBN:978-952-245-888-9

Karjalainen, V., & Saikku, P. (2011). Governance of integrated activation policy in Finland. In R. van Berkel, W. de Graaf, R., & T. Sirovatka (Eds.), *The governance of active welfare states in Europe*. RECWOWE (pp. 216–236). London: Palgrave Macmillan.

Kemshall, H. (2002). Effective practice in probation: An example of 'advanced liberal' responsibilisation?. *Howard Journal of Criminal Justice, 41*(1), 41–58.

Keskitalo, E. (2008). *Balancing social citizenship and new paternalism: Finnish activation policy and street-level practice in a comparative perspective*. Helsinki, Finland: Helsinki University Press.

Lantz, S., & Marston, G. (2012). Policy, citizenship and governance: The case of disability and employment policy in Australia. *Disability & Society, 27*(6), 853–867.

Lemke, T. (2001). The birth of bio-politics: Michel Foucault's lecture at the College de France on neo-liberal governmentality. *Economy and Society, 30*(2), 190–207.

Liebenberg, L., Ungar, M., & Ikeda, J. (2015). Neo-liberalism and responsibilisation in the discourse of social service workers. *British Journal of Social Work, 45*(3), 1006–1021.

Matarese, M. (2009, August). Help me help you: Reciprocal responsibility in caseworker-client interaction in a New York City shelter', Paper presented at the DANASWAC conference, Gent, BE.

Miller, P., & Rose, N. (2000). *Governing the present: Administering economic social and personal life*. Cambridge, UK: Polity Press.

Muncie, J. (2006). Governing young people: Coherence and contradiction in contemporary youth justice. *Critical Social Policy, 26*(4), 770–793.

Newman, J., & Tonkens, E. (2011). Introduction. In J. Newman & E. Tonkens (Eds.), *Participation, responsibility and choice: Summoning the active citizen in Western Eeuropean welfare states* (pp. 9–28). Amsterdam, NL: Amsterdam University Press.

O'Malley, P. (2009). Responsibilization. In A. Wakefield & J. Fleming (Eds), *The SAGE dictionary of policing* (pp. 277–279). London, UK: Sage.

Osallistavan sosiaaliturvan kokeilu 2018. (2018). Retrieved from https://thl.fi/fi/tutkimus-ja-asiantuntijatyo/hankkeet-ja-ohjelmat/osallistavan-sosiaaliturvan-kokeilu.

Peeters, R. (2017). Manufacturing responsibility: The governmentality of behavioural power in social policies. *Social Policy and Society*. Advance online publication. Retrieved from https://doi.org/10.1017/S147474641700046X

Pollack, S. (2010). Labelling clients 'risky': Social work and the neo-liberal welfare state. *British Journal of Social Work, 40*(4), 1263–1278.

Rose, N. (1990). *Governing the soul: The shaping of the private self*. London, UK: Routledge.

Rose, N. (2000). Government and control. *The British Journal of Criminology, 40*(2), 321–339.

Rose, N., O'Malley, P., & Valverde, M. (2006). Governmentality. *Annual Review on Law and Social Science, 2*, 83–104.

Sama, T. B., Lauronen, J-P., Karimo, A., Mäntyneva, P., Aaltonen, H., Hiilamo, H., Komp, K., & Moisio, P. (2017). Inclusive social security – ideas and models in Finland, The Netherlands, Denmark and Germany. Appendix in Neljä Osallistavan Sosiaaliturvan Mallia [Four Models for Inclusive Social Security in Finland]. Publications of the Government ́s Analysis, Assessment and Research Activities 18/2017. Retrieved from http://urn.fi/URN:ISBN:978-952-287-351-4

Scoular, J., & O'Neill, M. (2007). Regulating prostitution: Social inclusion, responsibilization and the politics of prostitution reform'. *British Journal of Criminology, 47*(5), 764–778.

Teghtsoonian, K. (2009). Depression and mental health in neoliberal times: A critical analysis of policy and discourse. *Social Science and Medicine, 69*(1), 28–35.

The basic income experiment. (2018). Retrieved from: http://www.kela.fi/web/en/basic-income-experiment-2017-2018.

Impact of neo-liberalism in Spain: research from social work in relation to the public system of social services

Impacto del neoliberalismo en España: investigación desde el trabajo social en relación con el sistema público de servicios sociales

Enrique Pastor Seller ⓘ , Carmen Verde Diego and Ana I. Lima Fernandez

ABSTRACT

After the economic crisis, neo-liberal policies in Spain established cuts in the public social welfare systems, which have had to face the increase in social demands from the population with fewer economic and human resources. The effects have been particularly hard on the population. The European Commission, in the *Commission Staff Working Document, Country Report Spain 2017*, notes an increase in inequality in Spain in spite of its macroeconomic improvement. The article summarises the impact that the economic crisis had on Spanish families and the austerity measures from the neo-liberal policies implemented by the government. Concerned by the social services' capacity to respond to them, the General Council of Social Work carried out Research Projects (2014–2015). Their analysis is presented here. The research started from 32,127 social workers, a confidence level of 95.5%, and a margin of error of ±3 in the worst-case scenario of $P = Q$. The sample comprised 2406 professionals. The results can be extrapolated to the totality of social workers in Spain and confirm the serious consequences the austerity measures have had on the population, social welfare systems and social workers who have dealt with neo-liberalism using social critical theory and militant practice.

RESUMEN

Las políticas neoliberales españolas, tras la crisis, han establecido recortes en los sistemas públicos de bienestar social que han tenido que afrontar el aumento de las demandas sociales de la población con menos recursos económicos y humanos. Los efectos han sido de extraordinaria complejidad para la ciudadanía y los profesionales del trabajo social, situación denunciada por la European Commission en la *Commission Staff Working Document. Country Report Spain 2017,* al constatar un incremento de pobreza, exclusión social y desigualdad entre ricos y pobres en España a pesar de los datos macroeconómicos. El artículo sintetiza el impacto que la crisis económica tuvo en las familias españolas y las medidas de austeridad de las políticas neoliberales implementadas por el gobierno. Preocupado por la capacidad de los

Servicios Sociales para responder a ellos, el General Council of Social Work from Spain llevo a cabo dos proyectos de investigación (2014 y 2015) con la finalidad de conocer el impacto de la austeridad en la ciudadanía, en los sistemas de protección social y en las intervenciones de los profesionales de los trabajadores sociales. El artículo presenta los resultados de ambas investigaciones empíricas basadas en la administración de un cuestionario validado a un universo de 32.127 trabajadores sociales, participando un total de 2406 profesionales del trabajo social en activo de toda España, muestra estratificada con un nivel de confianza del 95.5%, margen de error del ±3 y en el supuesto más desfavorable de P = Q, siendo sus resultados extra extrapolables a la totalidad de los trabajadores sociales en España. Los resultados constatan los graves efectos de la crisis en la ciudadanía, en los sistemas de protección social y en las intervenciones profesionales, los cuales han afrontado el neoliberalismo desde la teoría social crítica y una práctica militante.

The neo-liberal handling of welfare policies in Spain at the time of the economic downturn

The economic crisis of 2008 affected Spain deeply (as it did other countries in southern Europe such as Greece, Italy and Portugal). It was intensified by at least three circumstances: (1) economic growth sustained mostly by the long-term speculation of the real estate sector; (2) abusive banking practices, especially regarding housing and the marketing of high-risk financial products to small savers; and (3) cases of financial and political corruption and corporate crime (Council of the Judiciary, 2013; Villoría, 2015). All of the above resulted in a 'map of outrage' (Nofre, 2013) with hundreds of squares being occupied throughout Spain protesting 'against the financial coup d'etat', a movement that came to be known as the *Spanish revolution* (Antentas, 2017; Gerbaudo, 2017).

In this context, the economic crisis led to serious consequences, particularly in 2013, the year which was the subject of the *First Report on Social Services in Spain* (2014). Mass unemployment reached 26.94% in 2013 (according to the *Labour Force Survey*, NIS-National Institute of Statistics). The precariat (Standing, 2011) became widespread: the number of part-time employees rose to 2,730,000 in 2013, salaries decreased, labour conditions worsened and employment did not necessarily mean families could escape poverty (European Commission, 2017). Towards the end of 2013, there were 651,200 homes in which all active members were unemployed. Currently, this stands at *1,277,600 homes*, according to data from the *Labour Force Survey*.[1] That same year, there were 580,000 homes without any type of income: no salary, no subsidy from the social welfare system (unemployment benefit) and nothing from social services (FOESSA & Cáritas, 2013). This resulted in the global impoverishment of the population: 11,600,000 people lived on the poverty threshold in 2013 (FOESSA & Cáritas, 2013) and this figure has not stopped growing until it has reached 28.6% (European Commission, 2017). Certain groups suffered more than others: immigrants, the elderly, young people, women, and especially children, reaching 26.2% of all children in 2012 (González-Bueno, Bello, & Arias, 2012), a figure that has not stopped growing either, reaching 35% (European Commission, 2017; Save the Children, 2015), placing Spain as the second highest European country in child poverty, behind only Romania (38.1%).

An increase in social dualism in Spain has been confirmed (OECD, 2015; Oxfam, 2016; Saltkjel, 2017). As reported by the European Commission (2017), despite its macroeconomic improvement, Spain is the European country with the highest increase in social inequality between the rich and the poor in the last few years. It was hoped that given the family-oriented social model in this country, the Spanish government would deal with the impact of the economic crisis on poor and exhausted families by reinforcing the social welfare system. On the contrary, pressured by the European troika[2] (Salmon, 2017), the government amended the Spanish Constitution of 1978 to include a 'public spending ceiling' to avoid the 'embargo' (Art.135). These austerity measures were justified as being 'unavoidable', just like in other countries (Kelsey, Mueller, Whittle, & Khosranivinlk, 2016; Pentaraki, 2013) – even as rational and unquestionable 'austerity common sense', as Pentaraki (2018) would point. Funding and human resources were cut in public services, with limited replacement (1 replacement for every 10 retired civil servants). Essential public services such as healthcare, education and social services were privatised or 'externalised' to non-governmental organisations and businesses. Access to benefits, for example, those intended for dependent person, was restricted and the amounts were reduced from 2010 and particularly in 2013 (Deusdad, Comas-d'Argemir, & Dziegielewski, 2016). The solidarity of the social states was replaced with individual competitiveness, shifting the responsibility for maintaining welfare away from the government and onto the families. In particular, this 'refamilarisation' had a significant impact on women who found themselves having to do more care work after the crisis (Leon & Pavolini, 2014). The public were accused of having 'lived above their means' as a new austere moral attitude took hold (Kelsey et al., 2016; Lorenz, 2016), in an environment of punitive neo-liberalism (Davies, 2016).

Neo-liberal discourse justified the decrease in funding in social services in Spain, with its budget being reduced by 23% between 2011 and 2015. Meanwhile, the emergency social demands of the population grew; 182% in 2012, particularly in women and children (General Council of Social Work-GCSW).[3] Just as in other countries such as Greece (Pentaraki, 2017a), the impact the cuts have had on the municipalities, which are the main welfare providers, has been felt all over Spain (Pastor-Seller & Sanchez, 2014).

The austerity measures implemented by neo-liberalism affected the traditional role of social work in Spain, already described in the 1990s by De La Red Vega (1993). Its duties were to facilitate access to resources for the population with needs socially recognised as a public responsibility, to participate in the design and implementation of the government's social policy and, through that, to promote social justice. Neo-liberalism destroyed this social work function of mediation between public policies and private demands of the population (Lorenz, 2014). Its consequences were a fracture in social workers' own professional practice: on the one hand, they are prevented from responding to the needs of a society increasingly impoverished and, on the other hand, they were disabled, in their relational work with people, from defending citizens' rights (Lorenz, 2017) precisely in a moment when they needed more than ever to commit politically in their defence (Strier & Feldman, 2017).

In short, government neo-liberalism leads to situations of 'structural violence', not only because of the lack of protective policies to tackle the crisis but, paradoxically, by destroying those that already exist with austerity policies (Black, 2014). However, this situation is not unique to Spain. Rather, it is a result of global neo-liberalism, with increases in inequality and cuts in social expenditure (Davies, 2016; Fairclough & Graham, 2002; Hayes, 2017; Matsaganis & Leventi, 2014; Steinebach & Knill, 2017). In this context, social work, in its specific situations, faces difficulties due to increasing demand, a reduced ability to respond and the ethical commitment social workers have with the general public. These issues are discussed in the specialised literature (Aronson & Sammon, 2000; Baines, MacKenzie Davis, & Saini, 2009; Banks, 2009; Campanini, 2017; Colley, 2012; Dominelli, 1999, 2010; Ferguson, Lavalette, & Whitmore, 2005; Lorenz, 2017; Strier & Feldman, 2017; Wallace & Pease, 2011; Wronka, 2014).

Social welfare in Spain through GCSW established a broad strategy of ethical, political and social commitment to fight against neo-liberalism. Among other things, it is worth highlighting the work on two *Reports on Social Services in Spain* (Lima, 2014,2015a), which are the subject of this article.

Method

The results published in this article have been derived from research that aimed to analyse how neo-liberal policies have affected the social welfare system, its workers and the general public. These findings are based on the actual opinions of active social workers.

The article presents the results of two empirical research projects, hereinafter RSSS I, 2014 and RSSS II, 2015. These were based on a validated questionnaire given to 2406 active social workers from all over Spain, using a stratified and representative probabilistic sampling in all the autonomous communities in Spain and at a national level. To be more exact, the questionnaire was administered in two 'waves', based on a sample of 1361 in 2013 and 1045 in 2014, considering as the universal set the entire 32,127 active social workers in those years and association members in all state territory.[4] The sample provides a confidence level of 95.5%, the margin of error of ±3, and in the worst-case scenario of $P = Q$, its results can be extrapolated to all social workers in Spain.

The selection criteria for the participants were: (1) active social workers; (2) geographical representation of the whole of Spain; and (3) members of their respective territorial professional associations. For the results of the research to be extrapolated, a weighted proportionate stratified sampling was carried out according to the weight of social workers who were members of each professional association by the autonomous community.

All those participating were informed of the aims of the investigation and took part voluntarily and anonymously, meeting all the standards required of empirical research. The average duration of each survey was approximately 30 minutes.

The data were collected through surveys on the Internet using the social worker database of each of the professional associations. The first research (RSSS I) took place between May and July 2013 and the second (RSSS II) between May and September 2014. The questionnaire was initially validated after carrying out 80 surveys, with subsequent analysis of the answers in order to improve the final version. The data analysis was performed using the SPSS computer programme and Excel, using frequency analysis, contingency tables, comparison of averages and segmentation analysis. Contrasting of the most significant hypotheses was obtained using the chi-square test.

In both research projects, the validated questionnaires contained 76 questions (with some variations), organised in sections: (1) identification details of the social workers; (2) characteristics of the work done by the social workers; (3) characteristics of the users; (4) social workers' opinion about social services; (5) social workers' opinion about the handling of the economic crisis; and (6) social workers' outlook on the future and challenges to be faced. Specifically, in the RSSS II (2015), a new section was included regarding social workers' opinion about the local administration reform and it went into greater detail about what they thought of the austerity policies and how they related to the violation of the general public's social rights.

There is no knowledge of other empirical research carried out in Spain with such a high number of participating social workers or one in which the results can be extrapolated to the entire social worker profession of a state. This is empirical research which, among other benefits, stands out for its analysis of how the theoretical relationship between neo-liberalism and social work in Spain has been substantiated in professional working practice in this country.

Analysis and discussion of the results

Sample's socio-demographic data

With regard to the *socio-demographic characteristics of the participants*, it is noted that in Spain, as in other countries, social work is a profession largely dominated by females (83%), with an average age of active workers between 35 and 44. They work mainly in the public social services system (86.8%), particularly in social services at a municipal level. Only 9.6% work in private institutions and 3.4% in publicly owned companies which are privately managed. The latter were very scarce before the economic crisis. Comparatively, in the RSSS II (2015), although the data are similar, there is a clear loss of workers in public social services (86%) and their presence in private entities rises to 14%.

In addition, the high percentage of workers in municipal social services shows why 72% of social workers are against the local administration reform approved in 2013, describing it as 'bad' or 'very bad' (69%) as it reduced the benefits in municipalities with less than 20,000 inhabitants. They consider that it will take the service away from the ordinary citizen (74%), territorial inequality will increase as services are centralised again (79%), funding will worsen (64%), it will lead to an increase in cost (54%), coordination will become worse (51%), and social rights will be lost (70%) (RSSS II, 2015). Of course, in the end, this part of the reform was not implemented as the municipalities 'resisted' austerity measures (Medir, Pano, Viñas, & Magre, 2017).

Characteristics of social workers' work conditions

Regarding the *working conditions*, in the RSSS I, 2014, 33% of social workers claimed that in the previous year the number of workers in their department had decreased. There are significant differences between the two studies when talking about work overload: in the first (RSSS I, 2014), 73% of workers claimed they had to deal with a heavy or very heavy workload. This figure increases to 86% in the second study (RSSS II, 2015). 35% say they have to work longer hours on a daily basis (compared to 26% in RSSS I) and 61% do it at least once a week. Only 4% do not exceed their daily working hours. In addition, 45% of social workers declare that they do not receive any type of compensation for working longer hours.

The comparative analysis between both studies points to the slow decapitalisation in human resources of the social services system. This leads to poor working conditions for social workers as well as the slow but progressive trend towards outsourcing or privatisation of many social services, reported by 80.2% of those surveyed. With regard to this, 75.1% are against the combination of public/private funding systems in social services on the grounds that private management of social services will not ensure all citizens have right of access to them (57.8%) or that the quality of social services will decrease (52.8%). Additionally, 54% of those surveyed in RSSS II told us that the main problems are the high level of demand from the public and the limited resources available. Seventeen per cent refers to being saturated at work, reflected in a work overload and stress, and 9% complained of excessive bureaucracy in many of their daily tasks.

These figures are very relevant, as they shed light on the work overload facing social workers in Spain and the fact that they maintain levels of attention to the public due to their moral sense of responsibility despite receiving no compensation. They highlight the challenge social workers face in responding to more users within a system that is being reduced, working in worse and more stressful conditions, just as reported in Greece (Aronson & Sammon, 2000; Karagkounis, 2017; Pentaraki, 2017a, 2017b) and in Canada (Baines et al., 2009).

The results also show the reluctance of social workers to pass the responsibility of the State on to other private entities of charitable character, meaning social justice is replaced by charity (Barrera-Algarín, Malagón-Bernal, & Sarasola-Sánchez, 2013). They also show the tense situation in Spanish social work between 'accommodating' or 'resisting' austerity (Hyslop, 2018), which, as observed by Wallace and Pease (2011), is stuck in a perpetual crisis of resources and legitimacy. The results are consistent with the global changes arising in social welfare areas in the face of neo-liberalism (Harvey, 2005). This sector has to deal with the rise in poverty while the public sector is weakened, putting at risk the possibility of social services offering welfare to address the impact of the economic crisis ((Dominelli, 2010; Healy, 2008; Lorenz, 2005).

Changes in the characteristics of service users

The two studies (RSSS I and II) identified the *change in the population making demands, the type of demand that is most requested and the most affected groups*: 74.7% of social workers state that the crisis has led to an increase in demand. There are not only more habitual users, but also 'others who have never been to social services before'. About 43.4% of those taking part confirmed these changes as being 'considerable' and only 13.4% claimed that the population making demands 'had not changed'. Regarding the 'type of change', 45% of those interviewed said it corresponds to 'people who used to be middle class', 29% said 'people with no type of financial income' and

26% claimed it was 'younger people'. The impact the financial crisis has had on the impoverishment of the Spanish middle-class, young people and the children (European Commission, 2017; González-Bueno et al., 2012; Save the Children, 2015) is therefore laid bare through empirical research. There is also evidence of family solidarity in the Spanish family model being exhausted (Martinez Virto, 2014) in contrast to other countries with social models such as Scandinavia, in corroboration with other research (Belmonte-Martín & Tufte, 2017).

The most requested *type of demand* in RSSS I (2014) is in the category of 'dependency/elderly' (40.8%) and in 'poverty/exclusion and income security' (40%). The comparative analysis is very interesting as in RSSS II (2015) this order is reversed: 50% of those surveyed said 'poverty/exclusion and income security' was the most requested, while 'dependency/elderly' dropped to 26%. These results coincide with the cuts to benefits in the area of dependency and the fact that in 2014 these could no longer be requested, causing the drop in these figures and its direct effect on the results obtained. Regarding the *groups requiring most attention*, the two studies identified the 'average profile' of the person going to social services as 'female', between '36 and 50', with primary school studies, dependent children, unemployed, without benefits or with an average monthly income of between €300 and €500. This does not mean that they are always the beneficiaries of the benefits requested. However, it does show that it is still mostly women who go to social services to ask for aid, either for themselves or their families.

Applications and social services response

It is quite significant to establish the *reasons why people go to social services*. According to those surveyed, they come in the following order: requesting financial aid; requesting information and guidance; and requesting all types of assistance (RSSS I). In this regard, the comparative analysis is also significant as it shows that 'requesting financial aid' rises 5.6 points, while the 'request for information and orientation' drops 2.7 (RSSS II, 2015).

As expected, these results confirm how the impact of the economic crisis, which began in 2008, has gradually got worse as unemployment benefits for families have dried up. In this sense, the RSSS II study can already demonstrate how the crisis has spread and families have suffered as a result of the neo-liberal policies of the government, as revealed in other research on this matter (Martinez Virto, 2014).

In RSSS II (2015), the 'neglect' is shown in the percentage of requests classified by social workers as necessary which did not lead to benefits or services for the people requesting them, even though they had rights to them. Twenty-four per cent of those surveyed said that they could not determine how many, but 49% estimated that 50% or even more of those requests approved are not covered. Only 6% stated that this situation affected 10% of requests. According to those interviewed, the neglect was greater in 'psychosocial care', 'residential care' and 'legal protection'. In corroboration with other research (Baines et al., 2009; Pentaraki, 2017a), the 'map of neglect' demonstrates the inability of social services in Spain to respond to the general public due to budget restrictions as a result of the austerity measures, together with the abandonment of government functions in satisfying the needs of the users. When the social workers were asked the reason for this neglect, 49% regarded it as a question of finance, 17% blamed the lack of political interest in responding to the demands of the general public, 9% indicated the delays in evaluating the cases, and 7% mentioned the lack of coordination between the administrations as the main reason behind these shortcomings.

Quality of services provided

Regarding the quality of attention, those surveyed considered that it has significantly worsened since the start of the economic crisis (2009–2012) in the areas of 'dependence for the elderly', 'poverty/exclusion and income security' and 'dependency/disability' (RSSS I, 2014). These data reiterate the impact the cuts have had on the dependency system in Spain, as already commented above. The comparative analysis with the second study (RSSS II, 2015) confirms these results, but the deterioration of the quality of attention in 'poverty/social exclusion', followed by 'dependency/the elderly', are even more marked and 'care for females' appears for the first time. Once again, the inability of the social service to respond to the increase in poverty since 2013 and dependency with benefits already removed is demonstrated. As a result, the pressure austerity measures put on women as a group in the restructuring of the family in Spain is also evidenced.

The future of social services

Regarding the *future of social services*, 61% of those surveyed have a pessimistic view. The major concerns are the lack of funding for the system, especially regarding 'dependency' and 'childcare' (54%), and the organisational challenges in the areas of 'information', 'family support', 'psychosocial care' and 'prevention and social inclusion' (37%) (RSSS II).

The *challenges* to be faced in the future are these: ensuring that social services remain public (34%); overcoming problems of funding (20%); improving the quality of service (11%); and adapting to new requirements (10%) (RSSS II, 2015).

In both studies, social workers were asked about their *expectations for the own future*. Twenty-seven per cent of those surveyed in RSSS I (2014) were pessimistic, and this number increased to 38% in RSSS II (2015). The results reflect a certain feeling of demoralisation and burnout, with significant differences depending on age: 55% of social workers under 29 think that their work situation will improve over the next few years, while those over 46 are much more negative, with 63% thinking the opposite.

Government management of the economic crisis

When specifically asked about their *opinion on how the economic crisis has been managed*, an overwhelming 90% of social workers believe that the government has not taken into account the impact its cuts have had on social services. The research goal of finding out, through the social workers within the social services system, whether the impact of neo-liberalism and the austerity measures that followed it affected the general public is here clearly confirmed. This is particularly alarming when taking into account that those surveyed claimed that only 14% of actions implemented in the system are evaluated (RSSS II, 2015), which proves that the neo-liberal policies do not include a social analysis of the magnitude of the crisis. Seventy-four per cent of those surveyed believe that the government has not used all available resources to avoid the violation of human rights of its citizens, as established in the United Nations report (2011) which obliges the government to avoid social inequality, poverty and social exclusion. Seventy-one per cent know, in their professional environment, people who have lost access to social services as a result of the crisis. Eighty-eight per cent know people who have lost benefits and services, and 80% are aware of cases in which the increase of co-payments for services has had a very negative effect. In this regard, the RSSS II (2015) notes that 90% of social workers consider that the implementation of austerity measures violates the human rights of some people and 73% believe that these measures have a greater effect on the more vulnerable, especially children (according to 90% of social workers) and women (78%). Through these results, we can observe the social workers' rejection of neo-liberal reforms (Strier & Feldman, 2017), expressed particularly in the restructure of public services, opposition to the culture of privatisation that shifts public services to the finance market, and against the loss of social rights by the general public.

These results raise two important questions. Firstly, the 'proletarianisation' of social work, common in other countries (Pentaraki, 2017b) with a situation of austerity shared between workers and users: 'The concept of shared reality refers to situations in which the social worker helps the service user to deal with the adverse consequences of a socio-economic reality that they themselves also experience' (Pentaraki, 2017a, p. 7).

Secondly, the role of the social services in Spain in defending the rights of the public is expressed in both studies not only in the workplace as a 'resilient discourse in daily activity' as Hyslop (2018) would say, or true to Pentaraki's acts of micro-resistance (2017a), or founded on 'work ethics' (Banks, 2009; Colley, 2012); rather it spreads to the militant practice of social work in Spain.

The narrative of workers' impotence and resignation regarding social activism in the Spanish social service can be traced both individually and to the activities of the GCSW between 2011 and 2017, legitimated in the research reports, as it will be explained below. The organisation promoted and participated in the *Orange Tide*[5] shoulder to shoulder *with* the public. They carried out information campaigns, intensified their presence in the media, complained about the privatisation of social services[6] and defended public social services.[7] In this sense, social work in Spain does not have enough with simply implementing measures, but aspires to recover its main role in the design of social policies. It desires to recover that mediation role between the state and the public (Feldman, Strier, & Koreh, 2017; Lorenz, 2017; Strier & Feldman, 2017) that neo-liberalism took away from it. This can be observed, amongst other actions, in the meeting in 2015 between the GCSW and the Minister for Health, Social Services and Equality, where the GCSW demanded its presence in each and every advisory body related to social intervention, or that a State Pact is agreed defining social services as a fundamental citizens' right, guaranteed in the Constitution.[8] The GCSW also dedicated several issues of their journal *Servicios sociales y Política social* to the crisis, its impact and how social services could respond to the general public's problems in a neo-liberal climate.[9] They complained about the consequences of the austerity policies before the European Parliament, with social workers travelling to Brussels accompanied by users of the welfare system who had been victims of the cuts. They captured this whole experience in the documentary *Derechos sociales por la Dignidad* (Pi, Pecot, & Albarrán, 2015)[10] as a form of protest.

This critical and militant stance is evident in the results of the RSSS II (2015) study, where the vast majority of social workers (92%) recognise that they are aware of the social service demonstrations in Spain (*the Orange tide*) and almost half (47%) have actively participated in them. In addition, 69% view these actions by the GCSW favourably given they protest against government neo-liberalism, defend the dignity of the public and put social rights of the citizens before market interests (Lima, 2015b).

Finally, both studies (RSSS I and II) highlighted the tension in social welfare towards neo-liberalism (Baines et al., 2009; Dominelli, 1999, 2010; Ferguson, 2008; Ferguson et al., 2005; Strier & Feldman, 2017; Wallace & Pease, 2011) and the increase in ethical dilemmas for workers (Banks, 2009; Colley, 2012) in corroboration with Spanish research (Abad Miguélez & Martín Aranaga, 2015; Pastor-Seller & Sanchez, 2014). In similar terms, both studies draw attention to the criticism towards the break-up of social services, the rejection of privatisation and the defence of public social services.

Conclusions

The RSSS I (2014) and II (2015) studies highlight the precarious working conditions of social workers in Spain, the break-up of the public social welfare system, its progressive privatisation, the shortage of financial and human resources, and the deterioration in the quality of the services. All this is at the time when demand is highest, especially regarding 'financial aid' for middle-class families, people with no type of income and groups that are particularly vulnerable to austerity measures: the elderly, young people, women and children.

The results also show how families are struggling to cope after the restructuring of the family, neglect of welfare users and the inability of the social welfare system to satisfy the needs of the general public, in agreement with other research (Baines et al., 2009; Pentaraki, 2017a).

At the same time, they reveal Spanish social workers' awareness of government neo-liberalism and austerity and their predominant stance against them. The results confirm that workers have become aware of the effect neo-liberalism has on the public directly connected to the loss of democratic guarantees (Black, 2014; Hayes, 2017; Pastor-Seller, 2017) and, in the words of Lorenz (2017), a 'relational community'. The studies found that there was discomfort among workers between fulfilling their ethical commitment towards the general public, and satisfying a welfare-oriented social service and containing public outrage (Davies, 2016; Lorenz, 2016, 2017).

The way social welfare has faced up to neo-liberalism and austerity in Spain is not just with theoretical reports. As this empirical research shows, it is mostly based on critical professional practice and actions of militant activism in almost half of the Spanish social workers (47%). In addition, 69% approved the protest initiatives and socio-political commitment led by the GCSW, the administrative body that represents them.

Social workers in Spain have stood side-by-side with the general public, empowering the most vulnerable (Cree, 2013; Ferguson, 2013), restoring their dignity in the face of neo-liberal ideals and personal shortcomings (Hyslop, 2018) and defended their legitimacy to demand their social rights.

The research highlights that the concern of social workers as they come to terms with the breakdown of the welfare agreement (Fairclough & Graham, 2002) and the violation of citizens' human rights as a result of government neo-liberalism (Wronka, 2014) have become an opportunity of transformation for social work in Spain. Social workers are testing new professional approaches that are more progressive than the past individual care, such as community social work and radical social work, or anti-oppressive social work which also identifies with other parts of the world such as New Zealand (Hyslop, 2018), Greece (Karagkounis, 2017; Pentaraki, 2017a), Greece, Spain and Portugal (Ioakimidis, Santos, & Herrero, 2014), Israel (Strier & Binyamin, 2014), Ireland and Italy (Garrett & Bertotti, 2017).

The research results demonstrate the militant commitment of social workers at an individual level and the legitimation of the actions of their professional organisation, the GCSW, in their rejection of dominant discourses about the 'austerity common sense' (Pentaraki, 2018) and turning political their actions once more. Critical social work in Spain, in addition, presents political propositions to confront neo-liberalism. Probably, the main one is to guarantee citizens' social rights in the Spanish Constitution itself (which would entail its modification) through the strengthening of the public system of social services. Towards this goal, the GCSW is preparing a restructure of this system that will be presented before the end of 2018. Its main characteristics, amongst others, are enough budgets to meet the demand, to decrease the ratio of citizens covered by one social worker, universal basic income for each citizen, the figure of the social worker as the coordinating professional for the service users, etc.

It can be concluded, based on the results of the research detailed above, that the political social commitment of most social workers, the participation of half of the Spanish social workers in protests to defend social services and citizens' rights, and the approval of actions carried out by the administrative organisation, the GCSW, reflect a critical and militant social worker in Spain. This belongs to a process that has already been dubbed a 'new concept of social work in southern Europe' (Ioakimidis et al., 2014).

Notes

1. Press Release 27 July 2017. *Labour Force Survey*. Institute of Statistics. Retrieved from http://www.ine.es/daco/daco42/daco4211/epa0217.pdf.
2. European Commission (EC), European Central Bank (ECB) and International Monetary Fund (IMF).
3. The Spanish GCSW is an organisation comprising the professional bodies of social workers in Spain, representing more than 30,000 social workers.

   Expand in Press Release 21 November 2013: Social workers condemn the increase in demand for emergency social benefits while funding is cut. Retrieved from https://www.cgtrabajosocial.es/comunicaciones/los-y-las-trabajadoras-sociales-denuncian-el-aumento-de-la-demanda-de-ayudas-de-emergencia-social-mientras-se-recorta-la-financiacion/65/view.
4. The response was inferior to what was initially expected, probably due to the excessive caseload of the interviewees, as shown in the own research findings, where social workers report working beyond their office hours to meet the increasing demand.

5. After the *Movimiento de los indignados* (Taking to the streets) (15-M, 2011), other workers of different public social service systems in Spain started to protest along with the population, as equals, protesting against the austerity policies and defending public services. Each professional sector was assigned a colour, with social work being orange.

6. See release 4 April 2013: Social workers protest that the local administration reform will lead to the privatisation of primary care social services. Retrieved from http://www.cgtrabajosocial.com/comunicaciones/los-trabajadores-sociales-denuncian-que-la-reforma-de-la-administracion-local-permitira-privatizar-los-servicios-sociales-de-atencion-primaria/31/view.

7. Press Release 19 February 2013: Social workers demand that Congress, in the State of the Nation debate, commits to maintaining the public social welfare system. Retrieved from http://www.cgtrabajosocial.com/comunicaciones/los-trabajadores-sociales-exigen-que-el-congreso-en-el-debate-del-estado-de-la-nacion-se-comprometa-a-mantener-el-sistema-publico-de-servicios-sociales/20/view.

8. Press Release 3 March 2015: The General Council of Social Work meets with the minister Alfonso Alonso. Retrieved from https://www.cgtrabajosocial.es/noticias/el-consejo-general-del-trabajo-social-se-reune-con-el-ministro-alfonso-alonso/2645/view.

9. http://www.serviciossocialesypoliticasocial.com/. Particularly numbers 96, 103, 106, 108, 113.

10. Presented by Streaming, by the GCSW and the El Diario.es newspaper on 17 March 2015, followed by a very interesting debate. Retrieved from https://www.youtube.com/watch?v=d3IFUeKy0rl.

Disclosure statement

No potential conflict of interest was reported by the authors.

ORCID

Enrique Pastor Seller http://orcid.org/0000-0001-8693-5138

References

Abad Miguélez, D., & Martín Aranaga, I. M. (2013). El Trabajo Social ante la crisis. Nuevos retos para el ejercicio profesional de los y las trabajadoras sociales. *Cuadernos de Trabajo Social, 28*(2), 175–185.

Antentas, J. M. (2017). Spain: from the *indignados* rebellion to regime crisis (2011–2016). *Labor History, 58*(1), 106–131. doi:10.1080/0023656X.2016.1239875

Aronson, J., & Sammon, S. (2000). Practice amid social service cuts: Working with the contradictions of 'small victories'. *Canadian Social Work Review, 17*(2), 167–187.

Baines, D., MacKenzie Davis, J., & Saini, M. (2009). Wages, working conditions, and restructuring in Ontario's social work profession. *Canadian Social Work, 26*(1), 59–72.

Banks, S. (2009). From professional ethics to ethics in professional life: Implications for learning, teaching and study. *Ethics and Social Welfare, 3*(1), 55–63.

Barrera-Algarín, E., Malagón-Bernal, J. L., & Sarasola-Sánchez, J. L. (2013). La deconstrucción del Estado de Bienestar: Cambios en el ejercicio profesional de los trabajadores sociales y aumento del voluntariado social. *Cuadernos de Trabajo Social, 26*(1), 115–126.

Belmonte-Martín, I., & Tufte, G. C. (2017). Spain's and Norway's welfare regimes compared: An outcome-based evaluation of how welfare regimes influence the risk of poverty and social exclusion. *Journal of Powerty, 21*(4), 372–387. doi:10.1080/10875549.2016.1204647

Black, W. K. (2014). Spain rains on the austerity victory parade. *Challenge, 57*(2), 42–53. doi:10.2753/0577-5132570203

Campanini, A. (2017). Los trabajadores sociales y la práctica política en Italia. In E. Pastor-Seller (Ed.), *Sistemas y políticas de bienestar, una perspectiva internacional* (pp. 29–44). Madrid: Dykinson.

Colley, H. (2012). Not learning in the workplace: Austerity and the shattering of illusions in public service work. *Journal of Workplace Learning, 24*(5), 317–337.

Council of the Judiciary. (2013, April 25). *El CGPJ informa.* Retrieved from file:///C:/Users/Carmen/Downloads/EL%20CGPJ%20INFORMA%20(Nota%20Pleno%2025-4-2013).pdf

Cree, V. (2013). New practices of empowerment. In M. Gray & S. A. Webb (Eds.), *The new politics of social work* (pp. 145–158). Basingstoke: Palgrave MacMillan.

Davies, W. (2016). Neoliberalismo 3.0. *New Left Review, 101,* 129–143.

De La Red Vega, N. (1993). *Aproximaciones al Trabajo social.* Madrid: Siglo XXI.

Deusdad, B. A., Comas-d'Argemir, D., & Dziegielewski, S. F. (2016). Restructuring long-term care in Spain: The impact of the economic crisis on social policies and social work practice. *Journal of Social Service Research, 42*(2), 246–262. doi:10.1080/01488376.2015.1129013

Dominelli, L. (1999). Neo-liberalism, social exclusion and welfare clients in a global economy. *International Journal of Social Welfare, 8*(1), 14–22. doi:10.1111/1468-2397.00058

Dominelli, L. (2010). *Social work in a globalizing world.* Cambridge: Polity Press.

European Commission. (2017). *Commission staff working document. Country report Spain 2017.* Retrieved from http://www.obcp.es/index.php/mod.documentos/mem.descargar/fichero.documentos_2017-european-semester-country-report-spain-en_51b2d58d232E23pdf/chk.07600d6cf773cee15dbecb3552c8329f

Fairclough, N., & Graham, P. (2002). Marx as a critical discourse analyst: The genesis of a critical method and its relevance to the critique of global capital. *Estudios de Sociolingüística, 3*(1), 185–229.

Feldman, G., Strier, R., & Koreh, M. (2017). Liquid advocacy: Social welfare advocacy in neoliberal times. *International Journal of Social Welfare, 26*(3), 254–262.

Ferguson, H. (2013). Critical best practice. In M. Gray & S. A. Webb (Eds.), *The new politics of social work* (pp. 116–127). Basingstoke: Palgrave MacMillan.

Ferguson, I. (2008). *Reclaiming social work: Challenging neoliberalism and promoting social justice.* London: Sage.

Ferguson, I., Lavalette, M., & Whitmore, E. (Eds.). (2005). *Globalisation, global justice and social work.* London: Routledge.

FOESSA & Cáritas. (2013). *Desigualdad y derechos sociales. Análisis y perspectivas.* Madrid: Autor. Retrieved from http://www.caritas.es/imagesrepository/CapitulosPublicaciones/4551/Desigualdad20y20derechos20sociales.20VersiC3B3n%20digital.pdf

Garrett, P. M., & Bertotti, T. F. (2017). Social work and the politics of 'austerity': Ireland and Italy. *European Journal of Social Work, 20*(1), 29–41. doi:10.1080/13691457.2016.1185698

GCSW, Pi, V. (Producer), Pecot, G., & Albarrán, J. (Director). (2015). *Derechos sociales por la dignidad.* Spain. Retrieved from https://www.youtube.com/watch?v=a9poEy8RuQE

Gerbaudo, P. (2017). The indignant citizen: Anti-austerity movements in southern Europe and the anti-oligarchic reclaiming of citizenship. *Social Movement Studies, 16*(1), 36–50. doi:10.1080/14742837.2016.1194749

González-Bueno, G., Bello, A., & Arias, M. (2012). *La infancia en España: El impacto de la crisis en los niños.* Madrid: UNICEF.

Harvey, D. (2005). *A brief history of neoliberalism.* New York: Oxford.

Hayes, G. (2017). Regimes of austerity. *Social Movement Studies, 16*(1), 21–35. doi:10.1080/14742837.2016.1252669

Healy, L. (2008). *International social work: Professional action in an interdependent world* (2nd ed.). New York, NY: Oxford University Press.

Hyslop, I. (2018). Neoliberalism and social work identity. *European Journal of Social Work, 21,* 20–31. doi:10.1080/13691457.2016.1255927

Ioakimidis, V., Santos, C. C., & Herrero, I. M. (2014). Reconceptualizing social work in times of crisis: An examination of the cases of Greece, Spain and Portugal. *International Social Work, 57*(4), 285–300.

Karagkounis, V. (2017). Social work in Greece in the time of austerity: Challenges and prospects. *European Journal of Social Work, 20*(5), 651–665. doi:10.1080/13691457.2016.1255593

Kelsey, D., Mueller, F., Whittle, A., & Khosranivinlk, M. (2016). Financial crisis and austerity: Interdisciplinary concerns in critical discourse studies. *Critical Discourse Studies, 13*(1), 1–19. doi:10.1080/17405904.2015.1074600

Leon, M., & Pavolini, E. (2014). 'Social investment' or back to 'familism': The impact of the economic crisis on family and care policies in Italy and Spain. *South European Society and Politics, 19*(4), 353–369. doi:10.1080/13608746.2014.948603

Lima, A. (Coord.) (2014). *I report on social services in Spain.* Madrid: General council of social work from Spain.

Lima, A. (Coord.) (2015a). *II report on social services in Spain.* Madrid: General council of social work from Spain.

Lima, A. (2015b). Fighting against the fallacy: Social workers know that social development is not incompatible with economic development. *Servicios sociales y Política social, 32*(108), 21–44.

Lorenz, W. (2005). Social work and a new social order-challenging neo-liberalism's erosion of solidarity. *Social Work & Society, 3*(1), 93–101.

Lorenz, W. (2014). Is history repeating itself? Reinventing social work's role in ensuring social solidarity under conditions of globalisation. In T. Harrikari, P.-L. Rauhala, & E. Virokannas (Eds.), *Social change and social work. The changing societal conditions of social work in time and place* (pp. 15–29). Farnham: Ashgate.

Lorenz, W. (2016). Rediscovering the social question. *European Journal of Social Work, 19*(6), 4–17. doi:10.1080/13691457. 2015.1082984

Lorenz, W. (2017). European policy developments and their impact on social work. *European Journal of Social Work, 20*(1), 17–28. doi:10.1080/13691457.2016.1185707

Martínez Virto. (2014). *Crisis en familia: síntomas de agotamiento de la solidaridad familiar. VII Informe sobre exclusión y desarrollo social en España.* Madrid: FOESSA & Cáritas.

Matsaganis, M., & Leventi, C. (2014). The distributional impact of austerity and the recession in Southern Europe. *South European Society and Politics, 19*(3), 393–412. doi:10.1080/13608746.2014.947700

Medir, L., Pano, E., Viñas, A., & Magre, J. (2017). Dealing with austerity: A case of local resilience in Southern Europe. *Local Government Studies, 43*(4), 621–644. doi:10.1080/03003930.2017.1310101

Nofre, J. (2013). Cartografías de la indignación (2011–12). *Ar@cne, revista electrónica de recursos en internet sobre geografía y ciencias sociales, 169.* Retrieved from http://www.ub.edu/geocrit/aracne/aracne-169.htm

OECD. (2015). *Government at a Glance 2015.* Paris: Author. Retrieved from https://doi.org/10.1787/gov_glance-2015-en

Oxfam. (2016). *An economy for the 1%. How privilege and power in the economy drive extreme inequality and how this can be stopped.* Retrieved from https://www.oxfam.org/sites/www.oxfam.org/files/file_attachments/bp210-economy-one-percent-tax-havens-180116-en_0.pdf

Pastor-Seller, E. (2017). Mechanisms for participation in the public system of social services in Spain: Opportunities for the development of social work with citizenist approach. *European Journal of Social Work, 20*(3), 441–458. doi:10.1080/ 13691457.2017.1283588

Pastor-Seller, E., & Sanchez, M. (2014). Analysis and impact of the economic crisis and regulatory changes in the needs and benefits system municipal social services: Analysis case Spain. *Revista de Cercetare si Interventie Sociala, 47,* 7–31.

Pentaraki, M. (2013). If we do not cut spending, we well end up like Greece: Challenging consent to austerity through social work action. *Critical Social Policy, 33*(4), 700–711. doi:10.1177/0261018313489941

Pentaraki, M. (2017a). Practising social work in a context of austerity: Experiences of public sector social workers in Greece. *European Journal of Social Work.* Latest articles, 1–12. doi:10.1080/13691457.2017.1369396

Pentaraki, M. (2017b). 'I am in a constant state of insecurity trying to make ends meet, like our service users': Shared austerity reality between social workers and service users – Towards a preliminary conceptualisation. *The British Journal of Social Work, 47*(4), 1245–1261. doi:10.1093/bjsw/bcw099

Pentaraki, M. (2018), Austerity common sense and contested understandings of the austerity measures within a leadership of a professional association of social workers. *European Journal of Social Work.* Latest Articles. doi:10.1080/ 13691457.2018.1435507

Salmon, K. (2017). A decade of lost growth: Economic policy in Spain through the great recession. *South European Society and Politics, 22*(2), 239–260. doi:10.1080/13608746.2017.1301065

Saltkjel, T. (2017). Welfare resources and social risks in times of social and economic change: A multilevel study of material deprivation in European countries. *European Journal of Social Work.* Latest Articles. doi:10.1080/13691457.2017. 1320525

Save the Children. (2015). *Barómetro de la infancia. Pobreza.* Retrieved from https://www.savethechildren.es/barometro-infancia/pobreza-relativa

Standing, G. (2011). *The precariat: The new dangerous class.* London: BloomsburyAcademic.

Steinebach, Y., & Knill, C. (2017). Social policy in hard times: Crisis-coping strategies in Europe from 1976 to 2013. *International Journal of Public Administration, 40*(14), 1164–1174. doi:10.1080/01900692.2017.1317802

Strier, R., & Binyamin, S. (2014). El trabajo social en Israel, situación actual y desafíos. In E. Pastor-Seller & M. A. Martínez Román (Coords.), *Trabajo social en el siglo XXI: una perspectiva internacional comparada* (pp. 233–248). Madrid: Grupo 5.

Strier, R., & Feldman, G. (2017). Reengineering social work's political passion: Policy practice and neo-liberalism. *The British Journal of Social Work.* doi:10.1093/bjsw/bcx061

United Nations. (2011, March 17). *Report of the independent expert on the question of human rights and extreme poverty, Magdalena Sepúlveda Carmona.* A/HRC/17/34, 4–8. Retrieved from http://www2.ohchr.org/english/bodies/hrcouncil/ docs/17session/A-HRC-17-34.pdf

Villoría, M. (2015). Corruption in Spain. *Servicios sociales y Política social, 32*(108), 77–100.

Wallace, J., & Pease, B. (2011). Neoliberalism and Australian social work: Accommodation or resistance? *Journal of Social Work, 11*(2), 132–142. doi:10.1177/1468017310387318

Wronka, J. (2014). Human rights as the bedrock of social justice: Implications for advanced generalist practice. In K. Libal, S. Megan Berthold, R. Thomas, & L. Healy (Eds.), *Advancing human rights in social work education* (pp. 19–38). Alexandria, VA: Council of Social Work Education Press.

The neoliberal turn in Chilean social work: frontline struggles against individualism and fragmentation

El giro neoliberal en el trabajo social chileno: luchas contra el individualismo y la fragmentación desde la primera línea de intervención

Gianinna Muñoz Arce

ABSTRACT

In Chile, the right-wing dictatorship (1973–1990) implemented the first neoliberal 'experiment' in the world, affecting the development of social work in a traumatic way. More than 40 years after the coup, the inheritance from the dictatorship appears to still be blocking discussion and implementation of critical perspectives in social work. The inception of the Social Protection System in 2000 has contributed to reinforcing depoliticised and individually oriented approaches of social workers' interventions. However, practices of resistance to this apparent hegemonic order can also be detected and identified within social work. Drawing upon preliminary findings of an exploratory-sequential study, this article analyses the way in which neoliberal ideology has impacted contemporary Chilean social work and illuminates strategies employed by many in the profession to defy such constraining rationality.

RESUMEN

Durante la dictadura cívico-militar que tuvo lugar en Chile entre 1973 y 1990 se implementó el primer 'experimento' neoliberal en el mundo, el cual afectó de manera traumática el desarrollo del trabajo social. Más de 40 años después del Golpe de Estado, las herencias de la dictadura aun interfieren en la discusión e implementación de perspectivas críticas en trabajo social. Esto se refleja, por ejemplo, en los enfoques de intervención individualistas y despolitizados que ejecutan trabajadoras/es sociales en el marco del Sistema de Protección Social que comenzó a implementarse a partir del 2000. A pesar de ello, es posible detectar ciertos actos de resistencia que los/as trabajadores/as sociales ejercen frente a esta racionalidad hegemónica. Basándose en los resultados preliminares de un estudio exploratorio-secuencial sobre prácticas interprofesionales, este artículo analiza las maneras en las cuales el ethos neoliberal ha impactado al trabajo social chileno en el contexto contemporáneo e identifica estrategias empleadas por los/as trabajadores/as sociales para desafiar dicha racionalidad.

Introduction

Neoliberalisation has been defined by Harvey (2005) as a variant of liberal thought that exacerbates economic liberalisation through market freedom, deregulation and privatisation. Its emphasis on competition and individual responsibility has resulted in its installation as a hegemonic discourse on a global scale (Eagleton-Pierce, 2016). The hegemonic nature of neoliberalism lies in its capacity to penetrate not only the economic but also the cultural and social domains of life by colonising the common-sense way people interpret, live in and understand the world, operating as an ethic in itself (Boltanski & Chiapello, 2005; Butler, Gambetti, & Sabsai, 2016; Harvey, 2005; Venugopal, 2015).

The impacts of neoliberalism on social work have been studied worldwide in recent decades. In more developed countries, social work has been subjugated by the discourse of managerialism, an approach that, in the context of a declination of welfare provision, is based upon the assumption that better management will resolve a wide range of economic and social problems. Top-down interventions, emphasis on quantifiable measures, preponderance of evidence-based approaches, lack of engagement with social theory as well as a dominant emphasis on business thinking and technocratic skills, are some of the features of managerialism commonly identified in social work (Ferguson & Lavalette, 2006; Garrett, 2013; Rogowski, 2013; Thompson & Wadley, 2016, among others).

Neoliberalism has impacted Latin American social work in a different way. As welfare states have never existed in most Latin American countries, we are obviously not experiencing its progressive dismantling like our European colleagues. In Latin America, and especially in Chile, neoliberalism was imposed violently in the 1980s under the civic-military dictatorship lead by Augusto Pinochet (1973–1990), which destroyed the state's role in social policy. Particularly in Chile – perhaps because Pinochet's dictatorship has been defined as the bloodiest and longest dictatorship in Latin America (Amnesty International, 2013; Harvey, 2005; Klein, 2009) – a social trauma experienced by all society, including social workers, has accompanied the imposition of the neoliberal hegemony during the last four decades.

From a critical perspective, however, neoliberalism entails resistance. Neoliberal hegemony is not conceived as a space of oppression while practices of resistance happen outside of neoliberal domains. Neoliberalism and resistance are understood here as two forces dialectically interwoven, mutually imbricated (Moore, 1997). Following such an approach, this article examines how Chilean social work has been hit by the imposition of neoliberalism since the Pinochet era, and identifies, at the same time, some strategies that Chilean social workers have undertaken to counteract such a hegemonic rationale throughout the years. This paper analyses the current stage of social work from a past-present dialectic perspective (Benjamin, 1995; Pappe & Luna, 2001; Ridgway, 2015). This theoretical approach asserts that current events are founded by a 'historical heritage', which implies that clues to understanding the present can be found in the past. Following such an approach, This paper reveals past Chilean social work to find some keys to interpreting professional experiences faced by social workers today.

The first and second sections of the article describe the abrupt changes faced by social work because of the dictatorship and the imposition of the neoliberal model, and the development of the profession in such a context and during the first decade of the post-dictatorial period. To further examine the ongoing expressions of neoliberalism and resistance in Chilean social work, the third section discusses findings from research studying frontline social workers' experiences in implementing the Chilean Social Protection System (SPS), a social policy designed and funded by the World Bank and currently in force. To conclude, an overall analysis of frontline social workers' struggles against the individual and fragmented nature of neoliberal social policies is presented, discussing the relevance of the findings for Chilean and international social work.

Methods

This article discusses findings from a mixed methods research project examining the way in which Chilean social workers undertake interprofessional practices that underpin the implementation of the SPS. The study explores how Chilean social workers deal with neoliberal policy approaches and what strategies they have found to subvert and counteract such approaches in practice. It is an exploratory-sequential study consisting of three stages. This paper draws upon the findings produced in the first and second stages.

As the study has taken a critical historiographic perspective underpinned by the past-present dialectic perspective (Pappe & Luna, 2001; Ridgway, 2015), the first stage of research aimed to reconstruct the recent history of Chilean social work. It consisted of a literature review focusing on academic documents, written testimonies and dissertations produced by social workers since the beginning of Pinochet's authoritarian rule in the 1970s – that is, the beginning of the neoliberal 'experiment' in Chile. Social workers' experiences in implementing social policies and their attempts to resist the neoliberal rationale imposed during the dictatorial and post-dictatorial periods are discussed in this article's first and second sections.

The second stage of research consisted of six focus group interviews with frontline social workers who currently implement diverse social programmes forming the SPS (programmes targeting children, women, older and disabled people living in poverty). The focus groups were performed between January and April 2017 and took between 90 and 120 min each. Each interview consisted of between four and twelve participants, involving a total of 53 social workers. 43 of them were women and 10 were men. The majority of the participants graduated in the 2000s (38 of them). Only eight social workers graduated in the 2010s and seven of them in the 1990s.

The participants were recruited independently, aiming to include social workers implementing the diverse programmes derived from the SPS. Every social worker individually agreed to participate in the study and signed written consent. Data were analysed following the guidelines of thematic analysis proposed by Braun and Clarke (2006). Pseudonyms were used in this article to refer to the respondents. Ethical permission for the study was granted by the author's organisation.

Chilean social work and the neoliberal experiment

With the coup d'état and the establishment of the right-wing military dictatorship in September 1973, a radical transformation of Chilean society took place. The implementation of 'the first neoliberal experiment' (Harvey, 2005) entailed the imposition of a shock doctrine that has been identified as the most radical and abrupt neoliberal reform ever conducted in Latin America (Klein, 2009). Under the cloak of the military regime's law reforms, and following Milton Friedman's proposals, a free market reorientation of the Chilean economy was carried out, led by a group of young Chilean economists trained at the Department of Economics of the University of Chicago – the so-called 'Chicago Boys'. As in other parts of the globe also hit by the neoliberal wave, the Chilean state's functions were reduced, social expenditure was considerably diminished, universal social programmes became targeted and education, housing, pensions and health care services were privatised. The neoliberal shock in Chile was also related to the precarisation of labour, the weakening of labour rights and the prohibition and repression of collective action, which facilitated the process of the accumulation of capital and the re-redistribution to the rich (Harvey, 2005). In fact, the average household income of the richest 20% of the Chilean population was calculated to be 13.8 times higher than the poorest 20% in 1986, which placed Chile as one of the most unequal countries in Latin America (Meller,1996).

What is different in the Chilean neoliberal turn, if compared with other countries, is that the implementation of neoliberalism was produced through the violence of a dictatorship (Garretón, 2012). It resulted not only in drastic economic changes but also sudden and brutal ruptures in the social fabric and civic engagement. The neoliberal turn adopted under the dictatorial rule also aimed to destroy the foundations of the existing party political system, union movements and other social organisations by the fierce repression of all solidarities (Harvey, 2005). Tens of thousands of people who were linked to the political left were detained, tortured, killed or 'disappeared'. The total number of people officially recognised as 'disappeared' or killed between 1973 and 1990 stands at over 3000 and survivors of political imprisonment and/or torture at around 40,000 (Amnesty International, 2013).

The coup and subsequent neoliberal reforms abruptly changed Chilean social workers' situation. Schools of social work were closed during the first years of the dictatorship, due to the ideological nature of social work education at that time (Sepúlveda, 2016). Many social work academics and students were expelled, exiled and some of them are still registered as 'arrested-disappeared' (Chilean Social Workers Association, 2013). Some of the social workers' testimonies compiled by López (2010, pp. 122–123; 153–154) reflect how this abrupt neoliberal turn affected the profession's development:

> The dictatorship changed our lives and all we used to do as social workers, it all finished [...] all we had learnt from critical thinkers such as Paulo Freire, all our hope, all what we had built during the re-conceptualization process [...] the first months were overwhelming. I worked in a community centre, and the military forces set fire to our offices, because we trained community leaders to oppose resistance against Pinochet [...] One day they [the military forces] broke into my house, and I was with my baby [...] It was difficult to resist but the truth is that we were so convinced of what we did that we went ahead, without any doubt.

Social work was stripped of its university status in 1981, and as a consequence, curricula were redesigned in order to remove the theoretical and political content of training courses. New laws were created in the 1980s to restrict the manoeuvrability of social work professional associations (e.g. establishing the voluntary nature of professional affiliation, limiting the legal authority of associations to establish rules of ethical conduct for their members, among others). Social workers also were dispossessed from their positions as directors of state social services, which, before the coup, used to be exclusive occupations for them (Sepúlveda, 2016).

As the state's role was diminished and policy started to target individual users in the 1980s, those social workers who remained working for the state were hired exclusively to conduct surveys that aimed at targeting services users. The casework method became the dominant approach used by social workers at this stage, due to the suspicion that community intervention generated in the context of dictatorship (López, 2010). This turn towards an individual-based perspective in social work, functional to the neoliberal rationale imposed, was reinforced by the annihilation of the intellectual dimension of social work through 'the censorship of bibliography, the literal incineration of social work dissertations and professional manuscripts that were considered undesirable or subversive' (Castañeda & Salamé, 2014, p. 20). Among this so-called subversive literature, as the testimony of López (2010) illustrates, we found Paulo Freire's books on the pedagogy of the oppressed, the theology of liberation and diverse Latin American scholars that had built a critique against conservative and individualist social work and claimed the necessity of reconceptualising the profession from a radical perspective.

Despite the brutal repression of any act of community organising or political activism, the clandestine work of NGOs – funded at that time by international organisations related to the defence of human rights – played a crucial role in promoting community engagement and political action against the dictatorship. In such settings, many social workers clandestinely exerted resistance against Pinochet's rule and struggled for the return of democracy through the strengthening of community organisations and the promotion of popular education. Social workers, risking their lives, also played a key role in denouncing human rights violations during the military regime and working with victims and their families (Saracostti, Reininger, & Parada, 2012). The action of the strong citizen movements, supported by NGOs, allowed the end of the dictatorship through a plebiscite in 1988, which assisted the return of democratic regimes in 1990. The end of 17 years of Pinochet dictatorship was also understood as the beginning of a promising future for social work and proliferated great expectation and hope regarding the possibilities that democracy could offer in terms of reparation of trauma experienced by many in the profession (López, 2010).

Is happiness coming? Social workers in the post-dictatorial era

'Chile, happiness is coming' was the motto of La Concertación, the coalition that ruled the country for twenty years after the Pinochet dictatorship finished. The policy approach of La Concertación governments included a noticeable focus on economic growth and the restoration of a democratic ethos. Post-dictatorial governments took a major turn in social policy by increasing social expenditure and creating an array of new social programmes targeting people living under the poverty line and affected by special conditions (e.g. age, gender, ethnicity, disability). However, despite these and other relevant changes towards a social democratic approach on social policy, the post-dictatorial regimes did not alter the foundations of the neoliberal model imposed by the dictatorship (Garretón, 2012). Even more, some policies imposed during the military regime were accentuated during the post dictatorial era, such as privatisation and commodification of welfare services, targeting of service users and reduction of the state's role to regulate market functioning.

In fact, the maintenance of neoliberal precepts such as privatisation and commodification is expressed, for example, in the outsourcing of state social services that started in 1990. As the coverage of social policy increased considerably, the private sector (including profit and non-profit organisations – mainly NGOs) was involved for the first time in the implementation of state programmes. Since that time, NGOs have started to depend almost exclusively on the state's funds. This change in social services provision is relevant to social work, as the majority of Chilean social workers began to be employed by NGOs to implement social policies in the frontline (Rubilar, 2015; Saracostti et al., 2012).

The maintenance of neoliberal precepts during the post-dictatorial era is also expressed in the deregulation of the education system. Because of the proliferation of private universities during the dictatorship, the number of social workers has increased considerably since the early 1990s. Many schools of social work were created at that time and social work students augmented 356% between 1990 and 1999 (Rolando, Salamanca, & Aliaga, 2010). Each school of social work started to deliver its own curriculum, which also illustrates the way in which the free market ideology operates. The Chilean Social Workers Association took several years to recover from the consequences of repression suffered during the dictatorship, which hindered the possibility for it to have any influence in the design of the social work curriculum delivered by public and private universities at that time (Rubilar, 2015). This has resulted in a diversity of theoretical and ideological frameworks on Chilean social work training courses since the 1990s, implying that conservative, liberal, social democratic and critical perspectives started to co-exist in social workers' discourses in an eclectic and inconsistent way (Saracostti et al., 2012).

Currently there are 32 higher education centres delivering social work degree programmes throughout the country and the number of social workers who graduate each year is estimated at approximately 15,000. Chilean social workers exhibit a rate of employability of 80%, but their wages are comparatively much lower if compared with other university professionals (Rubilar, 2015). The dependence of social workers on NGOs as their main employer in Chile leaves them in a very unstable condition, as NGOs are also in a precarious situation due their almost exclusive dependence on state funds. As the Chilean state provides funds for a fixed term, NGOs cannot assure social workers' wages for longer periods than those initially agreed (generally 12-18 months) (López, 2010).

All the factors described above – deregulated professional training, increasing number of social workers and dependence on a fragile labour system provided by NGOs – have deteriorated Chilean social workers' labour situation. Such a precarisation leaves them in the condition of 'disposable workers' who are responsible for adapting themselves to the social policy market's rules (Harvey, 2005). As analysed in the following section, these factors are hindering the possibilities of social workers to develop a more reflective and critical approach in practice nowadays, which has been exacerbated since the inception of the SPS and the World Bank approach on social policy. Notwithstanding, and at the same time, the post dictatorial era has also brought opportunities for the reconstruction of the social work profession. Thanks to considerable efforts undertaken by academic and professional bodies to resist and reverse the impacts of the dictatorship in social work, university status was recovered in 2006 and the inclusion of social work as a research discipline in the National Commission for Scientific and Technological Research of the Chilean government was achieved in 2010. The latter enabled social workers to apply for state funding to conduct research, something unprecedented in the Chilean context. These improvements have raised expectations of many in the profession about the possibilities of increasing the legitimacy of social work and solidifying its role as an expert voice in social policy discussions (Saracostti et al., 2012).

The social protection system and social workers' struggles today

An important turn in the approach to social policy took place in 2000 when the SPS, designed under the guidelines of the World Bank, was launched by the Chilean state. The SPS, still in force, consists of a network of programmes designed to provide state protection over the life course of families and their individual members from an integrated social services approach. The creation of the SPS has been recognised as 'the new social policy approach' adopted in Chile, as its implementation demands multidisciplinary, cross-sectorial and inter-agency coordination of all existing social pro- grammes in each local area. Despite the novelty of such an approach in the Chilean policy context, neoliberal rhetoric remains untouched. Even more, it appears to have been exacerbated by the World Bank's framework (Campana, 2014). The World Bank approach of social risk has reinforced an idea of poverty understood as an individual problem, citizenship as a legal status and the statés and social workers' roles as protectors of people 'at risk' (Bentura, 2014). It has accen- tuated the principle of targeting adopted during the dictatorship, directing social programmes toward specific sectors of the population – those at risk of remaining outside the markets laws – assuming that risks and mechanisms of protection against them are individual responsibilities. Also, the SPS exhibits a noticeable focus on measurement of individual goals (for each family member) and on conditionality of social rights.

As Butler et al. (2016) state, those practices that designate sectors of the population as people at risk and in need of protection not only negate the capacity of those declared vulnerable to act pol- itically but also expand biopolitical forms of regulation and control. Conditionality of social rights underpinning the SPS is a clear example of that. Such a hegemonic approach of current social policies has situated social workers in a contradictory tension of emancipation and domination, where the desire to promote counter-hegemonic practices is in constant dispute with the logic of control under- lying the SPS. Most social workers, as a consequence, see themselves as hegemonic rhetoric appar- atus, who act as operators, propagandists and classifiers of the objective and material manifestations of subaltern groups. This makes social workers perceive themselves at a crossroads, because although they appear to be aware of the barriers to the promotion of emancipation within the context of the SPS, they also identify their professional limitations to cope with such an approach in practice (Bentura, 2014).

The following social worker's account illustrates such a view:

> I feel sometimes as a cop, controlling families. I would like to do things different with the families I work with. But I do not know how to do it, to be honest. I don't feel I have the tools to do it. I mean, I don't feel able to say, ok, let's organise the families, let's form an organised community able to fight for their rights. I know that this is important, but how? People don't want to participate, they all prefer you to visit them in their houses, everyone in her/his house. They don't even know their own neighbours, there is no collective interest [...] And the SPS goes in the same direction because it demands me to work only with families rather than community groups, watching if families fulfil what is expected to receive their money. It doesn't have any sense.
>
> (Ana, female SW qualified in the 2000s)

The quote above provides several keys to understanding the current stance of Chilean social work. First, we can observe the insecurity regarding professional capacities. The expansion of social work education and its deregulation, as discussed in the previous section, may be related to the perception of incapacity of social workers to address complex issues (Rubilar, 2015). The weakness of the theor- etical dimension in social work training is closely related to the depoliticisation of social worker prac- tices (Bentura, 2014) and loss of professional sense (Saracostti et al., 2012), as reflected in this social worker's account. It also suggests social workers' lack of methodological tools in reverting to fear and distrust in collective action reproduced within the Chilean population since the dictatorial period. Thus, social workers feel abandoned in their efforts to deal with the consequences of neoliberalism and overwhelmed by the magnitude of its rationale (Garrett, 2013). The quote also illustrates how neoliberalism exerts, as Bourdieu (2010) states, a mode of domination based on insecurity, which forces workers into submission, even into the acceptance of exploitation to some extent. It demonstrates the lack of hope exhibited in some of the participants' accounts, reflecting how neoliberal ideology –the SPS's individual-based approach of intervention – expands as a naturalised condition.

On the other hand, the implementation of the SPS demands social workers to establish interprofessional practices – relationships of collaboration with the diverse SPS programmes existing in each local area. However, given the precarious nature of social workers' labour conditions, the possibility of fulfilling such a task becomes difficult:

> There is a great professional turn-over because labour conditions are bad. So you coordinate actions with colleagues from other services, but if they leave you have to start all it over again […] the SPS rests on our responsibility as professionals […] if you have any complaint, there is a queue of colleagues waiting for your job.
>
> (Maria, female SW qualified in the 1990s)

> We don't have enough time to visit seventy-six families a week and also undertake actions of coordination with other programmes […] I know that what I do with these families is not enough, but I do not have time. Also, some families do not want anymore, I mean, they want the subsidy and ok, they do not want to grow further, so … Why is interprofessional practice important?
>
> (Tomas, male SW qualified in the 2000s)

As Boltanski and Chiapello (2005) assert, neoliberal functioning is founded on employee initiative and autonomy in the workplace – a 'freedom' that came at the cost of material and psychological security. With the implementation of the SPS, Chilean social workers are, perhaps more than ever, required to manage their practices on their own, as each social worker has his/her own families to intervene with and his/her own set of goals to be reached with each family member. Also, the idea of 'disposable worker' (Harvey, 2005), which is assumed by some social workers, serves to discipline them and leads to adjustments to their lifestyles and aspirations (Garrett, 2013). In addition, the latter quote also enables us to see how neoliberal rationality appears in a subtle manner, for instance blaming the poor for their poverty. This reflects how expansive the oppressive logic of neoliberalism is: even those exploited populations are able to stigmatise other exploited populations (Butler et al., 2016; Eagleton-Pierce, 2016; Venugopal, 2015).

The depoliticised and individual-based approach promoted by the SPS along with the precarious labour conditions experienced by frontline social workers and the possible insufficiency of theoretical training are interpreted here as some of the barriers to social workers developing a critical approach while implementing the SPS. The passive attitude observed in many social workers' discourses, their fear to introduce changes in practice and the lack of an emancipatory imagination illustrate the way in which neoliberalism – embedded in political violence resulting from the dictatorship – (Garretón, 2012) is still having an impact on Chilean social work. The fragmented and individualistic intervention approach of the SPS reinforces the neoliberal rationale and social workers appear to be trapped in that.

Notwithstanding, the 'new social policy approach' can also be a breeding ground for the emergence of forms of resistance to be exerted by social workers. As Butler et al. (2016) assert, the very recognition of the hegemonic nature of neoliberalism may serve the purpose of envisaging ways of resisting against it. The question that arises here is related to whether social workers can subvert the hegemonic order imposed by the dictatorship first and then reinforced by the SPS. We have found in this research three subtle but significant strategies of resistance exerted by some social workers in the current context of the SPS implementation: the re-activation of collective action, the use of professional discretion and the production of social work knowledge with political purposes. These can be labelled as subtle or minor acts of resistance (Strier & Bershtling, 2016) if compared with other research on resistance (Aronson & Smith, 2010, 2011; Carey & Foster, 2011; Thomas & Davies, 2005, among others); however, they are significant in the Chilean context given the traumatic consequences of the dictatorship in social work, the violent nature of neoliberalism imposition and the lethargy from professional bodies once democratic regimes recovered.

Waking up to collective action

All the social workers who participated in this study identified that the most difficult task for them was to go further with the individualistic approach of intervention provided by the SPS. It has been recognised that distrust and fear among the Chilean population are some of the consequences of the dictatorship (Garretón, 2012), and although social workers are also affected in these terms some of them are able to reverse these phenomena by activating collective powers. The following quote illustrates an isolated but significant experience accounted by a social worker, who understands the SPS's approach as an opportunity to revitalise social workers' collective action:

> [Interprofessional meetings enabled us] to realise that we were not alone. Then a colleague was bitten by a dog while doing a home visit, she did not have a contract so she had to pay the surgery and so on [...] As we already had met each other, organised ourselves and went to the Mayor to demand a contract for all of us and a refund for our colleague [...] The SPS obliged us to work together to connect programmes, but we used the instance not only to do bureaucratic coordination but specially to raise awareness and demand our rights as workers.
>
> (Laura, female SW qualified in the 2000s)

What we can see here is how social workers can use neoliberal orientations, forming interprofessional teams as demanded by the SPS for example, to counteract the very neoliberal rationale by gaining collective power and re-politicising professional action. From such a stand point, these social workers meet the challenge of identifying modes of vulnerability that inform modes of resistance, and, as Butler et al. (2016) claim, to resist those frameworks that aim to minimise forms of political agency. This is related to the self-perception of social workers as agents with power, an approach that can be enhanced by including critical approaches in professional training.

Professional discretion: integrated social services ... for what?

In a similar vein, we found recognition of professional discretion. It is seen as a strategy that enables social workers to counteract neoliberal rationality underlying social policy, which implies that social workers see themselves not as subaltern employees of the state but as actors able to dispute power in the frontiers of the state guidelines (Strier & Bershtling, 2016). Following this perspective, some social workers refer to themselves as 'the designers of social policy in the frontline', as referred by one interviewee. In this act of design or re-design of social policy in the frontline, social workers can recognise themselves as agents able to introduce changes in the intervention process:

> The [SPS's] guidelines indicate that I have to conduct eight sessions of a workshop with women [who have experienced domestic violence] but it is me who defines how the workshop will be approached. What I try to do is to provide support [as indicated], but I specially try to create awareness, showing them that if they work collectively, if they join feminist collectives, they can fight to avoid other women to experience the same, their daughters to experience the same [...] This is not indicated in the guideline, this is my own hallmark, because I believe in that [...] that is my way to raise myself against fragmentation and individualism of the SPS.
>
> (Katy, female SW qualified in the 2000s)

The use of professional discretion as a possibility to exert resistance against the hegemonic discourse of neoliberalism is closely related, as observed in the quote above, to a politicised way of understanding the professional role. Also, the recovery of the collective orientation of practice – which was a core element in the pre-dictatorial period of Chilean social work (Sepúlveda, 2016) – illustrates the envisaging of anti-hegemonic collectives as agents in the process of intervention (López, 2010). This means that the process of social work intervention is comprehended as a field inhabited by entangled power relations, tensions and frictions: in other words, by multiple manifestations of resistance. This is also depicted in the following quote:

> When the SPS started most of us felt afraid, because it implied joint working with other professionals that we never considered before. But now I think it is absolutely important [...] But the question is ... integrated social services, for what? [...] Is the integrated social services approach enough? I don't think so. I am convinced that we need to use coordination with other programmes or services to promote community bonds, to politicise

our practices with families [...] we created a blog to share experiences and a radio broadcasting [actions not requested by the SPS]. I think that is the only thing to fight against the [neoliberal] model, showing that things can be done in another way.

(Oscar, male SW qualified in the 2010s)

We can observe in these actions reported by the interviewees how social workers find alternative strategies to counteract individualism and fragmentation that underlie current social policies. The first motivation lies in the identity of social workers as activists, personally committed to transformation (Bourdieu, 2010; Butler et al., 2016). Then, the capacity of social workers to reflect on their practices and share these reflections emerges as another core element to reconstruct a critical appraisal of their professional role. Closely related to such an idea is the production of social work knowledge and its use for political purposes, as identified by some of the interviewees.

Making social workers' knowledge count

Resistance is always a form of challenging hegemonic power; hence the strategic knowledge of power is necessary for effective resistance. Theory enables social workers to be aware of inconsistencies and contradictions between their belief systems and social practices. As Garrett (2013) claims, in the current neoliberal world social workers need, perhaps more than ever, to comprehend how such a hegemonic order is produced in order to propose theoretically informed critical ways of thinking and working. Consistently with such a view, the third social workers' strategy to defy the constraining rationality of neoliberalism identified in the study relates to the foundation, production and dissemination of social work knowledge. This is a sensitive issue considering that the theoretical content of professional training was censured during the dictatorship and that it was reintegrated in a deregulated way during the post dictatorial era. The denial, rejection or dismissal of theory occurring in the previous periods appears to still have consequences in social workers' practices. However, some efforts to reverse such an anti-intellectual approach are also distinguished by one social worker:

Although it appears to be old-fashioned, I still meet colleagues that say 'one thing is theory and another is practice'. To me, the most basic act of resistance is to recognise that our action is not neutral, that we are not just implementers [...] This is why we started to give a theoretical background to our interprofessional meetings.

(Rosa, female SW qualified in the 2000s)

Another social worker reflects on the relevance of producing and sharing social work knowledge with emancipatory purposes:

We produced a seminar to enhance our capacity for critical reflection, we discussed about decolonial-feminist thought and interrogated our practices from such approaches. What are we doing with families? How coherent are we? Then we asked a university to help research and publish our experiences. Now we have been invited by the Regional Government to present our research to other professional teams and we see it as an opportunity to introduce alternative perspectives to work with families, as as first, to question the si s approach [publicly].

(Katy, female SW qualified in the 2000s)

Social workers' concern about understanding theory, producing own knowledge and disseminating alternative approaches is considered here as a counter-hegemonic act because it implies interpreting the professional position as an opportunity for struggling and engaging, as an activist, with the political purpose of social work. It implies having a broad vision of social transformation, revisiting the public dimension of social work that was so relevant for the profession in the previous stage of the dictatorship (López, 2010). This approach represents a way to reject being subject to the control of the SPS discourses and unsettle dominant power relations imposed by its practice guidelines.

These findings illustrate how some social workers attempt, through the implementation of subtle practices of resistance, to redesign hegemonic frameworks in their frontline interventions. The way in which Chilean social workers exert resistance coheres with the notion of 'deviant social work' proposed by Carey and Foster (2011), as such acts of resistance are individual and silent practices rather than collective and disruptive behaviours. Different from previous research on resistance, however, this study found that Chilean social workers do not develop strategic performances as suggested by Aronson and Smith (2010, 2011) nor use 'discursive resources' (Thomas & Davies, 2005) to resist the demands of the SPS. Chilean social workers do not need to justify their methodological decisions or publicly display an oppositional behaviour because the implementation of the SPS is not supervised or controlled by the Chilean state. Such a deregulation of social workers' practices in Chile, although it represents another expression of the radical nature of Chilean neoliberalism, is also, paradoxically, that which favours social workers' use of discretion in the form of resistance. Notwithstanding, it need to be recognised that such a space for discretion also entails risks, as practices of resistance conducted by the interviewees are still incipient, reactive and generally individual-based. This suggests the need for more reflection and collective engagement with critical perspectives of social work, to avoid pragmatic and non-idealistic versions of resistance that are also a reflection of the individual ethos of neoliberal colonisation (Carey & Foster, 2011).

Concluding remarks

The historical past of Chilean social work, its ruptures and continuities are signs, as Benjamin (1995) claims, that re-emerge as dialectical images in its present. Reiterations and regressions to its past show that social work is pendant and in process, an unfinished project. Historical and political fractures that have shaped Chilean social work over the last four decades emerge today as an inheritance that involves both neoliberal oppression and resistance against it. Such a professional inheritance places limits to social work, but, at the same time, provokes the creation of emancipatory strategies to contest the hegemonic order.

Despite the traumatic professional past and although neoliberalism is far from ending, social workers are called, from a critical perspective, to avoid a comprehension of neoliberalism from an ontological view that assumes it as an immutable phenomenon. This approach is relevant not only for Chilean social work but also for European social workers and other colleagues around the world who are being affected by the politics of managerialism which is subordinating professional agendas in the context of the dismantling of welfare states. As long as social workers understand themselves, as any other workers, as victims of a neoliberal rationale of precarisation and fragmentation, they will be able to recognise themselves as agents that need to think and act collectively, reconstructing confidence and connecting local experiences of resistance with other initiatives and social movements occurring at national and international scales.

Disclosure statement

No potential conflict of interest was reported by the author.

Funding

This work was supported by the National Commission for Scientific and Technological Research of the Chilean Government – CONICYT, Fondecyt Iniciación No.11160538.

References

Amnesty International. (2013). *Chile: 40 years on from Pinochet's coup, impunity must end*. Retrieved from https://www.amnesty.org/en/latest/news/2013/09/chile-years-pinochet-s-coup-impunity-must-end/

Aronson, J., & Smith, K. (2010). Managing restructured social services: Expanding the social? *British Journal of Social Work, 40*, 530–547. doi:10.1093/bjsw/bcp002

Aronson, J., & Smith, K. (2011). Identity work and critical social service management: Balancing on a tightrope? *British Journal of Social Work, 41*, 432–448. doi:10.1093/bjsw/bcq102

Benjamin, W. (1995). *La dialéctica en suspenso. Fragmentos sobre la historia* [Suspended dialectic. Fragments about history]. Lom: Santiago.

Bentura, P. (2014). *Los programas de transferencia de renta condicionadas como gestión neoliberal de la cuestión social* [Conditkional cash transfer programmes as neoliberal managment of social question]. *Servico Social e Sociedade, 117*, 94–121.

Boltanski, L., & Chiapello, E. (2005). *The new spirit of capitalism*. London: Verso.

Bourdieu, P. (2010). *Acts of resistance. Against the new Myths of our time*. Cambridge: Policy Press.

Braun, V., & Clarke, V. (2006). Using thematic analysis in psychology. *Qualitative Research in Psychology, 3*(2), 77–101. doi:abs/10.1191/1478088706qp063oa

Butler, J., Gambetti, Z., & Sabsai, L. (Eds.). (2016). *Vulnerability in resistance*. London: Duke University Press.

Campana, M. (2014). *Desarrollo humano, producción social de la pobreza y gobierno de la pobreza* [Human development, social production of poverty and poverty government]. *Trabajo Social, 16*, 79–89.

Carey, M., & Foster, V. (2011). Introducing 'deviant' social work: Contextualising the limits of radical social work whilst understanding (fragmented) resistance within the social work labour process. *British Journal of Social Work, 41*, 576–593. doi:10.1093/bjsw/bcq148

Castañeda, P., & Salamé, M. (2014). *Trabajo social chileno y dictadura militar* [Chilean social work and military dictatorship]. *Rumbo, 9*, 8–25.

Chilean Social Workers Association. (2013). *Trabajadores sociales detenidos desaparecidos*. Retrieved from http://www.trabajadoressociales.cl/provinstgo/actgremial27.php

Eagleton-Pierce, M. (2016). *Neoliberalism: Key concepts*. London: Routledge.

Ferguson, I., & Lavalette, M. (2006). Globalization and global justice. Towards a social work of resistance. *International Social Work, 49*(3), 309–318.

Garretón, M. (2012). *Neoliberalismo corregido y progresismo limitado: los gobiernos de la Concertación en Chile 1990–2010* [Amended neoliberalism and limited progressiveness: La Concertación governments in Chile 1990–2010]. Santiago: Clacso.

Garrett, P. M. (2013). *Social work and social theory. Making connections*. Bristol: The Policy Press.

Harvey, D. (2005). *A brief history of neoliberalism*. Oxford: Oxford University Press.

Klein, N. (2009). *The shock doctrine: The rise of disaster capitalism*. Toronto: Vintage Canada.

López, T. (2010). *El camino recorrido* [The way traveled]. Santiago: Libros de Mentira.

Meller, P. (1996). *Pobreza y distribución del ingreso en Chile* [Poverty and income distribution in Chile] (Working paper No. 32). Santiago: Cepal.

Moore, D. S. (1997). Remapping resistance: Ground for struggle and the politics of place. In S. Pile & M. Keith (Eds.), *Geographies of resistance* (pp. 87–106). New York: Routledge.

Pappe, S., & Luna, M. (2001). *Historiografía crítica: una reflexión teórica* [Critical historiography: A theoretical reflection]. Mexico: F.D.: Universidad Autónoma Metropolitana.

Ridgway, A. (2015). The past-present dialectic: A new methodological tool for seeing the historical dynamic in cultural historical research. In M. Fleer & A. Ridgway (Eds.), *Visual methodologies and digital tools for researching with young children* (pp. 55–72). Dordrecht: Springer.

Rogowski, S. (2013). *Critical social work with children and families. Theory, context and practice*. Bristol: The Policy Press.

Rolando, R., Salamanca, J., & Aliaga, M. (2010). *Evolución de la Matrícula Educación Superior de Chile 1990–2009* [Evolution of higher education enrolment in Chile 1990–2009] (Working paper No. 11). Santiago: Ministry of Education.

Rubilar, G. (2015). *Trabajo social e investigación social* [Social work and social research] (*Unpublished doctoral dissertation*). Universidad Complutense de Madrid, Spain.

Saracostti, M., Reininger, T., & Parada, H. (2012). Social work in Latin America. In K. Lyons, T. Hokenstad, M. Pawar, N. Huegler, & N. Hall (Eds.), *The Sage handbook of international social work* (pp. 466–480). London: Sage.

Sepúlveda, L. (2016). *Algunas reflexiones acerca del ejercicio profesional del trabajo social durante la dictadura militar* [Some reflections about social work during the military dictatorship]. In P. Vidal (Ed.), *Trabajo social en Chile: un siglo de trayectoria* (pp. 141–154). Santiago: Ril.

Strier, R., & Bershtling, O. (2016). Professional resistance in social work: Counterpractice assemblages. *Social Work, 61*(2), 111–118. doi:10.1093/sw/sww010

Thomas, R., & Davies, A. (2005). Theorizing the micro-politics of resistance: New public management and managerial identities in the UK public services. *Organization Studies, 26*(5), 683–706. doi:10.1177/0170840605051821

Thompson, L. J., & Wadley, D. A. (2016). Countering globalisation and managerialism: Relationist ethics in social work. *International Social Work.* Advance online publication. doi:10.1177/0020872816655867

Venugopal, R. (2015). Neoliberalism as concept. *Economy and Society, 44*(2), 165–187. doi:10.1080/03085147.2015.1013356

Social workers: a new precariat? Precarity conditions of mental health social workers working in the non-profit sector in Greece

Κοινωνικοί Λειτουργοί: Ένα νέο πρεκαριάτο? Οι συνθήκες επισφάλειας για τις/τους επαγγελματίες κοινωνικές/κούς λειτουργούς ψυχικής υγείας που εργάζονται στον μη κερδοσκοπικό τομέα στην Ελλάδα

Maria Pentaraki and Konstantina Dionysopoulou

ABSTRACT

Traditionally, in western countries, the social work profession primarily has come into contact with issues of precarity through the lives of service users. This paper introduces precarity in the social work scholarly literature as a feature of social workers' professional and personal lives. It draws from the findings of a qualitative small study of mental health social workers working in the non-profit sector in Greece. The findings reflect a picture of social workers experiencing precarious conditions as they have become part of the growing phenomenon of the working poor, surviving by loans, experiencing housing insecurity, reproductive insecurity, fuel poverty and unable to pay for their commuting expenses to and from work. Furthermore, the paper maintains that the expansion of the conditions of precarity to university-educated professionals, such as social workers, needs to be understood within an International Political Economy (IPE) perspective in order neoliberal capitalism which brings rising levels of inequalities to become a focus of intervention.

Περίληψη

Παραδοσιακά, ο κλάδος της κοινωνικής εργασίας έχει ασχοληθεί με το ζήτημα της επισφάλειας μέσα από τη μελέτη και τις παρεμβάσεις στις συνθήκες της ζωής των εξυπηρετουμένων. Η παρούσα μελέτη εισάγει στην επιστημονική βιβλιογραφία της κοινωνικής εργασίας την επισφάλεια ως στοιχείο που χαρακτηρίζει πλέον την επαγγελματική και προσωπική ζωή των ίδιων των κοινωνικών λειτουργών. Η εν λόγω μελέτη έγκειται στην παρουσίαση και αξιολόγηση των δεδομένων μιας μικρής ποιοτικής έρευνας που διεξήχθη σε κοινωνικές/ούς λειτουργούς ψυχικής υγείας που εργάζονται στον μη κερδοσκοπικό τομέα στην Ελλάδα. Τα ευρήματα αποτυπώνουν τις ιδιαίτερα επισφαλείς συνθήκες εργασίας και διαβίωσης των κοινωνικών λειτουργών, οι οποίοι έχουν γίνει μέρος του γενικότερου φαινομένου των φτωχοποιημένων εργαζομένων: Καλύπτουν τις βασικές για την επιβίωσή τους ανάγκες δανειζόμενοι/ες, ενώ παράλληλα βρίσκεται σε εντεινόμενη επισφάλεια ένα ευρύ φάσμα της ζωής τους, όπως η στέγαση, η αναπαραγωγή, η εξασφάλιση καυσίμων, αλλά και η κάλυψη των δαπανών μετακίνησης, ακόμα και προς τον τόπο της εργασίας τους. Επιπρόσθετα, η μελέτη υποστηρίζει ότι η επέκταση των συνθηκών επισφάλειας σε επαγγελματίες με πανεπιστημιακή εκπαίδευση -εν προκειμένω εξετάζονται οι κοινωνικές/οί λειτουργοί- και συνακόλουθα η δυσκολία άσκησης κοινωνικής πολιτικής υπό αυτές τις συνθήκες- πρέπει να γίνει κατανοητή μέσα από το πρίσμα της Διεθνούς Οικονομικής Πολιτικής, όπως αυτή χαράσσεται μέσα από τις επιταγές του νεοφιλελεύθερου καπιταλισμού. Στόχος είναι να αποτελέσουν πεδίο παρέμβασης οι παράγοντες που συντελούν στην αύξηση των ανισοτήτων και τον μαρασμό του κοινωνικού κράτους.

Introduction

Traditionally, in western countries, social workers have dealt directly or indirectly with the phenomenon of precarity through the lives of service users who lived in poverty (Parrott, 2014; Saar-Heiman, Lavie-Ajayi, & Krumer-Nevo, 2017; Shamai, 2017; Sheedy, 2013). They have also experienced dimensions of precarity through the poverty they experience as social work students (Gair & Baglow, 2017, and though insecurity and anxiety created through the neoliberal management conditions experienced in their professional lives (Duschinsky, Lampitt, & Bell, 2016; Seifert, Messing, Riel, & Chatigny, 2007; Smith et al., 2016).

However, during the last decade, in many western countries, including Greece, precarity as insecurity is being experienced by social workers not only in their professional lives but also in their personal lives (Pentaraki, 2017a). This had led to the phenomenon of shared austerity reality in which common insecure conditions are experienced both by service users and public sector social workers, albeit to different degrees (Pentaraki, 2017a). However, even though public sector social workers' lives have been adversely affected materially, the major issues identified centred around an existential insecurity related to the insecure social reproduction conditions that their children and their parents faced and their inability to help them out effectively. These experiences were constructed by the implementation of neoliberal austerity policies imposed to Greece by the TROICA, (a transnational decision making body comprised by the European Union, the European Central Bank and the International Monetary Fund) which reflected wider socio-economic global transformations (for a more detailed analysis see Pentaraki, 2013, 2015, 2017a, 2017b).

This paper moves the discussion forwards by focussing on precarity as experienced by social workers working in the non-profit sector in their own lives. By doing this it aims to explore increasing precarity amongst social workers; furthermore, it examines its consequences in their lives and then develops a conceptual framework to understand the origins, entrenchment and effects of precarity amongst social workers. It draws on findings from a small pilot study of mental health social workers working in the non-profit sector in Greece documenting their precarious experiences. However, this is part of a larger explorative study exploring the perceived impact of austerity measures and economic crisis on social workers in Greece. The decision to report on this subset of the sample was based on the consistent theme of being unpaid during the time of the interviews.

Before the research is presented, the paper will first briefly outline the socio-economic context of rising inequalities and then define issues of precarity.

Socio-economic context

During the last four decades the welfare state in western countries has faced reconfigurations along neoliberal lines such as social spending cuts and the transferring of welfare services from the state to the private sector (Harvey, 2005; Lorenz, 2017). These welfare reconfigurations have been extended since the 2008 global financial crisis, under the pretext of a crisis of public finances (Levitas, 2012; Pentaraki, 2013). Despite evidence that the crisis was primarily caused by financial capital's greedy and predatory practices of its banking sector, the welfare state was targeted. This was reflected by the transfer of public money from the poor to the rich in order to fund "the rescue of the world banking system, the bailout of corporations, and the salvage of the investment portfolios of the wealthy" (McNally, 2011, p. 5). These changes affected those employed in public services or in outsourced services as well as the quality of the provided services (Cunningham, Baines, & Shields, 2017; Pentaraki, 2017a, 2017b).

One of the countries that has been most seriously affected by neoliberal reconfigurations is Greece (Pentaraki, 2013, 2015, 2017a, 2017b). Despite evidence that the crisis in Greece and in other countries, e.g. Portugal, Spain, Italy and Ireland, was not caused by social spending, social spending cuts since the onset of the crisis have amounted to almost 60% in Greece (Karamessini, 2015). However, the effects have been magnified in Greece as elsewhere in southern Europe due to the familialist welfare state model (Papadopoulos & Roumpakis, 2013). Although, these issues are often presented by the mainstream media as being exceptional to Greece in order to make an argument that Greece brought this upon itself (Pentaraki, 2018a), there is no evidence to support this (Pentaraki, 2013). Fundamentally, the issues that Greece faces reflect wider socio-economic transformations experienced world-wide (Pentaraki, 2013, 2015, 2017a, 2017b, 2018a, 2018b; Pentaraki & Speake, 2015). For example, the context of rising global inequalities is reflected in the concentration of wealth in the hands of few. According to the international Anti-poverty Development Organization Oxfam Report (Oxfam, 2017) the eight wealthiest people in the world own as much wealth as half the world. Also, the Gini coefficient, which is an inequality measure used in economics, and intended to represent the income or wealth distribution of a nation's residents, reflects the almost universal rising level of inequalities world-wide (OECD, 2016). These increasing levels of inequality have led to rising levels of precarity, long characteristic of life in the non-west (Comaroff & Comaroff, 2012) that now have moved to the west and are not only experienced by marginalised population such as immigrants, unskilled workers and young people but also are now being felt by middle class university-educated professionals. In order to explore this further, the next section will outline the major scholarly work on precarity.

Defining precarity and precariat

Standing (2011) has popularised the term precariat in the academic literature. He presents precariat as a distinctive socio-economic group and "a class in the making" (Standing, 2011, p. 7). The composition of the precariat comprises an ever-growing number of people across the world who live and work precariously. They are usually employed in short-term jobs, without recourse to stable occupational identities, careers, stable social protection or relevant protective regulations. These insecure workers have no collective bargaining power and are being abandoned by the traditional working class organisations, most notably the trade unions.

The retrenchment of security (related to labour market, employment, job, work, skill production, income and representation) is a main dynamic of the process of precarisation. Migrants make up a large share of the world's precariat. Standing (2011) alludes to the precariat as being a distinct and separate group, contrasted to 'the salariat', a group that is often employed by the state in public administration and the civil service and is defined by secure employment, sick pay and paid holidays. However, this contrasted group does not seem to exist as much as Standing claims since social spending cuts have undermined public sector employment. In Europe, this consequence has effectively challenged the existence of the so called European Social Model (Hermann, 2014b).

Most of the scholarly literature, including Standing's work, uses the term precarious to describe atypical work such as short-term contract and casual work but, as Tompa, Scott-Marshall, Dolinschi, Trevithick, & Bhattacharyya (2007, p. 210) argue, "an exclusive focus on the nature of the labour contract obscures the fact that many labour-market experiences in the new economy of neoliberal capitalism – including those that fall under the banner of standard work – exhibit characteristics that could be experienced as insecure, and thus, potentially detrimental to health and well-being".

This paper moves beyond Standing's understanding of the precariat in a similar tradition to Vosko, MacDonald and Campbell (2009) and Tompa et al. (2007) amongst other scholars. It uses the term to discuss dimensions of insecurity that exist in *all* jobs such as social work jobs that have an occupational identity not just in atypical jobs (Tompa et al., 2007; Vosko, McDonald, & Campbell, 2009). It also extends the term precarity beyond the realm of work to discuss the consequences of insecure employment relations on workers' personal lives (Neilson & Rossiter, 2005).

Thus, in this paper 'precarious' is used to describe economic and social vulnerability and unstable, insecure, less protected work (Tompa et al., 2007). In line with this conceptualisation, precarity might be experienced differently and to varying degrees by different groups of people and to national contexts and welfare regimes. However, underlining these experiences is a generalised sense of insecurity due to material and psychological vulnerability resulting from neoliberal reforms. This can be observed even in countries such as Sweden. For example, Nässtrom and Kalm (2015) discuss that conditions of precarity have emerged in Sweden and in response to these 'The Precariat', an activist network, has been formed (Nässtrom & Kalm, 2015). Also, Andersen, Schoyen and Hviden discuss that even in Scandinavian countries neoliberal reforms have been implemented which have brought some rising levels of inequalities, insecurity and damage to the welfare state (Andersen, Schoyen, & Hviden, 2017).

The paper maintains that precarious conditions are embedded in the current structures of neoliberal capitalism (Casas-Cortés 2014; Kalleberg, 2009, 2011, 2013; Lee & Kofman, 2012; Mahmud, 2015; Millar, 2017).

Research study

This is a small qualitative pilot study which is part of a larger study exploring the perceived impact of austerity measures and economic crisis on social workers in Greece. The study reported here consists of nine face to face, in depth, semi structured interviews conducted between September and December 2012 with mental health social workers in the non-profit mental health sector. This homogeneity resulted in data saturation, as reflected in the consistent theme that emerged - that participants had not been paid for four months, on average, during the time of interviews thereby leading to experiences of precarity. The paper reports on their precarity.

The average length of each interview was 55 minutes. Each participant gave consent, having been informed about the research and potential publication of the content of the interviews and assured on matters of confidentiality and anonymity. Accordingly, their geographical locations were described in very general terms. Ethical research procedures were followed by the relevant university ethics committee.

The authors conducted the interviews in Greece, which were recorded, transcribed and then thematically organised by them to identify, categorise and analyse themes and patterns within the data (Braun & Clarke, 2006).

The non-profit mental health sector

All the participants worked in the non-profit mental health sector which emerged out of the psychiatric reform programme within a context of a neoliberal European agenda. More specifically they worked in mental health mobile units, residential care and day centres for mental health users with severe psychiatric disorders. A brief introduction of the reform programme provides context for the resultant precarity identified. The psychiatric reform programme was initiated in Greece in 1984 through the Commission of European Communities (EEC Regulation No 815/84) to address the inadequate functional capacity of the mental health system to meet mental health needs of the Greek population and provide effective community based services. However, this reform, implemented through the programme Psychargos, not only sought to address the needs of the mental health system through the advancement of de-institutionalisation and community mental health services but also to impose neoliberal funding models based on a competitive market agenda. This resulted in part of mental health service provisioning being outsourced/contracted out to private or non-profit organisations, which is a key feature of neoliberalism (Froud, Johal,

Moran, & Williams, 2017). This "new" sector was characterised by non-consistent funding. Similarly, instability in finances due to neoliberal restructuring has been identified in other western countries, such as Canada (Cunningham et al., 2017).

The mental health sector in Greece was one of the first state welfare provision services to be privatised/contracted out. Clearly, the outsourcing of state services (Evans, Richmond, & Shields, 2005) can be found across western countries and has expanded to cover a variety of public services such as social services, health, home care, and education (Harvey, 2005). It has been argued that the Psychargos reform programme has resulted in incomplete reform, as evidenced in the underdevelopment of sectorisation, adequate primary care policies, inter-sectoral coordination and specialised services – a difficult situation which is further undermined by the adverse impact of the current financial crisis (Giannakopoulo & Anagnostopoulos, 2016).

Participants

Participants were selected using convenience sampling. All participants were at the time of the interviews working at the non for profit mental health sector. The participants' ages ranged from 27 years to 32 years with an average age of 30 years. There were seven women and two men, all white and born in Greece. All participants were holders of an undergraduate social work degree, two had also a masters' level degree and five of the participants were on psychotherapeutic training programmes. The majority of them worked in the greater area of Athens. The social workers interviewed who did not work in Athens but worked in other cities also had urban, semi-rural and rural, and other remote settings in their area of professional practice. Their experience as mental health social workers ranged from three to six years. The average years of social work experience was 5.5 years. Their length of employment at the present employer ranged from one year to six years.

Their narrations of their experiences are utilised to provide testimony of the nature and impacts of precarity in their professional and personal lives. In order to provide anonymity for the participants they are provided with fictive names.

Findings

The findings present a picture of social workers living and working in increasing insecure and/or precarious conditions. The consequences of these experiences can cause emotional distress, anxiety and burn-out. Despite this insecurity/precarity, all the participants expressed a concern about the lives of the service users and the future of mental health services. Insecurity has been experienced as an all-encompassing phenomenon influencing all aspects of the social workers' lives, both personally and professionally. The findings are presented by focussing on the insecurity experienced by the participants 1) in their personal lives, and 2) in their professional lives.

Insecurity in participants' personal lives

The main theme that emerged is the impact on the social workers' of not being paid for many months. At the time of the interviews, none of the participants had been paid for a long time, on average for a period of four months. This non-payment/delay in payment has caused insecure conditions that have adversely affected the participants' material conditions and general well-being.

Deterioration of payment patterns and its consequences

It was reported by Eleni that despite the fact that difficulties in the consistency of payments existed previously, this is now the most difficult time. "We are four and half months unpaid […] this was not happening before to this extent […]. This is the most difficult time compared to previous times." The previous difficulties to which she alludes seem to be related to the outsourcing competitive based funding model, which did not have a continuous funding stream.

This delay in payment has changed the participants' living conditions adversely. They cannot afford the basic necessities of life, including housing insecurity and fuel poverty. Sofia, on this issue states:

> [...] I stay at my parents' home. This house is incomplete, it has no floors, it is not heated, [...] if I did not have this house I do not know if I could continue working given the way of payment and all of this situation [...] whenever we get paid a debt is redeemed, then there is not much money left for anything else, [...],

She continued to articulate the seriousness of the situation:

1. [I] just survive, every day is just work, home, home, work, which brings exhaustion, mental exhaustion [...]. The truth is that I'm [...] worried about it, I think it's serious, I think it's not just me, I'm facing it, and other people are confronted by it, I wonder where will it take us?

The above quotation reflects experiences of precarity surrounding both current survival needs and prospects for the future. Sofia explains that this is not only applies to herself for but also for the whole community. She highlights the critical supporting role of her family. This theme of the supporting role of families and friends was repeated by the other participants. Anna acknowledges their important role by stating "I cannot cope well, of course, without the help of my neighbours and my relatives, etc. [...]". However, Eleni was concerned for how long families and friends could provide help in the future:

> [...] things are more difficult than before as [my friend] cannot give me the money that she used to lend me. Just because the whole situation is more difficult than before because now she faces her own issues.

Although the help of families and friends was seen as invaluable, there was some embarrassment and sadness that the conventional intergenerational solidarity dynamics have been switched. This sense of embarrassment may suggest negative psychological consequences of the crisis to the participants. Dina stated:

> [I]t is really hard, what should I say, that parents [both sets] help? We [she and her husband] should be ashamed. They [the parents] contribute though [..] they live in a rural area [...] so they provide fruit, vegetables, meat. But this makes us sad since we should be helping them as they have already done their duty to raise us, but instead of this we still ask for their help.

Sofia could not take the stress anymore and was searching for alternative employment, but finding it difficult. Georgia also tried to make ends meet by having an additional job in the hospitality sector but the demands of working two jobs were very hard.

Concerns were not only about their future professional opportunities and development but also how these issues impacted these issues impact their personal lives and life course, including having children. These were clearly expressed by Dina when she said:

> Of course, there is no plan to have a child, even though I really wanted it, it is so scary [...]

In addition to the important issues of every day to day survival, such as heating and food, there were also reports of their inability to afford a range of other things such as travel expenses (including bus ticket to get to work), clothing expenses, social outings and gym membership. Combined, all of these reflect the deterioration of living conditions and quality of life.

All of these present and future concerns had created senses of 'going backwards' and an inability to progress and/or advance. This is articulated by Anna:

> Sometimes I have a feeling of regression. I have been working for so long now and instead of going forwards I am going backwards? This affects me emotionally too, way beyond [the day to day practical issues of survival].

Insecurity in their professional lives

The realities and feelings of insecurity experienced in their personal lives including those generated by not being paid for their work for months, are also intensified by other insecurities in their working lives as Petros expressed:

... I have experienced a great sense of abuse ... when you have people with mental health needs, it's too difficult ... This is too abusive and having to simultaneously manage all your own anxieties and all your own practical and operational needs, it is very, very abusive ... The difficulties are many when you have not been paid for five months. The time comes when you cannot put gas in your car or buy a bus ticket to go to work [Furthermore at work] ...

... there were too many times when we could not feed the patients, so simple, we could not pay the electricity in the residential home and there was a danger of not having electricity, we could not pay the pharmacy and the pharmacist was threatening to leave us without medicines, we were under the threat of eviction, and the police came with the eviction notice etc. [...]

Petros considers his life to be injured and thus grievable (Butler, 2009). The above quote clearly reflects the all-encompassing feeling of insecurity and precarity faced by participants as they try to deal with both their own material insecurity and the insecurities faced by service users. Dina expressed similar frustrations and concerns, particularly about the elimination of services provided to service users. Views that were reflected by all the participants. Trying to manage both sets of insecurity puts them in a position of double jeopardy (Abramovitz & Zelnick, 2010) and leads them to question the future of mental health provision at different levels. These conditions threaten not only the future of mental health services but also the mental health of the participants. This is clearly expressed in the following remarks by Petros:

From moment to moment anything can happen and at any particular time there might not be any mental health cover [...] this thing is too stressful. Every day needs a 'plan b' and a 'plan c' such as considering the possible re-institutionalisation of the service users [...], possible communication with their families, to come to collect them. Tomorrow it may be that the boarding school does not work [...]. This causes inconceivable anxiety, unbelievable anxiety, which has a catalytic effect on the quality of my life. Now I do not care about my income because my income was bad. ... the amount of burn-out is immense, immense, immense.

The participants also focussed on the precarity and the vulnerability of many service users and reported that they had a sense of both professional and personal responsibility to fill gaps left unfilled by family and health/social services. As the needs of service users have intensified in the economic crisis, so too have the pressures on social workers, professionally and personally, as they are stretched (sometimes to the limit) to meet these needs. For Sofia this has meant feeling obliged to work uncompensated beyond her contracted hours to meet her professional obligations to the service users. Several social workers expressed that they were overstretched and concerned that they were on the road to burn-out, yet felt that they had to continue. On the other hand, Anna described how she loved her work even though there was a voice telling her that "in this difficult times you cannot continue having the kindness to persevere (tin eugeneia)".

Discussion and conclusion

The findings present a picture of mental health social workers facing rising levels of insecurity in their personal and professional lives (Abramovitz & Zelnick, 2010; Pentaraki, 2017a). They reflect the situation of social workers being part of the growing phenomenon of the working poor (Pradella, 2015), experiencing multiple dimensions of insecurity: surviving on loans, experiencing housing insecurity, reproductive insecurity (Chan & Tweedie, 2015), fuel poverty and the inability to pay for their commuting expenses to and from work and so forth.

The participants discussed facing rising levels of insecurity/precarity due to the increased insecurity surrounding not only their own lives and professional employment but also the service users' lives (Abramovitz & Zelnick, 2010; Triliva & Georga, 2014), the lives of their family/friends, community (Kretsos, 2014; Papadopoulos & Roumpakis, 2013), future de-institutionalisation and the prospects for the mental health sector overall (Giannakopoulos & Anagnostopoulos, 2016). They have been managing primarily because of the support of their families and friends but now that almost everyone's conditions have deteriorated further their insecurity intensifies, the implications of which could be explored more in future research.

The findings reflect an increased sense of vulnerability as insecurity in everyday life (Butler, 2009; Casas-Cortés, 2014; Neilson & Rossiter, 2005), which emerge from the erosion of resources, policies and capacities that enable social reproduction (Papadopoulos & Roumpakis, 2013). This results in a generalised sense of social precarity, which emanates from the neoliberal undermining of collective security, solidarity and thus systems of social reproduction (Lee & Kofman, 2012; Lorenz, 2017; Lorey, 2015). This insecurity is all encompassing and inhabits the "microspaces of everyday life" (Ettlinger, 2007, p. 319). This, combined with the current socio-economic conditions, "leads to an interminable lack of certainty, the condition of being unable to predict one's fate or having some degree of stability on which to construct a life" (Neilson & Rossiter, 2005, p. 3).

The intensification of this insecurity is a reflection of the current socio-economic conditions (Bauman, 2013; Lorey, 2015; Mahmud, 2015; Pradella, 2015) from where the generalisation of employment insecurity emanates (Beck, 1992). The participants discuss how the conditions they experience leads them to an inability to plan one's life, which parallels the experiences of psychologists working in Community Mental Health Centres in Greece (Triliva & Georga, 2014, p. 149) who also experience the social milieu creeping into the psychotherapeutic relationship. Now it is not only immigrants, low skilled workers, young people, unemployed and service users who live in insecurity/precarity (Chan & Tweedie, 2015; Mahmud, 2015), it is also university-educated professionals such as social workers in Greece, teachers in England (Ferguson, 2017), adjunct academics in many countries in Europe and in the USA (Ivancheva, 2015; Pathe, 2014; Thorkelson, 2016) i.e. almost everyone on the planet (Lee & Kofman, 2012). The widening of social groups experiencing precarity reflects the global downwards convergence in terms of insecure working conditions and living standards overall (Hermann, 2014a, 2014b; Puig-Barrachina et al., 2014; Tompa et al., 2007). It also demonstrates the downward pressure on wages and jobs before and after the recent economic crisis. Instead of conditions in the global south improving, conditions in the global north have deteriorated (Comaroff & Comaroff, 2012). These conditions reflect what Neilson (2015, p. 195) calls the "absolute general law" of increased precarity within neoliberal capitalism. This is a feature of living in an age of insecurity (Elliott & Atkinson, 1999) which has been further intensified since the onset of the financial crisis.

The participants' precarious experiences are connected with both deteriorating material conditions and adverse psychological effects. Participants discussed feelings of abuse, embarrassment and sadness. These are emotions of insecurity affecting not only welfare professionals working in Greece but also employees working in public service delivery in countries such as England, which can be thought of as "emotions of austerity" (Clayton, Donovan, & Merchant, 2015, p. 24). Furthermore, the participants discussed fears for the future that prohibit them from making future plans such as having children. This reflects the observed wider trend of birth rates declining during economic recessions (Sobotka, Skirbekk, & Philipov, 2011). Other participants talked about how they experienced 'burn-out' in trying to ameliorate the increased level of insecurity that the service users experience due to the economic crisis. Such lack of security, stability and predictability in their day to day personal and/or working lives seem to relate to what Neilson (2015, pp. 184–185) called "Existential anxiety, and is understood as mental unease induced by the self-reflexive perception of life's precarious character, is intensified by the reality of deepening social and material precarity." These feelings can be related to the impact of the economic crisis, which Stolorow (2009) conceptualised as collective trauma, and allude to social workers being both wounded healers and fellow suffers (Golightley, 2017), as they experience the insecurities related to a shared austerity reality between themselves and the service users (Pentaraki, 2017a).

The participants were concerned about their own mental health and that of their service users. This concern reflects the general deteriorating conditions in Greece (see United Nations Human Rights, Office of the High Commissioner, 2015; Karamessini, 2015; Kokaliari, 2016; Economou, et al., 2016), which have led to the recognition by the UN Independent Expert Advisor that there is a humanitarian and human rights crisis in Greece (United Nations Human Rights, Office of the High Commissioner, 2015). As Salomon (2015) and others have contended, the denial of social rights under austerity has been substantial.

However, to recapitulate and conclude, these experiences reflect wider trends that are embedded in the current phase of neoliberal capitalism (Harvey, 2005). These experiences are primarily local manifestations of the global conditions of neoliberal capitalism and as such they have relevance for other countries. Furthermore, as the author has argued elsewhere (Pentaraki, 2017b, p. 1) "this understanding needs to inform the actions of social workers. It is important for these [experiences] to be contextualised within the socio-economic conditions in which they arise" in order for neoliberal capitalism to become a locus of intervention (Pentaraki, 2013; Pentaraki, 2017b, p. 1). Towards this end, internationally social work education needs to offer the critical resources necessary for social workers to understand the structural causes of precarity both in their own and service users' lives so they can become the locus of intervention. This can be achieved through the incorporation of an international political economy (IPE) perspective. The IPE perspective is key to understanding these dimensions of insecurity/precarity as reflecting wider trends, including the rising level of inequalities (Oxfam, 2017), degrading labour conditions (Puig-Barrachina et al., 2014; Tompa et al., 2007) and changing relationships between the state and welfare provision (such as social spending cuts and models of outsourcing). It also includes the roles of neoliberal transnational decision making bodies such as the TROICA (Pentaraki & Speake, 2015) in raising levels of precarity and poverty (Lorenz, 2017) etc.

However, the remit of this paper is not to analyse these trends in detail as they have been successfully analysed elsewhere (see amongst others Oxfam, 2017; Harvey, 2005; Pradella, 2015; Lorenz, 2017; Pentaraki, 2013; van Chung & van Oorschot, 2010). Its purpose is to introduce the discussion of the experiences and consequences of precarity in the lives of mental health social workers as an all-encompassing experience that affects both them and the service users, within the context of neoliberal capitalism. This aim is congruent with the critical tradition of the international tradition of social work, which seeks to unravel global oppressive structures and how they impact on the social work profession (Pentaraki, 2017b).

Thus, it expands the social work scholarly literature on poverty and insecurity (Parrott, 2014; Sheedy, 2013) by adding the discussion of these as they affect social workers themselves. The abuse and the insecurity felt by the participants moves beyond the suffering they experience due to the poverty of others (Smith et al., 2016) as it includes their own. In doing so, this paper creates intersecting links between the social work scholarly literature which examines the adverse impacts of neoliberal capitalism on social work (Aronson & Sammon, 2000; Baines, Davis, & Saini, 2009; Dominelli, 1999; Fabricant, Burghardt, & Epstein, 1992; Karagkounis, 2017; Pentaraki, 2017a, 2017b; Wallace & Pease, 2011) and the scholarly literature on precarity (Baines, Cunningham, Campey, & Shields, 2014; Baines, Cunningham, & Shields, 2017; Casas-Cortés, 2014; Cunningham et al., 2016; Mahmud, 2015). In particular, this research extends knowledge and understanding of precarious experiences previously related only to work in which marginalised populations, such as immigrants, youth or unskilled workers are engaged. But more importantly this paper introduces precarity in the social work scholarly literature as a feature of social workers' professional and personal lives. The study shows how the processes of precaritisation are expanding, as precarity is now also experienced by professionals such as social workers and service users.

The growing sense of insecurity/precarity due to the impact of the current economic crisis cannot be understood effectively without reference to the dominant neoliberal fiscal response to the last financial crisis. This response has included spending cuts on social services in which most social workers practice and of these the majority are women (Karamessini & Rubery, 2014). Future research needs to take this into account and explore gendered experiences of precarity (Vosko & Clark, 2009). Another interesting research area would be a comparative analysis of the experiences of social workers with professionals working in other sectors of the social services. Furthermore, a comparative perspective of precarity experiences in dissimilar countries (especially in welfare regimes and labour regulations) could provide a more nuanced approach in terms of the effects of neoliberal capitalism.

In general, the growing sense of insecurity/precarity due to the impact of the current economic crisis cannot be understood effectively without reference to the dominant IPE perspective of neoliberal capitalism that has governed the world during the last 40 years, in which it is argued that competitive markets are the most effective way of promoting well-being (Harvey, 2005). This claim is refuted not only by the experiences of this study's research participants in Greece but by the rising trends of global inequality.

This paper furthers the international debate about the devastating effects of austerity, which are multi-faceted, extensive and deep, and clearly undermine people's personal and social well-being, and the need to challenge them and fight for another society that centres around the needs of people, for the sake of the welfare state, the social work profession, the service users and social justice for all (Garrett & Bertotti, 2017; Pentaraki, 2013). A clear mandate for the social work profession towards this end is reflected in the statement against austerity by the International Federation of Social Workers (IFSW, 2016), produced while in Greece by the professional social work associations of Greece, Iceland, Ireland, Italy, Portugal, Spain and the UK. It is up to social workers, collectively and individually within and across countries and in collaboration with other progressive organisations, to make this mandate a reality (Pentaraki, 2013).

Disclosure statement

No potential conflict of interest was reported by the authors.

References

Abramovitz, M., & Zelnick, J. (2010). Double jeopardy: The impact of neoliberalism on care workers in the United States and South Africa. *International Journal of Health Services, 40*(1), 97–117.

Andersen, J, Schoyen, M, Hviden, B. (2017). Changing Scandinavian welfare states. In Taylor-Gooby, P., Leruth, B., & Chung, H. (Eds.), *After Austerity. Welfare State Transformation in Europe After the Great Recession* (pp. 89–114). Oxford: Oxford University Press.

Aronson, J., & Sammon, S. (2000). Practice amid social service cuts and restructuring: Working with the contradictions of small victories. *Canadian Social Work Review, 17*(2), 167–187.

Baines, D., Cunningham, I., & Shields, J. (2017). Filling the gaps: Unpaid (and precarious) work in the nonprofit social services. *Critical Social Policy*, 0261018317693128.

Baines, D., Cunningham, I., Campey, J., & Shields, J. (2014). Not profiting from precarity: The work of nonprofit service delivery and the creation of precasiousness. *Just Labour, 22.* Retrieved from http://justlabour.journals.yorku.ca/index.php/justlabour/article/view/

Baines, D., Davis, J. M., & Saini, M. (2009). Wages, working conditions, and restructuring in ontario's social work profession. *Canadian Social Work Review/Revue Canadienne de Service Social*, 59–72. Retrieved from http://www.jstor.org/stable/41669902

Bauman, Z. (2013). *Liquid modernity*. London: Wiley.

Beck, U. (1992). From industrial society to the risk society: Questions of survival, social structure and ecological enlightenment. *Theory, Culture & Society, 9*(1), 97–123.

Braun, V., & Clarke, V. (2006). Using thematic analysis in psychology. *Qualitative Research in Psychology, 3*(2), 77–101.

Butler, J. (2009). *Frames of war: When is life grievable?* London: Verso.

Casas-Cortés, M. (2014). A genealogy of precarity: A toolbox for rearticulating fragmented social realities in and out of the workplace. *Rethinking Marxism, 26*(2), 206–226.

Chan, S., & Tweedie, D. (2015). Precarious work and reproductive insecurity. *Social Alternatives, 34*(4), 5.

Chung, H., & van Oorschot, W. (2010). Employment insecurity of European individuals duringthe financial crisis: A multi-level approach. *Working paper on the reconcialiation of work and welfare in Europe. European Commission Sixth Framework Programme.* Retrieved from https://www.ssoar.info/ssoar/bitstream/handle/document/19796/ssoar-2010-chung_et_al-employment_insecurity_of_european_individuals.pdf?sequence=1

Clayton, J., Donovan, C., & Merchant, J. (2015). Emotions of austerity: Care and commitment in public service delivery in the north east of England. *Emotion, Space and Society, 14*, 24–32.

Comaroff, J., and J. L. Comaroff. (2012). Theory from the south: Or, How Euro-America Is Evolving Toward Africa. *Anthropological Forum: A Journal of Social Anthropology and Comparative Sociology 22* (2), 113–131.

Cunningham, I., Baines, D., & Shields, J. (2017). "You've just cursed Us": precarity, Austerity and Worker's Participation in the Non-Profit Social Services. *Relations Industrielles/Industrial Relations, 72*(2), 370–393.

Cunningham, I., Baines, D., Shields, J., & Lewchuk, W. (2016). Austerity policies,'precarity' and the nonprofit workforce: A comparative study of UK and Canada. *Journal of Industrial Relations, 58*(4), 455–472.

Dominelli, L. (1999). Neo-liberalism, social exclusion and welfare clients in a global economy. *International Journal of Social Welfare, 8*(1), 14–22.

Duschinsky, R., Lampitt, S., & Bell, S. (2016). *Sustaining social work: Between power and powerlessness.* Oxford: Palgrave Macmillan.

Economou, M., Angelopoulos, E., Peppou, L. E., Souliotis, K., Tzavara, C., Kontoangelos, K., & Stefanis, C. (2016). Enduring financial crisis in Greece: Prevalence and correlates of major depression and suicidality. *Social Psychiatry and Psychiatric Epidemiology, 51*(7), 1015–1024.

Elliott, L., & Atkinson, D. (1999). *The age of insecurity.* Verso.

Ettlinger, N. (2007). Precarity unbound. *Alternatives, 32*(3), 319–340.

Evans, B., Richmond, T., & Shields, J. (2005). Structuring neoliberal governance: The nonprofit sector, emerging new modes of control and the marketisation of service delivery. *Policy and Society, 24*(1), 73–97.

Fabricant, M., Burghardt, S. F., & Epstein, I. (1992). *The welfare state crisis and the transformation of social service work.* New York: Routledge.

Ferguson, D (2017). Homeless teachers: 'I wouldn't talk about it, I was so ashamed' Retrieved from https://www.theguardian.com/education/2017/may/23/homeless-teachers-ashamed-housing-crisis-professionals

Froud, J., Johal, S., Moran, M., & Williams, K. (2017). Outsourcing the state: New sources of elite power. *Theory, Culture & Society, 34*(5–6), 77–101.

Gair, S. & Baglow, L. (2017). Seeing it like it is: Australian social work students' experiences of balancing study, work, and compulsory field placement. *Australian Social Work,* Accepted for Publication. doi:10.1080/0312407X.2017.1377741

Garrett, P. M., & Bertotti, T. F. (2017). Social work and the politics of 'austerity': Ireland and Italy. *European Journal of Social Work, 20*(1), 29–41.

Giannakopoulos, G., & Anagnostopoulos, D. C. (2016). Psychiatric reform in Greece: An overview. *British Journal of Psychology Bulletin, 40*(6), 326–328.

Golightley, M. (2017). Social work under neo-liberalism: Fellow sufferer or wounded healer?. *British Journal of Social Work, 47*(4), 965–972. doi:10.1093/bjsw/bcx068

Harvey, D. (2005). *A brief history of neoliberalism.* Oxford: Oxford University Press.

Hermann, C. (2014a). Structural adjustment and neoliberal convergence in labour markets and welfare: The impact of the crisis and austerity measures on European economic and social models. *Competition & Change, 18*(2), 111–130.

Hermann, C. (2014b). Crisis, structural reform and the dismantling of the european social model(s). *Economic and Industrial Democracy,* 1–18, doi:10.1177/0143831X14555708

Ivancheva, M. P. (2015). The age of precarity and the new challenges to the academic profession. *Studia Universitatis Babes-Bolyai. Studia Europaea, 60*(1), 39–47.

IFSW (2016) IFSW Statement from The Solidarity Symposium on Social Work and Austerity. Retrieved from http://ifsw.org/news/ifsw-statement-from-the-solidarity-symposium-on-social-work-and-austerity/

Kalleberg, A. L. (2009). Precarious work, insecure workers: Employment relations in transition. *American Sociological Review, 74*(1), 1–22.

Kalleberg, A. L. (2011). *Good jobs, bad jobs: The rise of polarized and precarious employment systems in the United States, 1970s-2000s.* New York, NY: Russell Sage.

Kalleberg, A. L. (2013). Globalization and precarious work. *Contemporary Sociology, 42* (5)700–706.

Karagkounis, V. (2017). Social work in Greece in the time of austerity: Challenges and prospects. *European Journal of Social Work, 20*(5), 651–665.

Karamessini, M. (2015). The Greek social model: Towards a deregulated labour market and residual social protection. *The European Social Model in Crisis: Is Europe Losing Its Soul,* 230–288.

Karamessini, M., & Rubery, J. (Eds.) (2014). *Women and austerity: The economic crisis and the future for gender equality.* New York: Routledge.

Kokaliari, E. (2016). Quality of life, anxiety, depression, and stress among adults in Greece following the global financial crisis. *International Social Work*, 0020872816651701.

Kretsos, L. (2014). Youth policy in austerity Europe: The case of Greece. *International Journal of Adolescence and Youth*, *19* (supp. 1), 35–47.

Lee, C. K., & Kofman, Y. (2012). The politics of precarity: Views beyond the United States. *Work and Occupations*, *39*(4), 388–408.

Levitas, R. (2012). The just's umbrella: Austerity and the big society in coalition policy and beyond. *Critical Social Policy*, *32* (3), 320–342.

Lorenz, W. (2017). European policy developments and their impact on social work. *European Journal of Social Work*, *20*(1), 17–28.

Lorey, I. (2015). *State of insecurity: Government of the precarious*. London: Verso Books.

Mahmud, T. (2015). Precarious existence and capitalism: A permanent state of exception. *Southwestern University Law Review*, *44*, 699–726.

McNally, D. (2011). *'Global slump: The economics and politics of crisis and resistance'*. Oakland, CA: PM Press.

Millar, K. M. (2017). Toward a critical politics of precarity. *Sociology Compass*, *11*(6), e12483.

Näsström, S., & Kalm, S. (2015). A democratic critique of precarity. *Global Discourse*, *5*(4), 556–573.

Neilson, D. (2015). Class, precarity, and anxiety under neoliberal global capitalism: From denial to resistance. *Theory & Psychology*, *25*(2), 184–201.

Neilson, B., & Rossiter, N. (2005). From precarity to precariousness and back again: Labour, life and unstable networks. *Fibreculture*, *5* (022), 1–19.

OECD. (2016). *Income inequality remains high in the face of weak recovery*. Retrieved from http://www.oecd.org/social/inequality.htm

Oxfam. (2017). *An economy for the 99%: It's time to build a human economy that benefits everyone, not just the privileged few*. Oxfam GB for Oxfam International.

Papadopoulos, T., & Roumpakis, A. (2013). Familistic welfare capitalism in crisis: Social reproduction and anti-social policy in Greece. *Journal of International and Comparative Social Policy*, *29*(3), 204–224.

Parrott, L. (2014). *Social Work and Poverty*. London: Policy Press.

Pathe, S. (2014). *Homeless professor protests conditions of adjuncts*. Retrieved from http://www.pbs.org/newshour/making-sense/homeless-professor-protests-conditions-adjuncts/

Pentaraki M. (2013) "If we do not cut social spending, we will end up like Greece": challenging consent to austerity through social work action. *Critical Social Policy*, *33*(4), 700–711.

Pentaraki M. (2015). The executive committee of the Greek professional association of social work in an age of austerity: Examining its response. *European Journal of Social Work*, *18*(1), 140–155.

Pentaraki, M. (2017a). "I am in a constant state of insecurity trying to make ends meet, like our service users": Shared austerity reality between social workers and service users—towards a preliminary conceptualisation. *British Journal of Social Work*, *47* (4), 1245–1261.

Pentaraki, M. (2017b). Practicing social work in a context of austerity: Experiences of public sector social workers in Greece. *European Journal of Social Work*, Sept, 1–12.

Pentaraki, M. (2018a). Austerity common sense and contested understandings of the austerity measures within a leadership of a professional association of social workers. *European Journal of Social Work*, 1–12.

Pentaraki, M. (2018b). Social work practice of hospital social workers under the structural adjustment program in Greece: Social workers protecting the right to health care within the context of neoliberalism. *Czech and Slovak Social Work-reviewed scientific journal for fields of social work*, 18 (4), 7–20. Available at http://www.socialniprace.cz/soubory/sp4-2018_web-180831114230.pdf#page=62

Pentaraki, M., & Speake, J. (2015). Reclaiming hope within the geopolitics of economic bullying: The case of SYRIZA and post referendum Greece, AntipodeFoundation.org, 20 October, Retrieved from http://antipodefoundation.org/2015/10/20/reclaiming-hope-in-greece/

Pradella, L. (2015). The working poor in Western Europe: Labour, poverty and global capitalism. *Comparative European Politics*, *13*(5), 596–613.

Puig-Barrachina, V., Vanroelen, C., Vives, A., Martínez, J. M., Muntaner, C., Levecque, K., & Louckx, F. (2014). Measuring employment precariousness in the European working conditions survey: The social distribution in Europe. *Work*, *49* (1), 143–161.

Saar-Heiman, Y., Lavie-Ajayi, M., & Krumer-Nevo, M. (2017). Poverty-aware social work practice: Service users' perspectives. *Child & Family Social Work*, *22*(2), 1054–1063.

Salomon, M. E. (2015). Of austerity, human rights and international institutions. *European Law Journal*, *21*(4), 521–545.

Seifert, A. M., Messing, K., Riel, J., & Chatigny, C. (2007). Precarious employment conditions affect work content in education and social work: Results of work analyses. *International Journal of Law and Psychiatry*, *30*(4), 299–310.

Shamai, M. (2017). Is poverty a collective trauma? A Joint Learning Process with Women Living in Poverty in the City of Haifa in Israel. *British Journal of Social Work* Published Online 31 October doi:10.1093/bjsw/bcx116z

Sheedy, M. (2013). *Core themes in social work: Power, poverty, politics and values*. Maidenhead: McGraw-Hill Education (UK).

Sobotka, T., Skirbekk, V., & Philipov, D. (2011). Economic recession and fertility in the developed world. *Population and Development Review*, *37*(2), 267–306.

Smith, M., Cree, V. E., MacRae, R., Sharp, D., Wallace, E., & O'Halloran, S. (2016). Social suffering: Changing organisational culture in children and families social work through critical reflection groups—insights from Bourdieu. *British Journal of Social Work, 47*(4), 973–988.

Standing, G. (2011). *The precariat: The new dangerous class*. London: Bloomsbury Academic.

Stolorow, R. D. (2009). The economic crisis as collective trauma. *Trauma Psychology Newsletter, 4*(2), 5.

Thorkelson, E. (2016). Precarity outside: The political unconscious of French academic labor. *American Ethnologist, 43*(3), 475–487.

Tompa, E., Scott-Marshall, H., Dolinschi, R., Trevithick, S., & Bhattacharyya, S. (2007). Precarious employment experiences and their health consequences: Towards a theoretical framework. *Work, 28*(3), 209–224.

Triliva, S., & Georga, A. (2014). Austerity and precarity: The social milieu creeps into the psychotherapeutic context. *Rivista di Psicologia Clinica*, (1).

Vosko, L., & Clark, L. F. (2009). Gendered precariousness and social reproduction. In F. Vosko, M. MacDonald, & I. Campbell (Eds.), *Gender and the contours of precarious employment* (pp. 26–42). London: Routledge.

Vosko, L. F., MacDonald, M., & Campbell, I. (Eds.). (2009). Gender and the contours of precarious employment. New York: Routledge.

United Nations Human Rights, Office of the High Commissioner. (2015). *Greek crisis: Human rights should not stop at doors of international institutions, says UN expert*. Retrieved from http://www.ohchr.org/EN/NewsEvents/

Wallace, J., & Pease, B. (2011). Neoliberalism and Australian social work: Accommodation or resistance? *Journal of Social Work, 11*(2), 132–142.

Social work's 'black hole' or 'Phoenix moment'? Impacts of the neoliberal path in social work profession in Portugal

O momento 'fénix' ou 'buraco negro' do serviço social? Impactos do neoliberalismo na profissão de serviço social em portugal

Cristina Pinto Albuquerque 🆔

ABSTRACT

This article proposes a reflection about the transformation of social work practices in the context of a neoliberal path, particularly in Portugal. Within this context, social workers try to adapt their professional practices combining, by several processes, the core values and goals of the profession and the new demands of efficiency under the so called 'impact philanthropy' model. Several paradoxical effects derive from such changes. Not only relevant negative constraints and substantial transformations on the core goals of the profession are emerging, but also new forms of work are being shaped. So, are we witnessing a renewed opportunity to revalue social work (the 'Phoenix' moment) or an increased possibility of its depletion and emptiness (the 'black hole' moment)? To discuss this thesis are presented data from a study based on interviews with Portuguese social workers about the impacts of neoliberal management assumptions in their practices, as well as their processes of adjustment. Results show, in fact, many impacts (negative and positive) concerning the management of work processes and the conception of the practice's teleological basis and values. Additionally, adjustment processes or procedures ('tactical' or 'strategic' adjustment) used by professionals are identified.

RESUMO

O presente artigo propõe uma reflexão sobre a transformação das práticas do Serviço Social, particularmente em Portugal, sob influência do paradigma neoliberal. Neste contexto, os assistentes sociais tentam adaptar as suas práticas profissionais combinando, através de diversos processos, os valores e objetivos centrais da profissão e as novas exigências de eficácia sob o chamado modelo de 'filantropia de impacto'. Diversos efeitos paradoxais decorrem de tais mudanças. Não apenas constrangimentos negativos relevantes e transformações substanciais nos objetivos centrais da profissão emergem, mas também novas formas de trabalho se moldam. Deste modo, estaremos testemunhando um momento 'Fénix' ou um momento 'buraco negro' no desenvolvimento do Serviço Social? Para discutir esta tese serão apresentados dados de um estudo baseado em entrevistas a assistentes sociais portugueses sobre os impactos nas respetivas práticas dos pressupostos da gestão neoliberal, bem como nos processos de ajustamento que desenvolvem. Os resultados mostram, de fato, diversos impactos (negativos e positivos) na gestão dos processos de trabalho e na concepção da teleologia e dos valores da prática. Além disso, são identificados os processos de adaptação ('táctica' ou 'estratégica') utilizados pelos profissionais.

1. Introduction

The notion of 'neoliberalism', even despite its common present use, lacks consensus and is disputed by several analysts (Deeming, 2017). In fact, 'neoliberalism' is above all an unscientific classification. It is a kind of 'sponge concept' that allows aggregating, under the same classification, phenomena and dimensions with different senses and contents. Nevertheless, despite this constitutive imprecision, it is possible, according to several authors, to identify a set of traits, phenomena and effects recognisable globally under the label 'neoliberal' – and presented both in a critical or legitimating perspective.

Understanding neoliberalism and the current socio-political and economic project that it entails implies thus necessarily an extension of the analytical lenses that allow to embrace a vast and complex set of issues, simultaneously situated and global. It is a fact that historical, cultural and economic circumstances of a given geopolitical context influence the ways in which neoliberal 'reforms' are implemented and the depth of the impacts produced in their corresponding models of well-being and development. They are, to this extent, 'contingent on context' (McDonald, Harris, & Wintersteen, 2003), that is, related to a certain socio-political and ideological configuration existing in a given time/space. But they have also transversal and globalised features.

(a) Context and research arguments

In the present article, an assumption is made that neoliberalism is, in fact, a hybrid product resulting from the combination of different dimensions (economic, political, ideological and sociocultural) and consubstantiating an 'imaginary' spread throughout the world. It is the understanding of the impacts of this 'imaginary' in social work practices that will constitute the leading element of the article. It is assumed, therefore, that a certain 'neoliberal' narrative and ideology lead to mechanisms of rationalisation and 'disenchantment', to use a Weberian concept, that determine processes of transformation and adjustment in social organisations and in the values of social work.

Actually, as several studies seem to confirm, neoliberal perspectives affect, in a widespread and transversal way, the social work practised in several countries, although with some local variations. The diverse teleology of the profession and forms of contestation and/or adjustment in various welfare services to this 'new' path are, therefore, placed on the front page of the professional agenda and require social workers to increase reflexivity and critical awareness about the thresholds between what can and, above all, what must be done.

In the present article, we intend to discuss, from the perspective of ten social workers interviewed, the impacts of the managerial logic arising from the current neoliberal demands, in the structuring and readjustment of the social work processes and its practice purposes. The metaphor, expressed in the title of the article, aims to translate the two orientations coexisting and connecting in this adaptive process. On the one hand are the possibilities opened by the current paradigm for the transformation of the assumptions and procedures of social work practice, introducing dimensions of greater systematicity, comparability and evaluation – what can be translated metaphorically as 'the Phoenix moment' of social work by reference to the mythological bird with capacity to reborn invigorated of the own ashes. On the other hand lie the possibilities of dilution of fundamental values of social work, making the practice empty of basic guiding principles and hence diluted in concerns of administrative proofs of how to act and what results are obtained. The practice thus risks being a mere space for legitimising institutional objectives and consuming time and energy of social workers who, in addition, do not identify with what is asked of them. This possibility is metaphorically translated into the expression 'black hole', a cosmic property with a powerful gravitational force that causes a deformation and condensation in the continuous space–time. As physicists nowadays admit bodies that fall into a black hole do not disappear, but they become essentially different. The pressure on social work to respond quickly and effectively to the various issues with which it is confronted, proving its relevance and measurable results on a continuous basis, can indeed transform practice into something essentially different by reference to the core values of the profession.

The argument that is discussed in this article is how social workers stand at the confluence of these two orientations. How do they adjust their practices, whether in daily action (what we call tactics), or in a more structural and supra-organisational way (what we call strategic adjustment)? This adjustment can allow to respond to the new neoliberal ethos without forgetting the values and fundamental principles that structure traditionally the aims and the identity of the profession.

For many social workers, thinking about the impacts and arguments of macroeconomic policies and their political and ideological implications on welfare models seems to be at the antipodes of professional responsibility (Spolander, Engelbrecht, & Sansfaçon, 2015). This explains, in a way, the relative discursive and operational passivity recognised by the various studies, by reference to certain measures of neoliberal scope and their implications for professional practice, decision-making and the attainment of the core values of the profession (Gal & Weiss-Gal, 2014; Garrett, 2009; Spolander et al., 2015).

Actually, 'neoliberalism' translates primarily a particular world vision: a political-social 'imaginary' that determines priorities to be followed and shapes, accordingly, services and processes. It models also, consequently, the forms of acceptance and naturalisation of those priorities and its effects, presented as inevitable and functional. As Healy (2001) underscores, due to the profound transformation of western welfare states and the rise of new public management guidelines, contemporary social work is 'markedly different to its professional antecedents', implying new forms of engagement and critical reflection. It is thus fundamental that social workers understand and discuss their current practices, identifying not only the theoretical and axiological models that shape them, but also reflecting about how rhetoric and neoliberal policies affect the decisions and specificity of the profession (Ferguson, 2004; Ferguson, 2009; Ferguson, Lavalette, & Whitmore, 2004; Garrett, 2013; Schram & Silverman, 2012; Spolander et al., 2015) – in other words, assuming a critical perspective that doesn't forget the specific *loci* of professional practice.

This reflection is even more pertinent in countries such as Portugal where the level of illegitimate inequalities and poverty reach still unacceptable levels and where the breadth of the welfare state was late and in many areas residual (in Titmuss' perspective) and experimental, in parallel with a fragile economy. Indeed, the Portuguese case is paradigmatic for several reasons, even within the so-called countries of the South of Europe. The Welfare State was implemented belatedly (1974) after a period of conservative dictatorship and has been continuously recalibrated due to divergent pressures arising in particular from European integration and in the euro area. At the same time, organisations and some professionals maintained a limited perspective of the philosophy of social rights, reducing them to a mere benefit and to corporate logics inherited from the period of fascist dictatorship (1932–1974). The bureaucracy itself and the functional rigidity of services along with the supplementary function of the state (the so-called 'providential society' always had a crucial role) has always been evident, even though it has accentuated itself with right-wing governments and moments of financial rescue that the country has been experiencing (1977, 1983, 2011). Within this scope, the neoliberal markers have been progressively assuming a greater centrality and presence since the late 1990s. However, they were boosted in the last decade during the financial crisis post 2008 and the austerity policies imposed by the Troika between 2011 and 2014. Several authors have highlighted the effects of such policies in the Portuguese context, both in the transformation of life forms and in the welfare state, with implications that extend to other South countries and to the European Union itself (Jessop, 2002; Silva, 2002).

(b) General presentation of the study

In the present article, it is not possible to analyse the various implications and dimensions of the welfare reforms under way. Only some effects, evidenced by Portuguese social workers, are discussed concerning the transformation of their practices in various public organisational contexts (social protection, health and employment). To that end, ten in depth field interviews were conducted with social workers in front-line (3) and middle management (7) functions.[1]

The qualitative exploratory study highlights the diversity of the processes in course under the managerialism paradigm. First, its pernicious effects are explicit in line of other studies already carried out. Secondly, it is possible to identify the aspects that Portuguese social workers recognise as (potentially) positive in current management models. However, the goal was to go further than a mere diagnostic identification of impacts. It was also intended to identify the processes used for adjustment or ongoing professional reconstruction. In this context, it is possible to highlight different ways of adjustment to current changes, either in order to take advantage of them to achieve objectives of greater visibility and axiological affirmation of the profession, what is called 'strategic adjustment', or to pragmatically combine the demands of the daily practice with the perceived values of the profession, what is called of 'tactics adjustment'.[2]

(c) Structure of the article

The article is structured in two parts. First, is discussed the neoliberal 'social imaginary',[3] as well as the processes of diffuse rationalisation that it engages. Secondly, are presented the study results arguing the impacts of the social and political neoliberal imaginary in the practice of social work, and how it can 'dissolve' or 'recover' otherwise the symbolic anchors of the profession.

2. Neoliberalism as 'social imaginary'

The understanding of neoliberalism as a multifaceted and widespread phenomenon implies conceiving it as economic theory, ideology, political paradigm and social imaginary (Evans, 2010; Harvey, 2010; Spolander et al., 2015). Each one of these four dimensions acquires, in addition, different connotations depending on the geopolitical context in which they are expressed and the prioritised analysis angle. However, it is a fact that neoliberalism is much more than an economic doctrine. It is essentially a constructor of political discourses and the respective socio-ideological options and perspectives.

In effect, the association of certain current features (e.g. privatisation, withdrawal from the state in the provision of social services or competitiveness) with what is conventionally called neoliberalism seems to be scientifically and historically debatable. These traits were already present, one way or another, in Smith's or Stuart Mill's classic and reformist liberalism. For both, the road to equality and prosperity would only be ensured with the freedom of the market and a minimum of state interference. In this sense, the prefix 'neo' would translate essentially the evolution of such ideals embodied in capitalist functioning and exacerbated in a global context. It could be, thus, hypothesised that what seems to be indeed specific to the current moment is the dissemination of business rationalisation to all organisations and services outside the market, and in the processes of social functioning and thought. In other words, it is the levels and mechanisms of legitimation and wide diffusion of a 'productivist rationality' that are today unique and reticular.

'Neoliberalism' conceived as a 'social imaginary' is, in fact, perhaps the most globalised and profound feature of the phenomenon, contributing to enhance or justify its remaining dimensions. In fact, under the ambiguous adjective of neoliberal are aggregated a set of narratives that shape individual and collective behaviours and options, and, in parallel, contribute to the naturalisation and legitimation of certain socio-political intervention strategies, models of development and profound organisational reforms (Deeming, 2017; Ferguson, 2004).

Paradoxically, the deeper impact of the neoliberal narrative lies precisely in the incoherence between liberal discourses and current practices (Garrett, 2013): the dilution of the utopian sense of a better future that guided the modern project. As Wilkinson and Pickett (2009) have pointed out, 'for several decades, progressive politics have been seriously weakened by the loss of any concept of a better society' (2009, p. 240). Now, the promise of 'decent development' and progress shows, according to various data and analysts, its structural failure (Jessop, 2012; Piketty, 2014).

Still, even in the face of a global capitalist crisis scenario, as happened in 1930 and more recently in 2008, the idea that the system 'works' is not shaken in its essential pillars. As Jessop (2012) puts it, at such moments it seems to emerge essentially only a transmutation on the narratives: from a crisis 'in the system' to a crisis 'of the system' (p. 25). The possibility of profound reform is thus delegitimized and anchored above all in austerity programmes that tend to reconfirm principles.

That way, neoliberal imaginary persists and reinforces. In addition to influencing individual and collective values and practices, it determines a set of concepts of social functioning and legitimation of the associated narratives and assumptions.

A critical questioning of these assumptions presupposes, for instance, the emphasis on the idea that existing inequalities and the judgment about their (il)legitimacy do not arise – primarily – from the mere scarcity or lack of socioeconomic resources, but rather of multiple and interlocking processes of differentiated factors, themselves products and producers of complex forms of individual and collective organisation. Thus, it is particularly important to assess how current inequalities are analysed, understood and justified, politically and socially. It is such judgments that allow (or not) to base processes of social indignation that could trigger a socio-political critical action aimed to surpass illegitimate inequalities as a core aim of social work. Axiological rationality, translated into values and beliefs (individual and social) about what is considered socially and ethically (in)adequate, plays thus a central role in determining instrumental rationality.

Despite all the failed promises, contradictions and ruptures, the neoliberal socio-political imaginary has expanded throughout the world. In fact, it is presented currently not only as the sole possible narrative after 1989 but as the most effective for building more free and developed societies, thus justifying the 'good reasons' (Boudon, 2003) to be pursued and undeniable. Neoliberal discourse and imagery become thus a kind of 'common sense', a 'taken-for-granted consciousness of millions of people' (Ferguson, 2004, p. 1).

The central question that underlies this article is not however the understanding of the complex mechanisms of the current social indignation' numbness associated with this 'consensual' vision of the world, but rather of their respective effects on the practices and values of social work.

2.1. Impacts in social work

Several studies (Ferguson & Woodward, 2009; Lombard, 2008; Marobela, 2008; Spolander et al., 2014; Wastell, White, Broadhurst, Peckover, & Pithouse, 2010, among others) have shown that the impacts of neoliberal assumptions in social work practices are widespread and profound throughout the world, despite some local variations, both in the reconfiguration of public policies and in institutional management.

Although debates on the (il)legitimacy of social work and the question 'what is it for?' are not new in the history of the profession, perhaps in the present time unique elements are evidenced. The hypothesis argued is that the deepest and most complex of these elements is the possible antinomy between social work's axiological core and the current 'disenchantment of the world' (as Weber understands it) provoked by neoliberal 'rationalisation'.

Without the ability to generalise to all the fields of practice, there is evidence of generic 'disenchantment' traits on contemporary social work: the loss of a long-term temporal reference allowing the systematic transformation of life trajectories or political frameworks; the loss of a supra individual reference allowing complex and systemic understanding of social problems and its causes; the progressive loss of an argumentative universe associated with social rights and the fairness of decisions, to the detriment of their reasonableness and defensibility. Within this scope, the imagery of permanence can replace that of social change; the imaginary of effectiveness and results (read under the organisational prism, thus functional and immediate) can replace a priority concern with the process; the imaginary of individual responsibility can replace that of collective solidarity.

Data from the study conducted near ten Portuguese social workers put some light on the ongoing adjustment processes in several practice settings. The main idea is to understand how social workers can conduct and readjust their practices bounded by politics and orientations strange to social work's universe of sense and introduced by neoliberal imaginary.

3. Impacts and adjustments of social work practices in Portugal under the neoliberal social imaginary

The exploratory study is based in ten in depth field interviews, conducted with three social workers in front-line practice and seven in middle management functions. Considering the fields of practice that in Portugal are more affected by the current management paradigm – social protection (5 social workers), health (4) and employment (1) – we selected four public organisations (situated in Coimbra and Lisbon) and within them we asked for front-line and middle management social workers' voluntary collaboration. This convenience sampling doesn't allow data transferability to other practice fields and to other geographical contexts. Even so, although very limited, the conclusions of the study underscore relevant analytical clues to be explored in further studies, namely concerning the decision-making processes in diverse contexts and the argumentative readjustments. The interviews guide was structured in three global themes – (a) the impacts of management constraints in social work practices; (b) the adjustment processes; (c) the conceptions of the transformations ongoing in social work values. The data collected were analysed using thematic content analysis.

3.1. The impacts of the managerialism paradigm in social work practices

Several social workers interviewed recognise that professional daily practice is conceived today as an immense 'black hole', consumer of energies without producing significant results and potentially neutraliser of professional specificities. Social workers actually reveal feelings of 'deep loneliness', 'lack of hope', 'emotional and physical exhaustion', 'demotivation' ('it is not worth fighting for, I know I'm going to get upset and do not gain anything from it') and perplexity ('what is my role anyway?'; 'I no longer understand what I do and especially why I do it').

Similar results were obtained in other studies (Cowden & Singh, 2007; Jones, 2004, among others), revealing strong levels of dissatisfaction and stress among front-line workers as they feel that they work more for service performance than for an adequate response to clients. These risks are even more pronounced in contexts such as the Portuguese, where resources are scarce, inadequate or poorly distributed, in a scenario where, in fact, social services themselves are transmuted into replicas or hybrids of the corporate universe and lost part of their critical power and creativity when imprisoned in performance logics and contracts that are vital to their financial survival. As one social worker interviewed states, 'I feel that I am only working for the urgent and emerging'.

In truth, the increased demands for accountability, project applications and planning are not necessarily negative, as professionals interviewed have recognised, but only if they are envisioned as a means and not as an end in themselves. Focusing on performance can, in fact, divert attention away from fundamental but non-measurable aspects and keep professionals besides the core meaning of the profession (Webb, 2006). But it can engage also profitable and strategic opportunities, as professionals recognise.

In the study developed in Portugal, the various front-line professionals and middle managers consistently revealed aspects also evident in the other studies previously mentioned. In particular, (a) difficulties in work processes' management: lack of time; excessive bureaucracy; lack of proficiency in management language; lack of management skills among others; (b) transform-ation in the conception of the practice teleology and values: priority to results and procedural tasks; individualisation of social problems; priority to palliative care and placebo measures and standardized professional relationship with clients – a sort of 'fleeting empathy' as a social worker refers.

Nevertheless, the identified difficulties are accompanied, from the perspective of the interviewees, by 'gains' or factors to be strategically enhanced to overcome some constraints and to assure reor-ganisation and affirmation of Portuguese social work in political and scientific terms.

The feeling of being enslaved by an excess of bureaucracy, quantification and screening pro-cedures is reported by the totality of social workers interviewed. However, they also underline one aspect that has positive implications for social work's organisation and visibility in the various ser-vices: the creation of national Procedural Guideline Manuals. As they refer, although recognising that manuals make practice more standardised and rigid, they also open possibilities of greater 'security', comparability and crossover between services and case decisions, and serve to nullify, or minimise, what interviewed professionals called a previous 'excess of discretion' and 'bad practices' in various welfare services.

This possibility of decision comparability is extremely relevant, according to the perspective of interviewed social workers, not only to overcome suspicions of 'clientelism' and decisions only guided by their 'good sense' and intuition but also as a source of recognition and professional and scientific legitimacy. As a health sector middle manager states: 'It is important to implement a uniform reporting model and have comparable records to assert ourselves as a class'. This does not imply the defence of a standardised and mainly procedural practice, but rather a more planned and comparable one. In fact, the guidelines referred to in the manuals only ensure structural comparability, and do not override the substance of decisions and the uniqueness of case analysis.

For the large majority of middle managers contacted the margins of autonomy and power aug-mented within the managerial system – and that, not only due to the place of social work in the organisational structure of welfare public services – as a support service or intermediate manager – which is now more visible organically ('the opportunity is open!'), and the functions more clear, but also because their 'voice' is consequently more heard and respected.

Two reasons are pointed out to explain this perceived increased recognition of social workers by politicians and organisation managers. The first one is associated with a more demanding and qualified training (namely with the expansion, in Portugal, of masters and PhD degrees) and a more informed theoretical-operational framework. The second one is linked to the contribution of social work within the new management path. As stated, especially by middle managers, social workers are significantly well positioned to assure processes of information processing in the relation-ship and dialogue with increasingly informed and demanding populations. However, this can imply a new form of underground control of clients leaving behind substantive criticism concerning social policies and welfare goals. This aspect deserves thus a greater reflection of professionals so that their major visibility and functional power can be harnessed for the fulfilment of ethical and political purposes of social work in detriment of 'organisational peace'.

In contrast, it is possible to identify the rise of bureaucratic 'pinchers' and loss of autonomy in front-line work. Decision-making and evaluation processes are accompanied nowadays by the use of experts, most of whom are external to the social universe (managers, lawyers, judges, engin-eers), who seek to legitimize social workers' interventions and reports, so making interference at the heart of social work practice. This role is also often played in Portugal by the middle man-agers (social workers) who supervise and mediate between front-line social workers and top managers.

This process of constant assessment and revalidation of the work of front-line social workers, often implying the change of their own professional assessments, constitutes, as several middle managers interviewed stated, a new 'professional paternalism' not necessary and even 'dangerous' ('it is the front-line workers that know the real situations, I'm at the desk!'). As one of them declares,

I'm forced to act as if I don't have confidence in their [frontline professionals] work and so, many begin to disinvest ... in terms of writing and arguments. The losses and the work of all parts increases, results are not necessarily better.

A front-line social worker confirms 'our leaders respect our work but seek to influence our decisions, our opinions ... especially those that do not depend on the legislation'. In fact, this is associated with specialisation, hierarchical bureaucracy and the breakdown of work into small plots and tasks guided by precise guidelines that embody some of the fundamental organisational and processual changes.

This 'Taylorism breakdown' is presented, in public discourses, as a factor of effectiveness. Data show, however, an increase of repetitive tasks at different points of the circuit (constant revisions by peers and experts) and a loss of overall view, producing articulation difficulties and time losses – the paradoxes of a paradigm that defends 'specialisation' aiming to promote more integrated interventions.

In fact, interviewed professionals underline that social work in Portugal is still very far from a real integrated and reticular practice revealing the need to develop more collaborative strategies and shared experiences. Nevertheless, evidence show that the managerial demands increase the level of competitiveness among professionals with burdensome results for teamwork and quality of service.

The incentive to planning processes (work plans, SWOT analyses, monitoring grids, etc.) and use of ICT is considered by all the interviewed as a positive factor, but cannot constitute itself as a mere procedure, an additional task to be fulfilled, stripped of any practical effect. Several professionals referred to constant changes in levels of procedural urgency, revision of the calendars at the last moment, or change of rules without proper framing and monitoring, as factors that increase the inefficacy of services and personal attrition. A social security middle manager pointed out exactly this 'firefighter syndrome': 'we are systematically confronted with ultimatums of tasks that we have to do in the immediate, requests for data, statistics, last-minute situations', leading to 'constant tension and pressure that is translated in the lack of rigour of the final work and consequent feeling of frustration'.

3.2. Readjustment strategies: the 're-enchantment' of social work?

Beyond the diagnosis of the impacts of the neoliberal social and political imaginary on social work practice, the intention of the study is also to reveal how the social workers interviewed readjusted their practices and principles of action to the constraints associated with the new management paradigm – a readjustment involving various forms of resistance, tacit or explicit. In fact, social workers don't accept and adapt uncritically to the new constraints. They find different ways, some of them tacit, of combining and reconstructing both the response to managerial demands and the defence of social work's core values. In the study carried out, it is possible to identify two types of interconnected adjustment processes: a 'tactics adjustment' and a 'strategic adjustment'.

The first one acquires often surreptitious forms and allows managing, in the best way, an everyday practice corseted between management demands and attention to users' needs. As Certeau (1984) states, tactics adjustment 'is dispersed, but it insinuates itself everywhere, silently and almost invisibly, because it does not manifest itself through its own products, but rather through its ways of using the products imposed by a dominant economic order' (p. xii).

This kind of tactical adjustment is associated essentially with two aims: first, the recovery of time, from management tasks to the relationship and follow-up processes, and second, the breaking off of 'bureaucratic pinchers', from organisational walls to community engagement.

In the first case social workers refer to processes of faster registration (e.g. pre-written baseline texts adaptable to each situation); informal organisation of tasks within the team in periods of increased pressure; 'creaming' selection in the perspective worked by Lipsky (1980), or even working hours' extension, with important impacts in terms of burn-out feeling. These procedures allow to preserve or conquest, in some way, time to practise the 'real social work', the 'essence of professional work near clients and concrete-life settings', beyond management tasks and demands.

In the second case, social workers refer to the articulation with external partners and networks; parallel projects of community empowerment (sometimes as voluntary work); and social movements support or stimulus. As social workers state

> with this communitarian project I can surpass the boundaries and bureaucratic moorings of my organization and do what I think that it's really important to develop with populations. And I can do it because a great part of this work is invisible and cannot be controlled. I have to present results of course but I feel freer and more cooperative with clients. I feel more like a social worker.

The 'strategic adjustment' process is targeted towards the best use of the management transformations in progress to acquire greater power and recognition in organisations. This opens a new conception of 'activism' relatively unrecognised, as Healy (2001) underlines the strategic and intelligent use of the neoliberal path to promote the key role and aims of social work.

In the study developed in Portugal diverse strategies are referred to achieve this goal: (a) the establishment of working groups and reflection (in partnership with universities or consultants) for the creation of social work specific instruments of registration and evaluation; (b) the publication by social workers of study results and interventions' apprenticeship; (c) the association in discussion groups and scientific societies (e.g. the creation in course of the Scientific Society of Social Work) outside regular work organisations, as a strategy of lobbying and visibility; (d) the use of ICT to create (inter)national networks, blogs or other processes of 'making community'. More broadly, in Portugal, forms of resistance and professional affirmation are also associated with the ongoing creation of a Professional Order and the value of research as the foundation of academic and social recognition.

The strategic adjustment process is associated with larger forms of resistance to neoliberal imaginary allowing to preserve and defend the specific principles and values of the social work profession, namely using research skills and professional forums. The social worker's contribution to the evaluation of neoliberal social and political impacts and the transformation of social policies are important fields for social work aiming the preservation and concretisation of its core values. Moreover, the assertion of a consistent theoretical framework, coupled with an increasingly qualified training and research, the use of new technologies as a work tool, and enlarged partnerships and alliances can constitute as pillars of a (new) 'phoenix moment' of social work. 'Recognising the challenges from within, critical social workers can strengthen and diversify their capacity to forge critical approaches relevant to social work in the 21st century' (Healy, 2001, p. 1).

4. Final remarks

The current rationalising and standardised 'machine', expanded by the neoliberal imaginary, seems effective to create conditions to a 'crisis of the symbolic' of the professional social work universe. This does not mean that social workers do not continue to advocate a 'rational action based on values', in the Weberian sense, associated with social justice and human rights, but the conditions and content of work have shifted substantially. Social work's key values and commitment are currently confronted with many differentiated political and organisational assumptions. Social workers are increasingly confronted with the exigency to demonstrate simultaneously specific and generalist practice competencies, detailed knowledge of the practice field and managerial skills, in order to be competitive (Healy, 2001).

The neoliberal social and political imaginary, anchored in presuppositions of efficacy, rationality, rapidity, individualisation and assessment, and translated namely in organisational management demands, is in various aspects in dissonance with social work core values and principles of action (Amaro, 2015; Dominelli, 2009; Dustin, 2009; Evans, 2009; Gregory, 2007; Webb, 2006).

The adjustment of social workers to the new managerialism scenario often seems to translate mere acritical accommodation (Jordan, 2005). 'For some, following rules and being compliant can appear less risky than carrying the personal responsibility for exercising judgment' (Munro, 2011,

p. 5). However, as other recent studies (Aronson & Smith, 2010; Wallace & Pease, 2011) also show, in many situations and contexts social workers do not 'passively' accept current rules. On the contrary, they detour, using various strategies, the homogenising and performative service guidelines, either to preserve or affirm their professional identity or to ensure clients' well-being, assuming a sort of 'moral underground', as Lisa Dodson (2011) refers. Thus, the use of prudential judgement and discretion – elements of professionalism underscored by several authors (Evans, 2016; Lipsky, 1980, among others) – remain nowadays essential. Nonetheless, it is more 'discretion as used' than 'discretion as granted' (Hupe, 2013), putting in the foreground the responsibility and initiative of each professional to identify possibilities and to use them to assure the most fair response to clients' needs and rights.

The current transformation of social work is clear, but the interviewed Portuguese social workers reveal some critical adjustment processes that give good clues to understand the current possibilities of a more strategical and political-social work. A moment of reconstruction of contemporary social work is thus in process – a moment that does not imply necessarily a crisis of the symbolic and a loss of social work values, but the apprenticeship of new ways to achieve them, namely, maintaining the main axiological features of social work – the questioning of illegitimate inequalities and the demand for social justice – and building, in the same movement, more systematic and accountable responses. In the same way it is important to comprehend the impacts of neoliberal social imaginary in the concrete lives of citizens in distress and in the preservation of social justice. For this purpose not only is the individual commitment of social workers essential but also collective organisation (of populations and professionals themselves), ability to overcome immediacy and individualised responses, reflexivity in professional practice, and, above all, 'moral courage' (Banks, 2011).

At one time or another in its history, social work confronted itself critically with the paradoxes of its professional activity, often merely seeming to confirm the *status quo*. Critical and radical perspectives, particularly, provide a theoretical framework that could support a more interventionist structural approach in exposing inequalities and transforming policies and services and contributing to keeping alive the profession's central focus, its aims and values. But they also underscore the idea that an ethics of conviction, although necessary, is insufficient to question and supplant the present 'state of things'. In fact, currently, some decisions seem to be made more in terms of their defensibility than in their appropriateness and fairness (Parton, 1998). In this sense, an ethics of responsibility and justice must necessarily be coupled with convictions that engage processes of (re)awakening of social indignation and macro influence, understanding and revealing the systemic relationship between macroeconomic orientations, social demands and social justice expectations.

Notes

1. Mostly women (one man) and with more than ten years of professional experience.
2. Strategy and Tactics are used, in this article, in the perspective presented by Michel de Certeau in the 1980's (1984). He defines strategy 'as a calculus of force relationships when a subject of will and power [...]' can 'capitalize on its advantages, prepare its expansions, and secure independence with respect to circumstances' (p. xi). In contrast he understands tactics in a more labile way 'in which the weak are seeking to turn the tables on the strong". Tactics must depend on "clever tricks, knowing how to get away with things, the hunter's cunning, manoeuvres, polymorphic simulations, joyful discoveries' (p. xii).
3. Many authors used the term 'social imaginary' in very different ways (e.g. J. Thompson, J.M. Lacan, C. Taylor, among others). The concept used in this article is more associated with the perspective of Castoriadis (1975): each society constructs a meaning for itself, a singular way of living, conceiving and constructing its own existence in a particular historical time.

Disclosure statement

No potential conflict of interest was reported by the author.

ORCID

Cristina Pinto Albuquerque 🔟 http://orcid.org/0000-0003-4194-8554

References

Amaro, M. I. (2015). *Urgências e Emergências do Serviço Social: fundamentos da profissão na contemporaneidade*. Lisboa: UCE.

Aronson, J., & Smith, K. (2010). Managing restructured social services: Expanding the social? *British Journal of Social Work*, *40*(2), 530–547.

Banks, S. (2011). Ethics in an age of austerity: Social work and the evolving new public management. *Journal of Social Intervention: Theory and Practice*, *20*(2), 5–23.

Boudon, R. (2003). *Raisons, bonnes raisons*. Paris: PUF.

Castoriadis, C. (1975). *L'Institution imaginaire de la société*. Paris: Seuil.

Certeau, M. D. (1984). *The practice of every Day life*. Oakland: University of California Press.

Cowden, S., & Singh, G. (2007). The 'user': Friend, foe or fetish? A critical exploration of user involvement in health and social care. *Critical Social Policy*, *27*, 5–23.

Deeming, C. (2017). The lost and the new 'liberal world' of welfare capitalism. *Social Policy & Society*, *16*(3), 405–422.

Dodson, L. (2011). *The moral underground: How ordinary Americans subvert an unfair economy*. New York, NY: The New Press.

Dominelli, L. (2009). Repositioning social work. In R. Adams, L. Dominelli, & M. Payne (Eds.), *Social work: Themes, issues and critical debates* (pp. 13–25). Basingstoke: Palgrave Macmillan.

Dustin, D. (2009). *The McDonaldization of social work*. Oxford: Routledge.

Evans, P. (2010). Constructing the 21st century developmental state: Potentialities and pitfalls. In O. Edigheji (Ed.), *Constructing a democratic developmental state in South Africa potentials and challenges* (pp. 37–58). Capetown: HSRC Press.

Evans, T. (2009). Managing to be professional? Team managers and practitioners in modernised social work. In J. Harris & V. White (Eds.), *Modernising social work: Critical considerations* (pp. 145–164). Bristol: Policy Press.

Evans, T. (2016). *Professional discretion in welfare services. Beyond street-level bureaucracy*. New York, NY: Routledge.

Ferguson, I. (2004). Neoliberalism, the third way and social work: The UK experience. *Social Work and Society*, *2*, 479–493.

Ferguson, I. (2009). 'Another social work is possible!' reclaiming the radical tradition. In V. Leskošek (Ed.), *Theories and methods of social work. Exploring different perspectives* (pp. 81–98). Ljubljana. University of Ljubljana.

Ferguson, I., Lavalette, M., & Whitmore, E. (2004). *Globalisation, global justice and social work*. London: Routledge.

Ferguson, I., & Woodward, R. (2009). *Radical social work in practice: Making a difference*. Bristol: Policy Press.

Gal, J., & Weiss-Gal, I. (2014). *Social workers affecting social policy: An international perspective*. Bristol: Policy Press.

Garrett, P. M. (2009). Marx and 'modernization': Reading capital as social critique and inspiration for social work resistance to neoliberalization. *Journal of Social Work*, *9*, 199–221.

Garrett, P. M. (2013). *Social work and social theory*. Bristol: Policy Press.

Gregory, R. (2007). New public management and the ghost of max weber: Exorcized or still haunting? In T. Christensen, & P. Lægreid (Eds.), *Transcending new public management. The transformation of public sector reforms* (pp. 387–422). Surrey: Ashgate.

Harvey, D. (2010). *A brief history of neoliberalism*. Oxford: Oxford University Press.

Healy, K. (2001). Reinventing critical social work: Challenges from practice, context and postmodernism. *Critical Social Work*, *2*(1), Retrieved from http://www1.uwindsor.ca/criticalsocialwork/reinventing-critical-social-work-challenges-from-practice-context-and-postmodernism.

Hupe, P. (2013). Dimensions of discretion: Specifying the object of street-level bureaucracy research. *Zeitschrift für Public Policy, Recht und Management*, *6*(2), S425–S440.

Jessop, B. (2002). *The future of the capitalist state*. Cambridge: Polity Press.

Jessop, B. (2012). Narratives of crisis and crisis response: Perspectives from north and south. In P. Utting, S. Razavi, & R. Buchholz (Eds.), *The global crisis and transformative social change* (pp. 23–42). London: Palgrave Macmillan and UNRISD.

Jones, C. (2004). The Neo-liberal assault: Voices from the front-line of British social work. In I. Ferguson, M. Lavalette, & E. Whitmore (Eds.), *Globalisation, global justice and social work* (pp. 95–106). London: Routledge.

Jordan, B. (2005). New labour: Choice and values. *Critical Social Policy, 25*, 427–446.

Lipsky, M. (1980). *Street-level bureaucracy: Dilemmas of the individual in public services*. New York, NY: Russell Sage Foundation.

Lombard, A. (2008). The impact of social transformation on the non-government welfare sector and the social work profession. *International Journal of Social Welfare, 17*(2), 124–131.

Marobela, M. (2008). New public management and the corporatisation of the public sector in peripheral capitalist countries. *International Journal of Social Economics, 35*(6), 423–434.

McDonald, C., Harris, J., & Wintersteen, D. (2003). Contingent on context: Social work and the state in Australia, Britain and the United States. *British Journal of Social Work, 33*, 191–208.

Munro, E. (2011). The Munro Review of Child Protection Interim Report: The child's journey. Retrieved from https://www.gov.uk/government/publications/munro-reviewof-child-protection-interim-report-the-childs-journey

Parton, N. (1998). Risk, advanced liberalism and child welfare: The need to rediscover uncertainty and ambiguity. *British Journal of Social Work, 28*(1), 5–27.

Piketty, T. (2014). *Capital in the twenty-first century*. Cambridge: Belknap Press.

Schram, S. F., & Silverman, B. (2012). The end of social work: Neoliberalizing social policy implementation. *Critical Policy Studies, 6*(2), 128–145.

Silva, P. A. (2002). O modelo de welfare da Europa do Sul: Reflexões sobre a utilidade do conceito. *Sociologia – Problemas e Práticas, 38*, 25–59.

Spolander, G., Engelbrecht, L., Martin, L., Strydom, M., Pervova, I., Marjanen, P., ... Adaikalam, F. (2014). The implications of neoliberalism for social work: Reflections from a six-country international research collaboration. *International Social Work, 57*(4), 301–312.

Spolander, G., Engelbrecht, L., & Sansfaçon, A.P. (2015). Social work and macro-economic neoliberalism: Beyond the social justice rhetoric. *European Journal of Social Work*. doi:10.1080/13691457.2015.1066761

Wallace, J., & Pease, B. (2011). Neoliberalism and Australian social work: Accommodation or resistance? *Journal of Social Work, 11*(2), 132–142.

Wastell, D., White, S., Broadhurst, K., Peckover, S., & Pithouse, A. (2010). Children's services in the iron cage of performance management: Street-level bureaucracy and the spectre of Švejkism. *International Journal of Social Welfare, 19*, 310–320.

Webb, S. (2006). *Social work in a risk society*. Basingstoke: Palgrave Macmillan.

Wilkinson, R., & Pickett, K. (2009). *The spirit level: Why more equal societies almost always do better*. London: Allen Lane.

Romanian social workers facing the challenges of neo-liberalism

Asistenții sociali din România în fața provocărilor neo-liberalismului

Florin Lazăr ⓘ, Anca Mihai, Daniela Gaba, Alexandra Ciocănel, Georgiana Rentea and Shari Munch ⓘ

ABSTRACT

With a history of almost 90 years, professional social work in Romania once flourished up until World War II. The Communist Party disbanded the profession in 1968 and it was reinstated after the fall of the Iron Curtain in 1989. Within the context of the socio-economic transition from a centralised to a free-market economy, Romanian social policy and social work have evolved from a Marxist/socialist-type ideology, one that advocates for state intervention, to a libertarian/neo-liberal-type ideology, which promotes both state withdrawal from welfare provision and individuals taking responsibility for their own welfare. These two trends continue to co-exist subject to sometimes divergent forces such as international institutions and internal Romanian social pressures. Using a qualitative approach, we explore how Romanian social workers are adapting to the neo-liberal realities and identify three types of perceived challenges: 1. those related to regulation, 2. linked with collaboration in social work activity and 3. those related to the social worker-client relationship. Under neo-liberal pressures, the social worker's role of agent of social change becomes marginalised in daily practice, leaving little power to influence agency policies that negatively impact clients.

REZUMAT

Cu o istorie de aproape 90 ani, asistența socială profesionistă din România a cunoscut o perioadă de înflorire până la Al Doilea Război Mondial. Partidul Comunist a desfiintat profesia în 1968, aceasta fiind repusă în drepturi după căderea Cortinei de Fier în 1989. În contextul tranziției socio-economice de la o economie centralizată la una bazată pe piața liberă, politica socială românească și asistența socială au evoluat de la o ideologie de tip Marxist/socialist, care pleda pentru intervenția statului, la o ideologie de tip libertarian/neo-liberal care promovează atât retragerea statului din furnizarea bunăstării, cât și responsabilizarea individului de asigurare a bunăstării proprii. Aceste două tendințe continuă să co-existe, fiind influențate de factori uneori divergenți precum instituțiile internaționale și presiunile sociale interne din România. Folosind o abordare calitativă, explorăm cum se adaptează asistenții sociali din România la realitățile neo-liberale și identificăm trei provocări percepute: 1. cele referitoare la reglementări, 2. cele referitoare la colaborarea în activitatea de asistență socială și 3. cele referitoare la relația asistent social – client. Sub presiunile neo-liberale, rolul asistenților sociali de agenți ai schimbării sociale devine marginal în practica de zi cu zi, aceștia având puțină putere de a influența politicile organizației care au un impact negativ asupra clienților.

Introduction

The social work profession is constantly evolving in the context of changing public policies and of socio-economic dynamics (Jordan, 2007). Under the pressures of welfare retrenchment, social work core principles and values are questioned, as the quasi-continuous austerity (Pierson, 1998) during the last two decades has led to constant restructuring of welfare systems (Jordan & Drakeford, 2012).

Although some social work scholarship has focused on the evolution of these policy shifts in several European countries that experienced serious financial bailouts during the 2008–2010 economic crisis, such as Greece, Spain, Portugal, Ireland or Italy (Garrett & Bertotti, 2017; Ioakimidis, Santos, & Herrero, 2014; Jordan & Drakeford, 2012; Karagkounis, 2017), little is known about how social work in peripheral Eastern European countries, such as Romania, experienced the austerity years (Pop, 2013).

In this paper we briefly analyse recent developments in Romanian social policies and social work amid international neo-liberal influences. Then, based on qualitative data, we explore the activities of Romanian social workers employed by public local authorities that manage (mainly) cash benefits to find out how these policies affect everyday practice.

Neo-liberal influences upon social work practice

Neo-liberalism is based on the principles of the free market, strengthened by the opportunities created by intense globalisation. Supported by international agencies, such as the World Bank, International Monetary Fund (IMF) and the World Trade Organisation (Abramovitz, 2012), the neo-liberal ideology has gained ground through the implementation of some of its economic principles in USA, UK, Western Europe and throughout the world, as seen in the early 1990s (Ferguson, 2004).

After communism's fall, neo-liberal principles entered Romanian public policies (Pop, 2013). The degree and nature of states' restructuring in accordance with neo-liberal agendas have not been a world-wide uniform process. This has led to various debates about how the changes in social policies during the post-communist decades in Central and Eastern Europe should be interpreted. Polese, Morris, Kovács, and Harboe (2014) describe these debates as polarised: on the one hand, seeing the post-communist transformation, as a process of 'Europeanisation' that changes the regional welfare systems into a Western European model or, on the other, seeing them as a sui generis case of welfare provision. However, the authors contend that there is a growing consensus in the literature on the main commonalities in the way social policies have been implemented internationally. First, the 'individualisation of the social' (Ferge, 1997) is a common theme. States shun social objectives such as equality and social cohesion and limit intervention that protects against social risks, counting, instead, on families, civil society and the free market as first welfare providers. Second is an emphasis on cash transfers along with a contraction of social services. Third is the privatisation of social protection as a response to the alleged deficient market and governance mechanisms for addressing social risks. Lastly, the devolution of provision and financing of social services and benefits to the local level have led to diminishing quality and growing inequality in accessing social services.

In a review of the literature on the impact of neo-liberal ideology and policies on social work, Wallace and Pease (2011) identify two types of general concerns: (a) the macro-impact on the welfare state and a consequent reconfiguring of social work and (b) the micro-impact at the level of practice that leads to changes in social workers' roles, professional identity, skills and values. At the macro-level, there is a growing concern related to the loss of legitimacy of the welfare benefits and a compromise of social work's moral authority due to the emphasis on managerialism (associated with corporatism and privatisation) and marketisation (associated with individualism and consumerism). At the micro-level, a perspective substantially less researched, Wallace and Pease (2011) argue that social workers' activities tend to be rather negatively affected by managerialism and marketisation. The authors assert that there is a growing perception of a devaluation of social workers' skills and knowledge by the replacement with skills driven by the managerialist logic of efficiency, calculability, predictability and control, and a reconstruction of professional relationships with clients that undermines social workers' power to support their clients.

The change of focus from providing services to documenting the allocation of social benefits through excessive form-filling and reporting not only leads to a weakening of social workers' skills (Harlow, Berg, Barry, & Chandler, 2013) but may actually drive them to change employers, either by shifting toward the less bureaucratic private sector or by changing fields all together. Social workers' focus on case management and social risks reduction without addressing root causes can lead to recruitment and retention difficulties (Harlow, 2004).

Neo-liberalism and the development of social policy and social work in Romania

Social work in Romania was established as an academic domain in 1929 and saw much growth during the inter-war period. After World War II, in 1968 the communist rule dissolved social work practice and education for ideological reasons (Buzducea, 2009; Lazăr, 2015).

The field of social work was reintroduced in Romania at the academic level in 1990, but the regulation of the profession followed more than a decade later with successive laws of social assistance (in 2001, 2006 and 2011) regarding the organisation of cash benefits and social work services, the recognition of the statute of social workers (law 466/2004) and a code of ethics (Lazăr, 2015). Despite specific provision in the Law of Social Assistance 292/2011 requiring each of the 3,181 administrative units (Ministry of Regional Development and Public Administration, 2018) to have a social work service, in 2012 a deficit of 11,000 social workers in public social work services (at both local and county level) was registered; also, roughly 30% of the rural localities and 8% of small urban settlements had no social work department (Teşliuc, Grigoraş, & Stănculescu, 2015, p. 122).

Evolution of international organisations' influences since 1990

The international organisations (World Bank, IMF, EU) aiming to support Romania's transition to the market economy promoted solutions that added global neo-liberal pressures (Cahill, Cooper, Konings, & Primrose, 2018) to the negative social consequences of the economic contraction following structural reforms (e.g. increased poverty and social inequalities) in the first decade post 1989.

The World Bank was involved since the early post-communist period in the drafting of the first Romanian social welfare law in 1995. In the late 1990s to early 2000s, the United States Agency for International Development (USAID) encouraged and financed the efforts to regulate and establish a professional body of social workers (the Romanian National College of Social Workers was created in 2005) and the recognition of the professional statute of social workers. During the early 2000s the World Bank and IMF lessened their involvement as Romania had improved its economic performances and had started the process of adhering to the EU.

The European support was especially influential in reshaping Romanian social policy after the late 1990s with the beginning of the EU accession process. This, on the one hand, forced Romanian authorities to adopt specific legislation aligned with EU 'acquis communautaire' in the area of social policy and, on the other hand, financed various social programmes (mainly civil society organisations) through the EU structural funds (pre-accession until 2007 and through European Social Fund after 2007).

The European Union's effect on social policies manifested itself in a focus on individual responsibility for one's own welfare (e.g. the replacement of the social welfare means-tested cash benefit, created in 1995 under the guidance of the World Bank with a guaranteed minimum income – GMI – establishing community working hours for adult recipients since 2001) and a policy-focus change from poverty reduction to social inclusion.

However, at the end of the 2000s IMF and World Bank reignited an interest in the country as Romania faced the impact of the 2008 economic crisis. Thus, in 2010 austerity measures were implemented with some cash benefits cut by 15% or completely dissolved and subsidies related to social work services provided by NGOs ceased (Lazăr, 2015).

As of 2011, the World Bank supported the Romanian government in reforming the social assistance national programme to reduce fraud and increase efficiency (e.g. reduce expenses for social assistance) (Pop, 2013; World Bank, 2011). Currently, the World Bank's influence on the development of the social work profession remains strong, as its specialists are providing technical assistance and financial support in implementing major changes in the social assistance system in accordance with the National Strategy on Social Inclusion and Poverty Reduction 2015–2020, drafted with World Bank's support as well (Ministry of Labour, Family, Social Protection and Elderly, 2015).

Internal domestic factors and changes in social work practice

Approaches on the part of international organisations swung between a neo-liberal agenda (mainly from the World Bank, IMF and USAID) and a conservative-type welfare regime (Pop, 2013). The welfare state in most Central and Eastern European countries (Romania included) developed in a hybrid system, integrating elements from traditional models (Bismarckian and Anglo-Saxon) in their internal social, economic and political contexts (Fenger, 2007; Hemerijck, 2013; Kovács, Polese, & Morris, 2017).

One of the first signs of a neo-liberal turn was the push toward the privatisation of social work. Law 466/2004, art. 9 on the statute of social workers (developed with USAID support) stipulates that social workers registered with the National Register of Social Workers (n.d.) (administrated by the National College of Social Workers in Romania – NCSWR) with at least five years of practice experience are allowed to establish 'private individual professional practice offices', similar to the regulation in the United States (Lord & Iudice, 2012). The competition for the provision of private social services has been encouraged slowly but steadily since 1998, evolving from subsidies to NGOs (Law 34/1998) to concession, procurement (2001, 2006, 2012) and grant financing (2005) (Teşliuc et al., 2015, p. 106). Moreover, legislation governing social work from 2011 allows public authorities to contract/outsource the delivery of services to private agencies, NGOs or private practice offices. These measures lead to an uneven development of social services, favouring their growth in richer municipalities. The unequal distribution of services is one of the consequences of the state's withdrawal from ensuring social protection for all, as emphasised in the first and the third of the commonalities presented above (Polese et al., 2014).

A second sign of a neo-liberal agenda is seen in steps purportedly aimed to assure quality and control. A managerial perspective is reflected in the provision from law 292/2011 establishing a ratio of one social worker to 300 clients. At the end of 2017 (Decree no. 797, published in November 2017) supplemental regulations provided lower thresholds depending on the type of services/activities: one case manager for up to 50 cases in child protection, work with older people, persons with disabilities and foster carers, and up to 300 cash benefits claimants.

However, while the primary focus of work is on social assistance benefits, among the responsibilities of those working at local level are the identification of needs, testing the means, drafting and implementing intervention plans, to monitor active cases, to develop strategies to address the identified needs of individuals from the community or of the community at large. As such, the social worker may assess the situations of the 300 benefits claimants in this highly regulated field, but not have time to address the underlying causes of their situations.

The status of the social inspectors was enhanced in 2016 (Ordinance no. 82/2016), gaining more authority to (a) verify the public and private social service providers and (b) check the social assistance benefits transfers in order to eliminate any case of error and fraud. But standardisation and control over practice in order to ensure economic efficiency, although it aims at helping clients (Gray, Dean, Agllias, Howard, & Schubert, 2015), leaves little room for social workers' judgement and discretion, potentially resulting in harm to service users (Ferguson, 2004).

These changes are impacting the activities of Romanian social workers as they feel they do not have enough time for working directly with clients. Moreover, two thirds of social workers perceived that their caseload had increased in the previous two years and one third believed that monitoring and supervision/control increased, whilst 40% reported a decrease in financing of social work programmes in the previous two years (Lazar, Dégi, & Iovu, 2016).

Given the focus of the literature on the disadvantages of a neo-liberal approach exacerbated by austerity measures (Jordan & Drakeford, 2012) and the challenges previously reported by Romanian social workers (Lazar et al., 2016), our qualitative study aims to explore the tension between professional values, standards and goals versus managerial preferences related to legal regulations and dominant ideology communicated through policy formation.

Methods

The data presented below is part of a research project examining the workforce of social work professionals in Romania.

We explore the daily work challenges (e.g. stressful aspects of job-related activities and main obstacles) faced by Romanian social workers employed in the public social services departments within public local authorities. We interpret the findings against the neo-liberal influences discussed above, with the aim of identifying links associated with this ideology and the stressful obstacles that social workers encounter in their daily activities.

This study received ethical approval from the University and was endorsed by the Executive Committee of the National College of Social Workers in Romania.

The data analysed for this study were collected through 10 semi-structured, face-to-face interviews with social workers employed in the public services for social work within their local councils/municipalities. Enrolment in the study occurred during the 11-months recruitment period from September 2016 through July 2017 using a snowball sampling approach: (a) we contacted social workers from the researchers' professional network and recognised by the local social work community, requesting they recommend social workers for interviews; (b) we mailed formal letters (especially to public institutions) inviting social workers to participate in the research; and (c) we included an optional item in our online questionnaire inviting respondents to provide their contact information for possible participation in the qualitative part of the study.

The audio-recorded interviews lasted an average of one hour. The interview guide covered themes such as working conditions, professional relationships, professional development and work-life balance. The average age of the respondents was 42, (ranging between 31 and 55 years old), employed as social workers for an average of 10.5 years (min. 4 – max. 18). All the respondents were women who had studied social work in Romania, with three of them employed in the field before graduating with a social work bachelor's degree. The respondents worked in different counties in rural (3 respondents) and urban areas (7 respondents).

Interviews were transcribed verbatim and two of the researchers, including the researcher who conducted the interviews, conducted the thematic analysis and coding. We used thematic analysis to analyse the major themes found within the data set (Boyatzis, 1998; Braun & Clarke, 2006). Given the exploratory purpose of our study, the themes were derived directly from the interviews, using an inductive thematic analysis approach (Vaismoradi, Turunen, & Bondas, 2013). MS Word was used for identification of themes and MS Excel for managing the corresponding quotes. The two coders independently coded each of the interviews line-by-line to develop a coding tree. These two investigators met regularly to discuss and reconcile the codes into higher order analytic concepts, resulting in three main categories.

Results

Social workers reported that their employment in public social services posed stressors that severely challenged their daily professional practice: lack of resources for meaningful intervention; insufficient collaboration with other institutions; tangled and uncorrelated legislation; and misunderstanding of the roles and tasks of social work (on the part of clients, external institutions and even other departments within the social worker's host organisation).

The central three themes that illustrate these challenges as described by the participants are: (a) obstacles and stress related to regulation, (b) limits of collaboration in social work activity and (c) the social worker-client relationship. To protect anonymity, we use 'Q' to indicate the interviewer's question and 'A' to represent the respondent's answer, followed by the respondent's number of years of professional social work practice experience.

Obstacles and stressful aspects related to regulation

Participants articulated that they were under constant pressure from regulation (e.g. laws, decisions, orders, norms, standards, procedures and other legal documentation). This normative approach to social work regulated every step of the intervention, which then limited their intervention process and their professional discretion by increasing the focus on compliance to reporting procedures.

Some respondents identified regulations as obstacles to effective intervention, leading to stress. In most interviews, social workers consider that the legislation they use in their daily work is changing too often, which makes it difficult to implement, and also that it is too restrictive, not leaving much room for the social worker's discretion:

> A: Legislation … is restrictive, we don't have too many loopholes to read beside the letter of the law. Therefore, we need to apply the law as it is and it doesn't provide too many solutions. [18 years of practice]

Others consider that the legislation should be simplified, made more specific and coherent:

> A: For instance, for social support benefit [guaranteed minimum income], the income is granted starting with the 1st of the next month; for supplementary allowance, you establish the right with the date of the submission of the request; for kindergarten tickets, there are also [other rules]; there are a few more issues because, you establish, not sure when, after the child fulfils the criteria, he goes to the kindergarten and all that. And you, working like this with all the laws, you start to wonder: but in that case, [in the law] how is it or [what should be done] in the other case!? But a consistent legislation would be good. [4 years of practice]

Some respondents discussed that they feel discouraged from innovating and looking for new resources or developing new social work activities or seeking out funding opportunities due to the great and increasing legislative instability. Some respondents reported that the ambiguities in understanding how to adhere to certain regulations led to informal cooperation between peers, creating an informal group of professionals from different localities with similar positions, whose members meet and discuss how certain provisions are to be implemented.

In addition to instability and the red tape generated, another perceived limit of the existing regulation is its exclusionary effects. One experienced respondent (15 years of practice) identified that the current social policies produce social exclusion because of the uneven distribution of social work services at the local level (for example in rural areas or small towns). Respondents explain this shortage of public social services by mentioning the lack of financial, human and material resources. They perceive that decision-makers do not find it necessary to employ more social workers to provide social services, due to the allegedly low number of clients. In the meantime, social workers are facing high workloads, keeping them busy responding to incoming requests from service users and only seldom screening new cases/applicants.

Some of the respondents also viewed political influences as obstacles mainly because they (a) allow no or limited space for innovation and creativity to design services adjusted to the local needs, (b) perpetuate a low profile of the profession, as most of the decisions are imposed top-down, without real consultation with the grass-roots social workers and with no clear political commitment towards social workers, and (c) are used as tools for stimulating the electorate in elections' periods, when more votes to support the status quo are needed:

Q   Are there any other stressful activities on your job?
A   Hmm … the ones strictly connected to these hasty activities, 'let's do something, to obtain political capital', near events of political nature … [11 years of practice]

The social worker employed in the mayor's office, especially in the communes, is responsible for the allocation of social benefits for the clients who may not be aware of procedures to allocate social benefits. As a result, it may appear to the clients as though the mayor decides who receives the benefits or the services. Thus, the allocation of social benefits to clients, some of whom live in poverty, may have unintended political consequences.

In small cities or rural areas, where the 'social assistance department' is integrated within the city hall and several formal leaders of the community have conflicting political perspectives (i.e. are members of different parties), social workers are caught between the quintessential 'rock and a hard place'; at times the social workers must convene several community leaders to make decisions together in difficult cases concerning children:

I faced reservation from my superior, especially last year during pre-electoral campaign, […], when [another informal leader] and himself, [the latter] who was running for office, […] hold different [conflicting] political opinions. So, I couldn't include both [in a meeting] without upsetting my superior. [6 years of practice]

Other challenges that social workers perceive as obstacles in their daily practice include: (a) the preference for top-down management decisions, which affects the productivity and loyalty of professionals; (b) the employment of personnel without social work education for positions requiring qualified social workers; (c) lack of services in the rural areas or small cities, where the needs are perceived to be higher than in larger cities, where there are more social and economic opportunities; and (d) lack of flexibility (and resources) to generate needs-based social services.

Limits of inter- and intra-institutional collaborations

Interviewees, ideally, viewed collaboration with colleagues from other departments in the same or other institutions as a positive, desirable activity. However, this is seldom the case in practice since sometimes collaborations are impeded either by bad administrative organisation or by the more general undervaluing of social work.

Some social workers mention a weak inter-institutional collaboration, as suggested by a social worker with 15 years of practice experience:

There is no common vision, every director of GDSWCP [General Directorate on Social Work and Child Protection] has his/her own vision, similar to the situation of the mayors […] maybe the Agency for Payments and Social Inspection [APSI] has another vision and there is not always consensus [between the GDSWCP director] with the ones from APSI.

Most of the respondents described the shortage of social workers to design, elaborate and deliver the social services as an obstacle to their collaborative work. Support from colleagues might also be limited due to heavy workloads caused by understaffing and insufficient number of qualified social workers. These factors increase stress for less experienced social workers, who might not always have access to supervision and, instead, have to rely on their colleagues or expertise:

[…] especially when you are new to the job, it is absolutely necessary for [the other team members] to help you and guide you because no matter how much you read the legislation … this is something that happened to me too … no matter how thoroughly you read a new law or set of laws that you need to work with, their interpretation is strenuous and requires work experience. That's a must, ok? [6 years of practice]

Even though human interactions may be generally positive within the employee's? institution, collaboration with other offices (from the same institution) may be described as limited. Thus, despite colleagues being friendly to the social worker, the social worker's assigned roles are perceived rather negatively as their job connotes an allocation of existing funds and not collecting them (i.e. is an expenditure of public resources):

> First of all, the social work department brings no money, no funds, and although the [financial]value of social benefits is relatively small, all the time, when we go to meetings [...] it's obvious that we want something. One time, in a discussion with my superior she told me: 'You, tell me, what do you want? Well, every time you come, you want something.' [4 years of practice]

In this context, one may feel that one's work is not valued, that one's proposal to offer support to citizens in the locality is draining the budget and, therefore, one should keep all requests to allocate resources to a minimum.

Obstacles and stressful aspects related to the social worker-client relationship

Our analysis revealed that the focus on the social worker–client relationship, the hallmark of the social work profession, remains paramount among social workers' concerns. However, most of those interviewed mentioned having experienced stressful situations in their relationships with clients, which can be viewed from either a structural or an interpersonal standpoint.

Most of these tensions seem to be fuelled by the macrosocial obstacles to practice previously identified in this paper (e.g. the overall resource scarcity, the difficult collaboration with other departments and professionals on specific cases). Several social workers highlighted their limited power to help certain clients, while at the same time acknowledging the wider societal determinants that lead to a lack of sustainable solutions for most of the social problems at the local level. For example, one social worker (13 years of experience) mentioned the scarce local employment opportunities available to clients, which links to wider societal phenomena such as the high migration of the youth, leaving behind an ageing population among whom persons who are 45–50 years old and low-skilled predominate.

The respondents questioned the 'one size fits all' poverty-alleviation policy without taking into consideration the varying living contexts (e.g. the differing needs in urban areas vs. the rural areas, the possibility to labour the land in agricultural areas vs. in mountain where fewer opportunities exist).

From an interpersonal point of view, several social workers felt that their clients' expectations of them were too high. This, coupled with clients' frequent unwillingness to fully cooperate and participate in the intervention processes (e.g. clients failing to provide documentation according to agreed deadlines resulting in cessation of benefits) were mentioned by social workers as barriers to successful work or as major sources of occupational stress. One exasperated respondent explained:

> And I have clients from years and years and I consider I explain pretty clear and [in ways that they can understand], which are their responsibilities, for example. Working the hours, with working all the needed hours in a month, because if not, you get suspended [from receiving the GMI] even for one-two missing days; with bringing the documents, every 3 months because this is written in the law, [...] there are clients who for years don't get used to this procedure. And they think that it will be overlooked, I mean [they say things like] `what if I haven't brought it last month and I bring it this month why do you have to suspend me? [4 years of practice]

Most of the interviewees reported problems related to an excessive workload caused by the deficient organisation of social work at all levels. Bureaucratic and overly complicated procedures for benefits allocation (e.g. extensive paper work, end of month reporting) are labour-intensive, at the expense of building relationships with clients and developing social services. For example, because of the limited time available for each client, counselling sessions tend to become brief, on-the-spot interventions on urgent or crisis matters, without attention to a more sustainable long-term counselling plan.

Some respondents consider that clients become dependent on welfare benefits and suggest that these benefits could be allocated on a temporary basis, while the savings are invested in social services. This perspective on the benefits allocation reveals the social workers' expectations that their clients become more pro-active in identifying formal solutions to their financial problems outside the state's support.

The social worker – client relationship is marked by the tension between the state's responsibility to protect its citizens and the individual's responsibility to provide for themselves. These perspectives emerge from the social workers' discourses: on the one hand, some have more understanding of the clients' situations, identifying reasons outside the clients' control, while, on the other, some favour restricting social benefits in order to encourage recipients to find formal work.

Discussion

We explored how Romanian social workers employed in public welfare offices (an under-investigated population) are adapting to the neo-liberal realities. The 10 social workers interviewed conveyed their subjective experiences of challenges related to regulation, collaboration in social work activity and the social worker-client relationship. The focus on managerialist logic is considered to be one feature of the neo-liberal approach that negatively impacts social work practice (Wallace & Pease, 2011). Extensive regulation, as a sign of managerialism, seems to be the most stressful aspect of neo-liberalism for social workers in the context of increased workloads and tightened budgets in the last few years (Lazar et al., 2016). Resources are insufficient to properly address clients' needs and add to the challenges faced by frontline social workers and generate tensions between the structural constraints (e.g. unequal access to and reduced funding for social services, low wages of social workers, uncoordinated social policies) and professional ethical imperatives (e.g. to adjust the intervention to the needs of the client/community to allocate resources for prevention of social problems, promote social justice, anti-discriminatory practice, self-determination, fighting social inequalities), as also seen in Ireland and Italy (Garrett & Bertotti, 2017).

The focus on paperwork alongside tighter eligibility criteria for benefits are other features of a neo-liberal perspective (Ferguson, 2004) pointed to also by Romanian social workers in this study, who claim they spend too much time reporting and monitoring clients' compliance with rules and procedures. Our findings are consistent with previous studies that have identified social workers' focus on processing of paperwork to be related to the management of cash benefits (Matarese & Caswell, 2017) and the increasing monitoring and surveillance of claimants of welfare benefits (Fletcher & Wright, 2017). Overly-bureaucratic work amid changing regulations and rather limited resources contributes to maintaining the focus of social workers in public welfare offices on allocating financial benefits, rather than delivering expert social work services through specialised social work skills/professional competences (e.g. psychosocial counselling). We argue that the social workers in our sample perceive themselves as street-level bureaucrats in charge of implementing national regulations and less able to exert their role of agents of social change (Garrett, 2014; Noordograaf, 2016).

Social workers in our sample are aware of the structural determinants of clients' vulnerability revealing critical reflection and understanding of the society (Ioakimidis et al., 2014). The 'blaming of the poor' (Abramovitz, 2012) is observed among a small number of social workers in our sample, but the Romanian media is 'scapegoating' some social assistance clients who 'sneak between the cracks' of the system (i.e. making fraudulent claims) and wrongly deem all clients 'undeserving' (Chelcea & Druță, 2016).

Our findings on the challenges faced by social workers in everyday inter-institutional collaboration suggest that joint working in concrete activities is undermined by the social workers' mistaken identity on the part of decision-makers as well as other co-workers. As Wallace and Pease (2011) pointed out, devaluation of social work is a challenge stemming from the managerial and neo-liberal focus, but, more broadly, also a sign of the struggle for recognition (e.g. identity work) carried out by social workers in a changing environment. Moreover, in the Romanian context, this misrecognition could also be exacerbated by the corruption of some local public officials (e.g. decision-makers and politicians) when employing staff without social work qualifications to conduct roles usually reserved for professional social workers.

The negative political influence was also underlined by social workers in our sample who pointed to the use of social assistance benefits for political gains but also the challenges for social work practice as a result of conflicting political views of local leaders. This was also identified in the Southern/Latin Rim welfare states (e.g. Italy), marked by clientelism in the provision of social entitlements to specific interest groups (Ferrera, 1996).

The interactions between the social worker and the client are determined by regulations, as the rights and obligations of both parties are specified in legal documents. For the social workers in this sample, it seems that some challenges arise from their own expectations regarding the behaviour of the clients (e.g. to be actively involved in the process or to comply with social workers' recommendations), which is to be found in other areas of practice as well such as child protection, juvenile justice and mental health (Liebenberg, Ungar, & Ikeda, 2015). The interplay between structural constraints and social work ethics and values seems to contribute to the emergence and constant widening of an underlying tension of the social worker–client relationship, creating a gap between what social workers can do and what they are expected to do, a tension that is very well explained by social work's location 'at the juncture of the individual and society' (Abramovitz, 2012, p. 42).

The limitation of the small sample size leads us to refrain from generalising the challenges faced by social workers identified in this study. Our sample comprised only women and it is possible that male social workers might have had different perspectives on the stressful aspects of their work. Social workers from other types of localities than those represented in this sample (e.g. villages or small cities) may find differing or additional obstacles to practice, resulting in other sources of stress. Despite these limitations, we believe that the rich findings obtained in this exploratory study are useful as a first step in understanding the impact of neo-liberalism on Romanian public welfare social workers and perhaps on social work practice in other countries as well.

In conclusion, our study begins to illuminate some of the specific ways in which neo-liberalism has impacted social work practice in Romania. Alongside established factors such as the managerialist focus, increased bureaucracy and workload and devaluation of social work practice, we identified the negative role of political actors in the context of reinstatement of the profession, the continuous tension between client and agency accountability that social workers experience and the on-going fight of Romanian social workers to bring about the social change that inspires them in their daily work. Moreover, our study highlights the risk of *self*-devaluation for social workers in local welfare offices facing multiple challenges. Social workers need to be consulted more often in the process of decision-making and have more opportunities to better adjust resources to the needs of the communities and clients in order to provide better services as they are the experts of policy implementation. Supervision could be one of the strategies to reduce job-related stress experienced by social workers as a result of various constraints (Kadushin & Harkness, 2014), while on an individual level social workers need to create self-care strategies that would allow them to better adapt to everyday obstacles/stress (Wagaman, Geiger, Shockley, & Segal, 2015). Future research could focus more on the impact of the changing policies on social work practice, on how networking among social workers contributes to addressing clients' needs and on how to find a balance between bureaucratic procedures and professional discretion in delivering social services of high quality.

Acknowledgment

This research was conducted in partnership with the National College of Social Workers of Romania with financial support from the Romanian National Authority for Scientific Research and Innovation, CNCS – UEFISCDI, project number PN-II-RU-TE-2014-4-2322/361/2015.

Disclosure statement

No potential conflict of interest was reported by the authors.

Funding

This research was conducted in partnership with the National College of Social Workers of Romania with financial support from the Romanian National Authority for Scientific Research and Innovation, CNCS – UEFISCDI, project number PN-II-RU-TE-2014-4-2322/361/2015.

ORCID

Florin Lazăr http://orcid.org/0000-0002-4078-0617
Shari Munch http://orcid.org/0000-0002-4491-3480

References

Abramovitz, M. (2012). Theorising the neoliberal welfare state for social work. In M. Gray, J. Midgley, & S. A. Webb (Eds.), *The Sage handbook of social work* (pp. 33–50). London: SAGE Publications Ltd.
Boyatzis, R. E. (1998). *Transforming qualitative information: Thematic analysis and code development.* Cleveland: Sage.
Braun, V., & Clarke, V. (2006). Using thematic analysis in psychology. *Qualitative Research in Psychology, 3*(2), 77–101.
Buzducea, D. (2009). *Sisteme moderne de asistenţă socială. Tendinţe globale şi practici locale* [Modern social work systems. Global trends and local practices]. Iasi: Polirom.
Cahill, D., Cooper, M., Konings, M., & Primrose, D. (2018). *The SAGE handbook of neoliberalism.* London: SAGE.
Chelcea, L., & Druţă, O. (2016). Zombie socialism and the rise of neoliberalism in post-socialist Central and Eastern Europe. *Eurasian Geography and Economics, 57*(4–5), 521–544.
Fenger, H. M. (2007). Welfare regimes in Central and Eastern Europe: Incorporating post-communist countries in a welfare regime typology. *Contemporary Issues and Ideas in Social Sciences, 3*(2).
Ferge, Z. (1997). The changed welfare paradigm: The individualization of the social. *Social Policy & Administration, 31*(1), 20–44.
Ferguson, I. (2004). Neoliberalism, the third way and social work: The UK experience. *Social Work & Society, 2*(1), 1–9.
Ferrera, M. (1996). The 'Southern model' of welfare in social Europe. *Journal of European Social Policy, 6*(1), 17–37.
Fletcher, D. R., & Wright, S. (2017). A hand up or a slap down? Criminalising benefit claimants in Britain via strategies of surveillance, sanctions and deterrence. *Critical Social Policy, 38*(2), 323–344.
Garrett, P. M. (2014). Re-enchanting social work? The emerging 'spirit' of social work in an age of economic crisis. *British Journal of Social Work, 44*(3), 503–521. doi:10.1093/bjsw/bcs146
Garrett, P. M., & Bertotti, T. F. (2017). Social work and the politics of 'austerity': Ireland and Italy. *European Journal of Social Work, 20*(1), 29–41. doi:10.1080/13691457.2016.1185698

Gray, M., Dean, M., Agllias, K., Howard, A., & Schubert, L. (2015). Perspectives on neoliberalism for human service professionals. *Social Service Review*, *89*(2), 368–392.

Harlow, E. (2004). Why don't women want to be social workers anymore? New managerialism, postfeminism and the shortage of social workers in social services departments in England and Wales. *European Journal of Social Work*, *7*(2), 167–179.

Harlow, E., Berg, E., Barry, J., & Chandler, J. (2013). Neoliberalism, managerialism and the reconfiguring of social work in Sweden and the United Kingdom. *Organization*, *20*(4), 534–550.

Hemerijck, A. (2013). *Changing welfare states* (1st ed.). Oxford: Oxford University Press.

Ioakimidis, V., Santos, C. C., & Herrero, I. M. (2014). Reconceptualizing social work in times of crisis: An examination of the cases of Greece, Spain and Portugal. *International Social Work*, *57*(4), 285–300. doi:10.1177/0020872814524967

Jordan, B. (2007). The political, societal and economic context of practice. In M. Lymbery, & K. Postle (Eds.), *Social work: A companion to learning* (1st ed., pp. 11–19). London: SAGE Publications Ltd.

Jordan, B., & Drakeford, M. (2012). *Social work and social policy under austerity*. London: Palgrave Macmillan.

Kadushin, A., & Harkness, D. (2014). *Supervision in social work*. New York: Columbia University Press.

Karagkounis, V. (2017). Social work in Greece in the time of austerity: Challenges and prospects. *European Journal of Social Work*, *20*(5), 651–665. doi:10.1080/13691457.2016.1255593

Kovács, B., Polese, A., & Morris, J. (2017). Adjusting social welfare and social policy in Central and Eastern Europe: Growth, crisis and recession. In P. Kennett, & N. Lendvai (Eds.) *Handbook of european social policy* (pp. 194–217). Cheltenham: Edward Elgar.

Lazăr, F. (2015). Social work and welfare policy in Romania: History and current challenges. *Visioni LatinoAmericane*, *13* (Numero Speciale), 65–82.

Lazar, F., Dégi, C. L., & Iovu, M. B. (2016). *Renașterea unei profesii sau despre cum este să fii asistent social în România?* [Rebirth of a profession or what is like to be a social worker in Romania]. Bucharest: Tritonic. Retrieved from http://api.components.ro/uploads/12c6a09675620f589055800ba6ceceee/2017/02/Rena_terea_unei_profesii_sau_despre_cum_e_sa_fii_asistent_social_in_Romania.pdf

Liebenberg, L., Ungar, M., & Ikeda, J. (2015). Neo-liberalism and responsibilisation in the discourse of social service workers. *British Journal of Social Work*, *45*(3), 1006–1021.

Lord, S. A., & Iudice, J. (2012). Social workers in private practice: A descriptive study of what they do. *Clinical Social Work Journal*, *40*(1), 85–94. doi:10.1007/s10615-011-0316-7

Matarese, M. T., & Caswell, D. (2017). "I'm gonna ask you about yourself, so I can put it on paper': Analysing street- level bureaucracy through form-related talk in social work. *British Journal of Social Work*, *0*, 1–20.

Ministry of Labour, Family. Social Protection and Elderly. (2015). National strategy on social inclusion and poverty reduction 2015–2020. Retrieved from http://www.mmuncii.ro/j33/images/Documente/Familie/2016/StrategyVol1EN_web.pdf

Ministry of Regional Development and Public Administration. (2018). Clasificarea UAT-urilor din Romania [The Classification of Territorial Unit Administration (UAT) from Romania]. Retrieved September 4, 2018, from http://www.dpfbl.mdrap.ro/nr_uat-uri.html

National Register of Social Workers. (n.d.). Retrieved from http://www.cnasr.ro/module/registru-cnasr/doi/1

Noordegraaf, M. (2016). Reconfiguring professional work changing forms of professionalism in public services. *Administration & Society*, *48*(7), 783–810.

Pierson, P. (1998). Irresistible forces, immovable objects: Post-industrial welfare states confront permanent austerity. *Journal of European Public Policy*, *5*(4), 539–560. doi:10.1080/13501769880000011

Polese, A. Morris, J. Kovács, B., & Harboe, I. (2014). 'Welfare states' and social policies in Eastern Europe and the former USSR: Where informality fits in? *Journal of Contemporary European Studies*, *22*(2), 184–198.

Pop, L. (2013). The decoupling of social policy reforms in Romania. *Social Policy & Administration*, *47*(2), 161–181.

Teşliuc, E., Grigoraş, V., & Stănculescu, M. (Eds.). (2015). Studiu de fundamentare pentru Strategia naţională privind incluziunea socială şi reducerea sărăciei 2015–2020. Retrieved from http://documents.worldbank.org/curated/en/465051467995789896/pdf/103191-WP-P147269-Box394856B-PUBLIC-Background-Study-ROMANIAN.pdf

Vaismoradi, M., Turunen, H., & Bondas, T. (2013). Content analysis and thematic analysis: Implications for conducting a qualitative descriptive study. *Nursing and Health Sciences*, *15*(3), 398–405.

Wagaman, M. A., Geiger, J. M., Shockley, C., & Segal, E. A. (2015). The role of empathy in burnout, compassion satisfaction, and secondary traumatic stress among social workers. *Social Work*, *60*(3), 201–209.

Wallace, J., & Pease, B. (2011). Neoliberalism and Australian social work: Accommodation or resistance? *Journal of Social Work*, *11*(2), 132–142.

World Bank. (2011). PROJECT APPRAISAL DOCUMENT ON A PROPOSED LOAN IN THE AMOUNT OF EURO 500 MILLION (US$710.4 MILLION EQUIVALENT) TO ROMANIA FOR A SOCIAL ASSISTANCE SYSTE MODERNIZATION PROJECT. Retrieved from http://documents.worldbank.org/curated/en/338351468094453173/pdf/582800PAD0P1211e0only1910BOX358351B.pdf

Mind your own business: technologies for governing social worker subjects

Sköt dig själv: teknologier för styrning av socialarbetarsubjekt

Marcus Lauri 🆔

ABSTRACT

A vast body of research has demonstrated negative effects on social work following from a neoliberalisation of the welfare state. This article explores some of the ways in which such neoliberalisation may be carried out and maintained, by shaping social workers subjects in ways that make them compliant in such a scheme. From interviews with social workers in Sweden, an analysis of budget governing, individual wage negotiations, the client contractor model and social worker supervision shows that such governing technologies may accentuate an individual, competitive and detached subject. This may in turn produce loyalty to individual selves and management, which risks undermining the formation of a social worker subject who is willing to stand shoulder to shoulder with both their co-workers and their clients.

ABSTRAKT

Omfattande forskning har visat hur nyliberaliseringen av välfärdsstaten fått negativa effekter. Denna artikel undersöker olika sätt som gör att socialarbetare formas för att göra dem medgörliga i en sådan omdaning. Genom intervjuer med socialarbetare i Sverige analyseras hur budgetstyrning, individuell lönesättning, beställar-utförarmodellen och socialarbetares handledning kan bidra till att skapa en individualistisk, konkurrensinriktad och likgiltig socialarbetare. Detta kan i sin tur skapa lojalitet med självet och ledningen vilket riskerar att underminera ett socialarbetarsubjekt som står på klientens och sina medarbetares sida.

Introduction

The effects on human life stemming from the last few decades of neoliberalism have been investigated in a wide variety of social science research that illustrates how welfare services such as social work have been subjected to rationalisation, standardisation and austerity. While standardisation, specialisation and other practices associated with the contemporary organisation of social work may have their benefits, several studies show that the recent decades of neoliberal welfare-state reorganisation have resulted in serious limitations for social work and suffering for both clients and social workers (cf. Kamali & Jönsson, 2018). While research that highlights the effects for social workers – like a faster pace of work, stress and alienation – is important, I argue that we must also look beyond these effects and focus on *how* such a transformation may be carried out and maintained (Oksala, 2013, p. 39). If the question of 'how' is not analysed, it is likely that resisting and changing such developments will prove more difficult. In a similar fashion, Pollack and Rossiter (2010, p. 167) advocate analysing social work and argue that we must:

> Challenge market rationalities and the ways in which our subjectivities as professionals and clients are organized around these logics and are disciplined in accordance with the neoliberal subject.

Historically, social work in welfare states has been characterised by a struggle between the subjugation and emancipation of clients (Penketh, 2000; Qvarsell, 1993). While such struggles still exist, the space for radical, critical and emancipatory approaches in social work practice seems to be diminishing (Butler & Drakeford, 2001; Ferguson, 2008; Harlow, Berg, Barry, & Chandler, 2013; Lauri, 2016; Rogowski, 2010).

While many individuals identify to some degree with their profession, it is often argued that social workers have a strong professional identity and make great use of their selves in their work (cf. Sheppard & Charles, 2017). Furthermore, social work is arguably a highly political endeavour because of its outspoken purpose of liberation and creating social and economic equality (IFSW, 2014). At the same time, social work may also be considered an endeavour that reproduces the social order and unequal relations of power (Payne, 2016). Such a dual understanding of social work makes an analysis of social workers' subject formation particularly important. If social workers are subjected to governing in ways that shape their subjects in accordance with the needs of contemporary modes of power, it is likely that this will undermine their willingness to criticise and challenge injustice and inequality. Consequently, the aim of this article is to analyse how contemporary neoliberal governing may shape social worker subjects and to deliberate on what this may mean for the relationship and identification with clients, co-workers and management. The questions guiding the analysis are: What subjectification effects may arise from the assemblage of governing analysed? What are the political implications that may follow from such subjectification effects?

Method and data

This article builds on selected interviews from a previous study (Lauri, 2016) in which 24 in-depth semi-structured interviews were conducted with social workers in six municipalities in Sweden.[1] The interviews followed five major themes: the reasons for becoming a social worker, their working environment, their degree of influence in their work, conflicts at work and their future as social workers. In this article, twelve out of those 24 interviews are selected for analysis because they provide accounts of the four technologies chosen for this analysis. The selection of technologies was made from the theoretical considerations chosen for this article (see following sections) and suggestions from previous research. The selected twelve interviewees work at eleven different organisations in municipal social services in three different municipalities in two urban regions. The organisational units of their employment range from work with child protective services, adolescents, substance abuse, financial support, disability assistance (LSS[2]) and employment. The interviewees are referred to by pseudonyms.

The fact that the accounts were gathered from a variety of locations and areas of specialisation suggests that their experiences cannot be regarded as either a general tendency in any particular social work specialisation or that they are unique to any one location. It does, however, allow the analysis of experiences from a multitude of sites and settings. Still, the empirical material analysed in this article is limited and the analysis is exploratory. Consequently, the results should not be considered definitive answers but an attempt to point towards indications of potentially problematic governing technologies and their subjectification effects.

An assemblage of governing

A governmentality approach allows for attention to the wide variety of 'things' at play that enable and mediate the exercise of power (Walters, 2012, p. 62): the assemblage of 'institutions, procedures, analyses and reflections, calculations, and tactics' (Foucault, 2007, p. 108). The exertion of power – governing – thus refers not only to laws and regulations or command and control operations (Collier & Ong, 2005, p. 13), but to all sorts of 'arrangements' to meet 'this or that end' (Foucault, 2007, p. 99). Directing attention to how such arrangements shape subjects to become amenable to governing, a governmentality approach entails an understanding of governing as a practice that far exceeds formal juridical-administrative institutions (Foucault, 1984, p. 64; Walters, 2012, p. 2). This understanding of subjects is based on the assumption that subjects do not exist *a priori*; they are not an inherent essential quality, but rather the effect of power (Foucault, 1980, p. 98). The deployment of such an assemblage of governing arrangements means that those subjected to them are not always aware of what they are subjected to (Foucault, 2007, p. 105). An important reason for this has to do with the political rationalities embedded in the exertion of this kind of power, those dominant logics embedded in discourse that characterise any given society, which frames the intelligible and sayable (Brown, 2006).

To operationalise my governmentality approach, I use three analytical concepts: rationalities, technologies and effects (Bacchi, 2009). *Rationalities* focus on the production of knowledge that shapes the understanding of reality and thus affects the knowledgeable; what is understood as reasonable in a particular context. *Technologies* refer to practical methods, techniques and institutions that enable the governing of human conduct, while *effects* refer to how human subjects are constituted, shaped and maintained by the interpellation of power. Consequently, the analysis focuses on select rationalities that define problems and make certain practices in social work seem to be logical responses to such problems. The practical arrangements – technologies – used in relation to such rationalities in the context of social work are analysed, along with the subjectification effects this may produce in the encounter between social workers, management and clients. Analysing rationalities and their connection to technologies points to the inseparability of knowledge production and power, i.e. through the truth effects of dominant discourses and the subsequent alignment of what we believe to be true with what benefits the exercise of power (Dean, 2010). As such, a governmentality approach makes possible an inquiry into the interaction between power and knowledge, between self and state regulation and the subsequent legitimisation of power and the social order.

Analysing neoliberal governing assemblages

Brown (2015) argues that neoliberalism entails the economisation of social relations. The dominance of a neoliberal political rationality means emphasising ideals such as productivity, efficiency and self-sufficiency, which may conflict with and subsequently undermine ideals of quality, equality, care and solidarity (Brown, 2006, p. 694, 2015, p. 10; Dean, 2010). Following this theoretical cue, in the following sections I will analyse two technologies related to economics in contemporary social work: (a) budget governing and (b) individual wage negotiation. Following Foucault's understanding of the intermeshing of power/knowledge, Collier and Ong (2005, p. 12) argue that neoliberal governing assemblages should be analysed in relation to the regulation of knowledge production. For this reason, I have selected two additional technologies for analysis: (c) the client–contractor model (a.k.a. the purchaser–provider split) and (d) so-called social worker supervision, to explore the possible ways in which this may shape the knowing and reflexive social worker.

Budget governing: producing cost-awareness and competition?

Budget governing is a technology that entails allocating financial resources to separate units within the same social work office, often coinciding with the now widespread specialised organisation of social work according to 'particular' social problems (Grell, Ahmadi, & Blom, 2013). It also entails giving the manager of each unit individual responsibility for not exceeding the budget. The installation of any technology should be understood as a response to a perceived problem (Bacchi, 2009). Presumably, decentralising fiscal responsibility is founded on a rationality that there is a *lack* of cost-awareness and fiscal prudence in social work and that installing such a technology will generate greater cost-awareness and financial 'care'.

How can this be understood from the perspective of a social worker? Interviewee Olivia tells me that the 'managers protect the budget, because if they can't meet the budgetary target, they're out head-first' and will be replaced by someone fiercer. Such claims have also been reported in an interview study by Astvik (2014), in which managers report that it is common knowledge, although not openly discussed, what happens to a manager who cannot meet their targets: they are out. As budget responsibility is decentralised to mid-level managers, they are given more formal authority to keep costs down, but at the same time they do not have the authority to exceed the budget targets, or even to voice critique, as they seem to run the risk of losing their jobs if they do not comply with the protocol. Whether such a threat is a reality or not, or whether it is common practice to fire managers in this way, is not the scope of this analysis. Rather, the narrative (or knowledge) of such a risk conveyed here illustrates that some social workers experience it as a fact, which may work as a way to make understandable and legitimise an austerity scheme, thus producing acceptance and functioning as a tool of self-governing.

Decentralising the responsibility for scarce resources may also produce competition. Interviewee Emma tells me that:

> The colleague I was supposed to make the house call with had to commit the child since the mother turns out to be homeless because of a denial from another division of the social services of her application for housing.

The demand for each unit to tend to its own budget may hamper cooperation between the different social work units and undermine a holistic approach to clients' needs. Interviewee Gabriel, who works with clients struggling with substance abuse, tells me that:

> Every unit, every manager has, which I can understand, a responsibility for their budget. But that leads to financial austerity [...] [and] a lot of discussions about who is supposed to pay. We have two managers with their separate little budgets [...] so it becomes unwieldy because you can't get those things to work, quite simple matters really. We deal with treatment, treatment facilities and such. Then maybe these people need a place to stay during the assessment. Then it's financial support who's supposed to take care of that, to approve it. If they don't, or if things don't work out, and they have no housing for a week or so before treatment, they abscond. They have a relapse and they're gone.

The conflict over 'who is supposed to pay' makes social work more complicated and may force social workers to care more about financial matters than clients. Narrow frames for spending, decentralised budget responsibility and punishment for exceeding budgets may thus generate a conflictual and competitive working environment within which each unit is shaped to 'mind its own business'. This may produce compliance in an austerity scheme, but arguably it also undermines the willingness of mid level managers to voice critique. As the cost-awareness produced by budget governing trickles down to the individual social worker due to their proximity to managerial authority, it may become part of common-sense discourse about social work. Interviewee Felicia responds to a question about her ability to make individual decisions on treatment:

> And then she [the manager] said, 'but hold it now,' like, 'how did you reason here?' like 'no, this is too much' or 'it costs too much' so in that case you might have to back off a bit. [...] Yes, we know more, so she trusts our appraisal on most of the cases. However, she might question it from, like, cost and that we should think about not having, oh, what is it she says ..., LEON,[3] I think: lowest effective level of care. It's something she learned on some kind of course, and it's pretty good to think like that. I don't know the complete philosophy behind it, but, but, that we should not take care of, I mean, care for people more than they need.

Although Felicia says that the manager admits to her knowing more about the case and about social work, the manager nevertheless alludes to the rationality of cost-awareness and of not providing more expensive care than a client needs. What a client needs, however, does not necessarily have a fixed answer; rather, it is dependent on context, dominant forms of knowledge and political priorities. From the rationality expressed by Felicia, it seems as though cost-awareness can shape the assessment of needs in a way that makes cheaper alternatives and limits to support seem reasonable.

One way of handling the conflicts that may arise from having your assessment overruled by management is to allude to a rationality of individual responsibility. Felicia tells me that an old man ...

> ... wanted to stay home and take 'time off' from rehab, where he is right now. And I didn't agree that he should because a week ago he drank when he stayed home. [...] eventually I felt like, why should I sit here and, like, he's a grown man, he's twice as old as I am, and he can choose for himself really. [...] instead, he should be held responsible for his own actions. At the same time, I have to explain to him that we're paying for this, you can't just go home and do what you want; in that case, you'll have to declare that you don't want the treatment anymore and, like, leave.

Although she argues that there is a risk of relapse if this client takes time off from rehab, Felicia also expresses the rationality of choice, individual responsibility and cost-awareness. It seems that the rationality displayed here says: you cannot go home because we are paying for your treatment; if you intend to have a relapse, be responsible about it, tell us right away and renounce your place on the programme.

A rationality by which fiscal matters seem to override matters of care is something that interviewee Nora also tells me about.

> Staying sober and off drugs, maybe even improved housing, and feeling better, that's a positive result to me, but when you read the meeting documents then it's all about the budget. The budget is in balance, then it's like 'who cares what happens to the clients?'

Nora is referring to management's talk about positive results in staff meetings, where the attention to the budget being in balance seems to have given the term 'positive results' a distorted meaning. On a similar topic, interviewee Beatrice tells me that in her municipality the management introduced a zero-sum game to remedy their budget deficit. This meant 'No new commitment of care for children may be initiated until another is finished, so that money may be released.' and Beatrice says: 'it's completely sick!' and dishonouring the 'claim to work in the best interests of the child or from individual assessments'.

These selected examples suggest that budget governing augments a focus on financial prudence and cost-awareness and that this may produce internal competition over resources and hamper a holistic and careful approach to clients. Such a governing technology may escape critique from managers due to the imminent threat of losing one's job (whether factual or not) and a common-sense rationality of cost-awareness. Budget governing is thus a technology that can lead to the prioritisation of fidelity to budget targets at risk of overriding other rationalities of resource allocation and attention, such as clients' needs or quality of support and care (Schröder, 2014). Competition between units may also divide social workers and undermine the formation of a subject that is oriented towards a collective. In addition, it is also a technology that may allow local politicians to escape criticism by decentralising the delicate decisions about how to prioritise scarce resources to mid-level managers (Mutvik, 2014).

Individual salaries: producing individual performance and submission?

Within several professions in Sweden, there is a long tradition of collective bargaining over salaries. Under such a system, salaries are typically negotiated between central union representatives and employer organisations, or the local union and the employer. However, over the past couple of decades, more and more employers have introduced individual negotiations over wages, sometimes with the connivance of unions. The extent to which such a technology is widespread in Swedish social work is not the scope of this analysis; rather, I intend to deliberate upon the possible effects it may produce in terms of shaping social workers subjects. Individual salaries arguably allude to a market rationality of performance and competition, under which individual financial rewards are expected to encourage workers to strive for improvement and perfection in their performance. The installation of such a technology should be understood as a response to a perceived problem of lack of efficiency in production, as any policy is a response that originates in a particular but seldom explicitly voiced representation of a problem (Bacchi, 2009). While the empirical support for enhanced performance is slim (Lapidus, 2015; Nilsson & Ryman, 2005), the technology of individual negotiation for wages may have other effects. Interviewee Rosa argues that your salary is dependent on your obedience and believes that it is a practice installed to divide and conquer. From word of mouth, she has been told that giving 'upwards-nudges' of affirmation to the management and 'being nice' have been included in the formal criteria for wage negotiation at her workplace. She reflects: 'Being nice!? What the hell does that mean?' What is meant by being nice is not clear, but Rosa is outraged over what I interpret as a demand to be 'civilised' and to avoid direct criticism of management. Rather, positive affirmation is encouraged. Another interviewee, Ylva, elaborates on the reasons behind the culture of silence at her workplace:

> This thing with individual salaries and that it's more and more about your individual performance, and that's about being loyal to the manager. [...] And I was told that I couldn't have more of a raise because I wasn't loyal to the operation.

According to Ylva, the negotiation of individual salaries is a practice that produces loyalty to management by stifling protest – a culture of silence. She had been told by her manager that voicing opinions about strenuous working conditions at staff meetings created unrest and harmed her co-workers and that this was an expression of disloyalty. Olivia has a similar experience:

> If you sit and whine during coffee and say that you have too much to do, you induce a bad atmosphere. It doesn't support an increased wage.

Not only may individual negotiations for salary produce a performance-oriented subject, as Olivia, Rosa and Ylva have argued, it may also stifle critique and enhance loyalty to management. In their study of social workers, Astvik, Melin, and Allvin (2014) met similar experiences. Those who protest say they are seen as troublemakers and that they have internalised a sense of being a tiresome burden to others (Astvik et al., 2014, p. 59). In addition, Ylva argues that individual salaries create an atmosphere of secrecy and says: 'Now, no one wants to disclose to others what they earn'. Lapidus (2015) points to a similar tendency and argues that individual wages may undermine workers' solidarity and cohesion (see Nilsson & Ryman, 2005 for an overview and similar conclusions).

Individual salaries are thus arguably a governing technology that is based on a notion – or problem representation – that workers are performing below their potential. The installation of individual salaries thus alludes to a rationality of individual salaries → competition between individuals → enhanced individual performance, i.e. a technology that produces competing individuals who strive to display their individual performance. Because performance is linked to wage negotiations with management, it is likely to be oriented towards the priorities of management and displayed accordingly, rather than towards peers or clients. As argued above, this may also be interpreted as a technology for stifling social workers' protest by shaping subjects loyal to management, which may undermine the formation of a critical and collectively oriented social worker subject.

Client–contractor model: producing a competitive and distant knower?

The client–contractor model (a.k.a. purchaser–provider split) is a business model introduced into the organisation of welfare provision in order to produce market-like competition between care providers. Its basic principle is to separate the work of assessment and 'purchase' from social work provision (Gleghorn, 1995). This technology is arguably based on a rationality that public service is somehow defective in terms of production and that the installation of this approach will increase efficiency and flexibility and improve quality (Gleeson & Knights, 2006; Jacobsson, 2002; Ranson, 2003). Regardless of whether such promises hold true or not, Rosa tells me what this division of labour has meant for her:

> I'm becoming more or less an administrative clerk. The idea is to make quick assessments, approve some kind of treatment. We're not supposed to engage with clients. That's the idea.

This division of labour means that social workers in municipal social services primarily engage in the assessment of clients but not in their further counselling or treatment, which is carried out by external providers, either municipal or private. Tina, who works in another organisation with this division of labour, says that her work primarily entails 'handling invoices, making contracts, you're so far away from contact with [clients]'.

These accounts suggest that, for those who work in the social services, the client–contractor model has reduced the time spent with clients. Social worker Donna[4] describes her experience in the following terms:

> The social services are divided into 'client' and 'contractor' [...] A thorough work for change, however, demands continuous contact, something which a social worker does not have the time for.

According to Donna, the reduced time spent with clients undermines a thorough work for change because such work demands continuous contact. This is an effect that has been highlighted elsewhere; for example, Gleghorn (1995) argues that such a model has problems dealing with the complexity of social problems and also points to effects like the fragmentation of social work, inflexibility and superficial assessments. Following an evaluation of the implementation of a client–contractor model in a Swedish municipality, Billquist and Gustafsson (2002, p. 9) put it bluntly: 'it was not good for anyone'.

Regardless of whether this technology actually produces efficiency, flexibility or higher quality (which seems unlikely), I want to concentrate on the alterations in the forms of interaction between social worker and client and how this may affect knowledge production. Witnessing the predicament of the client at first hand places a social worker in an ideal position to understand the effects of political and social structures, argue Daniel and Wheeler (1989). Similar arguments have been put forward for understanding the critical and structural approach to social problems that developed in the British and North American settlement movements in the late nineteenth century. It is believed that it was due to their proximity to suffering (they lived in community houses with their 'clients') that such knowledge about social problems was produced (Hugman, 2009; Pettersson, 2001). Interviewee Ylva ponders the effects of this practice:

> The social worker ends up further and further away from the client and then you can no longer *see* the individual, and that makes it easier to make those difficult decisions [...] because you can't see their suffering.

Arguing that the client contractor model makes it harder to 'see' the individual is something I interpret as a loss of the basis for complex knowledge production that can develop from witnessing suffering and injustice up close. Ylva argues that the distance produced by this practice makes it easier to make difficult decisions. This suggests that the technology of separating those who decide upon the allocation of public resources from clients makes austerity easier to implement because it produces a more distant and detached social worker subject. Such a method of organising work may shape social workers into less 'caring' subjects, which arguably makes it less discomforting to condition, reduce or deny claims for support. In fact, Olivia tells me, 'once a manager told me that this *is* the purpose of dividing us into clients and contractors!'

Similarly to budget governing, research also suggests that the client–contractor model produces competition for resources within the organisation (Jacobsson, 2002), and Lundström's (2011) research on Australian social work suggests that this model gave management an opportunity to hire less qualified labour for the assessment of clients' needs because they made less of a 'fuss'.

The accounts of Rosa, Tina, Donna, Ylva and Olivia taken together suggest that knowledge production founded upon both the social work profession and proximity to clients' suffering are important for understanding clients' predicaments and their origins. To determine the extent of this technology in Swedish social work, or whether it is increasing, is not the scope of this analysis. Rather, it is about highlighting the potential subjectification effects that may emerge from a client–contractor model. Although the empirical material is limited, in light of the analytical framework and other research into the matter, I would argue that reducing the time spent with clients and cultivating a culture of competition may shape a social worker subject who knows less, and therefore may care less, about clients' complex problems. There is also a risk that this may undermine the formation of a critical social worker subject and, due to the fragmentation of work, the sense of constituting a collective of social workers.

Regimentation of individual supervision: disciplining a reflexive subject?

Individual supervision for social workers is a long-standing tradition in social work (Kadushin & Harkness, 2014). In a Swedish context, its most common expression entails a practice in which the social worker sees an external counsellor for the purpose of unburdening and self-reflection and it is highly cherished by social workers (Höjer, Beijer, & Wissö, 2007). The shape and content of this supervision has largely been defined by the profession and is often characterised by long-term commitment and a psychoanalytical approach (Payne, 1994).

Previous surveys suggest that a majority of Swedish social workers are offered supervision, although there may be signs of a gradual decline (Höjer et al., 2007; Vision, 2013). Previous studies have suggested that managers rarely intervene in the content or aim of this supervision (Egelund & Kvilhaug, 2001), but in my interviews, I have found examples that suggest something different. Tina told me:

Tina:	The supervision is strictly about legal aspects.
Interviewer:	You mean the supervision you're getting, is about …
Tina:	Yes, legal matters.
Interviewer:	Okay, I was under the assumption that supervision was like a kind of, to relieve the socially burdening aspects of being a social worker, sort of. Isn't that what it's meant to be?
Tina:	Yes, that's what it's supposed to be, and I believe that's what is *has* been, and then we had a period of no counselling at all and now it's with a juridical consultant. Like, on legal matters.

Tina has experience of social work supervision undergoing changes. In her case, it has manifested as the shift from a free modus of reflection to supervision on legal matters. Another interviewee, Simon, told me that his supervision had been altered as well. At his workplace, he was used to choosing the counsellor who performed the supervision, but recently management had decided to change this and engaged counsellors who were not psychotherapists, but rather counsellors who use CBT and behavioural analysis instead of a psychoanalytical approach. 'She [the manager] just decided, we were not allowed to take part in it. […] this is worthless, it's not counselling.' As opposed to a psychoanalytical approach, CBT focuses more on the present and, according to Binkley (2011), its popularity comes not only from an understanding that 'it works' and that it is cheaper, but also because it alludes to the idea that mental health is the result of individual cognitive attitudes. Binkley argues that CBT fits well into a happiness discourse, which helps to shape individual subjects as responsible for constant self-control and self-improvement (see Ahmed, 2010 for similar conclusions).

Tina also told me of a previous experience when she worked at financial support:

Interviewer:	But did you have counselling at the other places as well?
Tina:	Mm-hm, at financial support I did and then our deputy manager was present.
Interviewer:	Why?
Tina:	To monitor, I suppose. Because our counsellor, she was quite troubled, because she had a plan about, like, how to do the counselling and what it was okay to discuss. So when we wanted to talk about something [else], she always had to ask her [the deputy manager], and if she wasn't there she had to, well, what could she say, is this okay or not?
Interviewer:	So the manager had decided what it was okay to talk about during counselling?
Tina:	In principle yes, and she was present most of the time, which of course made it impossible to talk about …
Interviewer:	But how did that feel?
Tina:	You felt constrained, like, monitored.

The few examples presented here suggest a particular interest from management in social workers' supervision. Deciding who does the supervision, with what theoretical approach and what is allowed to be talked about seems like a desire to manage the reflections and emotions that arise from engaging in contemporary social work. In their survey, Höjer et al. (2007) concluded that supervision is highly cherished and intensely defended by social workers but, similarly to the quotes above, there were reports of management intervention. Others reported that their supervision was terminated altogether, officially for reasons of austerity. Yet others reported that management had changed their supervision from external to internal, which was assumed to restrict the space for critical reflection and discussion. This was due to internal supervision often being performed by members of the management as opposed to external supervisors who are not directly employed by the organisation and thus have no formal ties with it (Höjer et al., 2007).

In light of such accounts, and in connection with previous sections on management efforts to stifle protest via economic sanctions and rewards, the examples of management's attempts to control supervision presented above may be understood as an effort to manage dissatisfaction among social workers. Whether this should be understood as a technology to handle rising discontent in an era of neoliberal austerity is not possible to discern from such a limited sample. However, I would argue that, if social workers are given a sanctuary space to reflect on any kind of displeasure, this may very well spur the formation of a critical subject. Given the rising discontent with the developments in social work during the last couple of decades, it is not unlikely that a need has developed for new technologies to handle this (Lauri, 2016). Controlling supervision by having managers present, by restricting the topics allowed for discussion and by focusing on CBT, 'superficial' matters may arguably be an attempt to undermine the formation of a wilful and critical social worker subject and produce an understanding that the key to their grievances can be found in themselves.

Concluding discussion

From my analysis of the four technologies above: budget governing, individual wage negotiation, the client–contractor model and social worker supervision, I suggest that they may be seen as a neoliberal governing assemblage with the ability to shape social workers into individualised, competitive and detached subjects. Interviewee Maude sums up the developments she has witnessed:

> Many of us feel bad, we're stressed [...], and the atmosphere in the group is deteriorating, and we also have a high personnel turnover. Then it's easy to start guarding your own because we all have so much to do, so you're, like, well it all divides us, and people lose the energy to engage in trying to improve things or engage with the union, because the only thing that you're occupied with is your cases and keeping your head above water.

The analysis and this quote from Maude suggest that, under current conditions, the interviewed social workers become detached from both peers and clients and instead tend to become loyal to their rationalised selves and to management – minding their own business. Olivia deliberates on her long experience of social work and explicitly says that she 'mourns the [loss of] collegiality' and Emma, who has only been working for a couple of years, says she will quit in the near future because 'under these circumstances' she's afraid she will 'become an unsympathetic person.' It seems as though she is afraid of what she will turn into (i.e. how her subject will be altered) as a result of working under current conditions.

An effect that may arise from detachment towards clients is that it obscures the context of which any individual is part, which makes it easier to embrace a neoliberal discourse of austerity and individual responsibility and to understand clients' predicaments as the result of poor choices (Bauman, 1998; Brown, 2015; Garrett, 2010; Wacquant, 2009).

Loyalty to management seems to be further augmented by punishing protest and rewarding silent performance. The conflict between protest and loyalty to management is not a new one. However, the particular rationalities and technologies examined here arguably display unique qualities that may be assigned to contemporary neoliberalism. This suggests that an individualised culture of silence may be established through such neoliberal governing assemblages, which is likely to hamper the formation of a critical social worker subject. While Rosanvallon (2008) argues that contestation and protest over perceived inequalities are fundamental to achieving change, Rancière (2006) proposes understanding democracy as a process rather than a condition. From such a perspective, criticism and protest against perceived injustices and those who exercise power is essential for the development of democracy. Brown (2015) argues that the market logics and individualisation that constitute the political rationality of neoliberalism make it difficult for citizens to establish a *collective* political subject, which leaves limited space for citizens to unite into a *demos*. If this is indeed true for social work, the analysis suggests that the process of shaping social workers into individualised, competitive and detached subjects, silent and loyal to management, has serious effects. It suggests that the formation of a critical *collective* social worker subject willing to protest against inequality and injustice is undermined.

While my interviews suggest that neoliberal governing assemblages may have the effect of producing such submission and compliance, for some of those who have uncovered and called out such a scheme, it has produced awareness and resistance outside of the traditional arenas of the workplace and unions. They have shared with me stories about their activist work in 'clandestine' networks that cut across union membership and social service offices and about their efforts to escape the surveillance and repression of current governing assemblages. This suggests that, although neoliberal governing assemblages may have problematic subjectification effects, they are not an all-engulfing and flawless machine. Hardt and Negri (2004) argue that a collective subjectivity can develop in radical spaces by challenging structures of power and, indeed, some of the critical accounts in this analysis suggest that some social workers respond to neoliberal governing assemblages by developing new techniques and collective subjects of resistance. Let us hope they will persist.

Notes

1. The strategy for selection was strategic. I wanted to gather accounts from a wide variety of sites and organisational settings, and I used several approaches to find respondents, such as contacting unions and management in the social services in different parts of the country, through national social worker networks and personal acquaintances. The interviews were recorded and transcribed between 2012 and 2015.
2. Law on support for disabled people.
3. LEON refers to the management rationality 'lowest level of effective care' used in some contexts like the Norwegian healthcare services (Holm, Mathisen, Sæterstrand, & Brinchmann, 2017).
4. This quote is from a social worker whom I interviewed but collected from a post on the website of a network of critical social workers (Nu Bryter vi tystnaden, 2015).

Acknowledgments

I wish to thank the interviewees for sharing their thoughts and critiques on this matter.

Disclosure statement

No potential conflict of interest was reported by the author.

ORCID

Marcus Lauri ⓘ http://orcid.org/0000-0002-3620-7105

References

Ahmed, S. (2010). *The promise of happiness.* Durham, NC: Duke University Press.

Astvik, W. (2014). *Lojal, lydig och tyst: Om nya styrsystem, decentraliserat ansvar och bristfällig dialog i socialtjänsten konferensen. Välfärd och Framtid på ABF i Stockholm 15–16 mars 2014.* Stockholm: Nu Bryter Vi Tystnaden.

Astvik, W., Melin, M., & Allvin, M. (2014). Survival strategies in social work: A study of how coping strategies affect service quality, professionalism and employee health. *Nordic Social Work Research, 4*(1), 52–66.

Bacchi, C. L. (2009). *Analysing policy: What's the problem represented to be?* Frenchs Forest: Pearson.

Bauman, Z. (1998). *Work, consumerism and the new poor.* Buckingham: Open University Press.

Billquist, L., & Gustafsson, G. (2002). En oreflekterad omorganisation. Socionomens forsknignssupplement nr 14. *Socionomen, 8*(14), 1–10.

Binkley, S. (2011). Happiness, positive psychology and the program of neoliberal governmentality. *Subjectivity, 4*(3), 371–394.

Brown, W. (2006). American nightmare: Neoliberalism, neoconservatism and de-democratization. *Political Theory, 34*(6), 690–714.

Brown, W. (2015). *Undoing the demos: Neoliberalism's stealth revolution* (1st ed.). New York, NY: Zone Books.

Butler, I., & Drakeford, M. (2001). Which Blair project? Communitarianism, social authoritarianism and social work. *Journal of Social Work, 1*(7), 7–19.

Collier, S. J., & Ong, A. (2005). Global assemblages, anthropological problems. In A. Ong & S. J. Collier (Eds.), *Global assemblages: Technology, politics, and ethics as anthropological problems* (pp. 3–21). Malden, MA: Blackwell Publishing.

Daniel, P., & Wheeler, J. (1989). *Social work and local politics.* London: Macmillan Education and British Association of Social Workers.

Dean, M. (2010). *Governmentality: Power and rule in modern society* (2nd ed.). Thousand Oaks, CA: Sage.

Egelund, T., & Kvilhaug, A. (2001). Supervisionens organisering. *Socialvetenskaplig Tidskrift, 3,* 180–198.

Ferguson, I. (2008). *Reclaiming social work: Challenging neo-liberalism and promoting social justice.* Los Angeles, CA: Sage.

Foucault, M. (1980). *Power/knowledge: Selected interviews and other writings 1972–1977* (1st American ed.). New York, NY: Pantheon.

Foucault, M. (1984). *The Foucault reader.* New York, NY: Pantheon Books.

Foucault, M. (2007). *Security, territory, population: lectures at the collège de France, 1977–1978.* New York, NY: Picador.

Garrett, P. M. (2010). Examining the 'conservative revolution': Neoliberalism and social work education. *Social Work Education, 29*(4), 340–355.

Gleeson, D., & Knights, D. (2006). Challenging dualism: Public professionalism in 'troubled' times. *Sociology, 40*(2), 277–295.

Gleeson, M. (1999). Service disputes cause had publicity und loss of trust. *Professional Social Work, 2*(12), 6.

Grell, P., Ahmadi, N., & Blom, B. (2013). Hur inverkar organisationsstrukturen på socialtjänstens klientarbete?: en sammanfattning av kunskapsläget. *Socialvetenskaplig tidskrift, 20*(3–4), 222–240.

Hardt, M., & Negri, A. (2004). *Multitude.* New York, NY: Penguin Press.

Harlow, E., Berg, E., Barry, J., & Chandler, J. (2013). Neoliberalism, managerialism and the reconfiguring of social work in Sweden and the United Kingdom. *Organization, 20*(4), 534–550.

Holm, S. G., Mathisen, T. A., Sæterstrand, T. M., & Brinchmann, B. S. (2017). Allocation of home care services by municipalities in Norway: A document analysis. *BMC Health Services Research, 17*(1), 1–10.

Höjer, S., Beijer, E., & Wissö, T. (2007). *Varför handledning?: handledning som professionellt projekt och organisatoriskt verktyg inom handikappomsorg och individ och familjeomsorg.* Göteborg: FoU i Väst.

Hugman, R. (2009). But is it social work? Some reflections on mistaken identities. *British Journal of Social Work, 39*(6), 1138–1153.

International Federation of Social Work. (2014). *Global definition of the social work profession.* Retrieved from http://ifsw.org/get-involved/global-definition-of-social-work/

Jacobsson, B. (Ed.). (2002). *Organisationsexperiment i kommuner och landsting.* Stockholm: Santérus.

Kadushin, A., & Harkness, D. (2014). *Supervision in social work* (5th ed.). New York, NY: Columbia University Press.

Kamali, M., & Jönsson, J. H. (Eds.). (2018). *Neoliberalism, Nordic welfare states and social work: Current and future challenges.* London: Routledge.

Lapidus, J. (2015). *Social democracy and the Swedish welfare model: Ideational analyses of attitudes towards competition, individualization, privatization* (Dissertation). Göteborgs universitet, Göteborg.

Lauri, M. (2016). *Narratives of governing: Rationalization, responsibility and resistance in social work* (Dissertation). Umeå universitet, Umeå.

Lundström, T. (2011). Om senmodernitet, riskbedömningar och social barnavård. In I. Höjer & S. Höjer (Eds.), *Familj, vardagsliv och modernitet* (pp. 101–114). Göteborg: Göteborgs universitet/Institutionen för socialt arbete.

Nilsson, T., & Ryman, A. (2005). *Individuell lön - lönar det sig?: fakta och tro om individuell lönesättning*. Stockholm: Arbetslivsinstitutet.

Nu bryter vi tystnaden. (2015, January 25). Veckans brott: Utredare, inte socialarbetare. Retrieved from https://nbvt. wordpress.com/2015/01/25/veckans-brott-utreda-och-administrera-framfor/

Oksala, J. (2013). Feminism and neoliberal governmentality. *Foucault Studies, 16*, 32–53.

Payne, M. (1994). Personal supervision in social work. In A. Connor & S. Black (Eds.), *Performance review and quality in social care* (pp. 43–58). London: Jessica Kingsley.

Payne, M. (2016). *Modern social work theory* (4th ed.). New York, NY: Oxford University Press.

Penketh, L. (2000). *Tackling institutional racism: Anti-racist policies and social work education and training*. Bristol: Policy.

Pettersson, U. (2001). *Socialt arbete, politik och professionalisering: den historiska utvecklingen i USA och Sverige*. Stockholm: Natur och kultur.

Pollack, S., & Rossiter, A. (2010). Neoliberalism and the entrepreneurial subject: Implications for feminism and social work. *Canadian Social Work Review, 27*(2), 155–169.

Qvarsell, R. (1993). *Skall jag taga vara på min broder?: tolv artiklar om vårdens, omsorgens och det sociala arbetets historia*. Umeå: Institutionen för idéhistoria, Univ.

Rancière, J. (2006). *Hatred of democracy*. London: Verso.

Ranson, S. (2003). Public accountability in the age of neo-liberal governance. *Journal of Education Policy, 18*(5), 459–480.

Rogowski, S. (2010). *Social work, the rise and fall of a profession*. Bristol: Policy Press.

Rosanvallon, P. (2008). *Counter-democracy: Politics in the age of distrust*. Cambridge: Cambridge University Press.

Schrøder, I. M. (2014). *Budgetblikket i socialt arbejde med udsatte børn og unge*. Frederiksberg: Professionshøjskolen Metropol/Institut for Socialt Arbejde.

Sheppard, M., & Charles, M. (2017). Personality in those entering social work training in England: Comparing women and men. *European Journal of Social Work, 20*(2), 288–296.

Vision. (2013). *Stolthet och profession: En rapport om arbetsvillkoren för socialsekreterare och biståndshandläggare i socialtjänsten*. Stockholm: Author.

Wacquant, L. J. D. (2009). *Prisons of poverty* (Expanded ed.). Minneapolis: University of Minnesota Press.

Walters, W. (2012). *Governmentality: Critical encounters*. London: Routledge.

Neoliberalisation, the social investment state and social work

Nyliberalisering, den sosiale investeringsstaten og sosialt arbeid

Edgar Marthinsen

ABSTRACT

This article focuses on the challenges to social work evolving from two major discourses contributing to the common sense contextualising social work within the new spirit of capitalism and the governing of the soul. Beside neo-liberal ideas and values challenging social work values and the welfare state, the question is also about managerialism. To what extent is the social worker able to contribute to liberating, reflexive critique, or exert pastoral power? I have chosen to see how the idea of the social investment state may be linked to Rose's and Foucault's ideas about expanding governmentality and end my discussion by relating to some of the early writing on social work's challenges in confronting ideas and practices interpreted as neoliberalisation moves.

SAMMENDRAG

Denne artikkelen fokuserer på utviklingen av velferdsstaten og sosialt arbeids rolle. I diskusjonen om hvordan nyliberalismen utfordrer sosialt arbeid reises i tillegg spørsmål ved betydningen av ledelsestenkning og teknologi. I artikkelen utforskes det hvordan ideen om den sosiale investeringsstaten kan forstås i lys av Rose og Foucaults begrep om en ekspanderende styringsskikk. Videre ses det på hvordan en rekke nyere tekster har drøftet de utfordringer som sosialt arbeid møter i det vi forstår som nyliberale samfunnstrekk. Intensjonen er å vie oppmerksomheten til noen av de motsetninger som oppstår når sosialt arbeid møter en ekspanderende nyliberal tankegang der det skal utøves. Innledningsvis fokuseres det på hvordan vi kan forstå nyliberalisme og hvordan velferdsstaten synes å bevege seg mot en sosial investeringsstat. Videre synliggjøres det hvordan sosialt arbeid synes å ha tilpasset seg og endret seg som praksis i de siste tiårene

Each individual ... an active agent in the maintenance of a healthy and efficient polity, exercising a reflexive scrutiny over personal, domestic, and familial conduct ... for their own welfare, that of their families, and that of society as a whole. (Rose, 1999, p. 228)

The Trondheim conference on Social Work and Neo Liberalism in April 2016 focussed on neoliberalisation as a movement and a dominant discourse rather than a complete project. This article focuses on central transformations of the welfare state and the role of social work. Two major discourses seem to contribute to the 'common sense' (Gramsci, 1971), the first contextualising social work within the 'new spirit of capitalism' (Boltanski & Chiapello, 2007) and the second within the 'governing of the soul' (Rose, 1999). Beside neo-liberal ideas and values challenging social work values and the welfare state, the question is also about managerialism and technology (Garrett, 2005). To what extent is the social worker able to contribute to liberating, reflexive critique – or are they being disciplined to exert pastoral power? I have chosen to explore how the idea of the social investment state may be linked to Rose's and Foucault's ideas about expanding governmentality and end my discussion relating to some recent writing on social work's challenges in confronting ideas and practices interpreted as neoliberalisation moves. To some extent, this may be read as a conflict between managerial and professional values, although this is not necessarily the case. There is no intention to give a review of the expanding literature on neoliberalism, society and social work, but to give attention to some of the conflicts embedded in an expanding neo-liberal mindset dominating the context of social work.

The rhetoric in play in the discourse on neoliberalisation should rather be interpreted alongside the concept of instrumental and strategic communication according to Habermas (1990), and not as a communicative action. Interests are always embedded within any ideology and the neoliberal discourse is not separable from the expansion of commodified markets where profit is paramount.

The first part of the article focuses on neoliberalism and how the welfare state is moving towards a social investment state. The second part gives a brief discussion of changes during the last generations of social work, and then how the recent changes seem to affect social work and its practices.

Neoliberalisation

Neoliberal policies are characterised by an emphasis on a remaking of the state, a bigger role for the market and an insistence on individual responsibility (see the article by Garrett in this issue). Some stress that the state works to serve in the interest of neoliberal politics promoting monetary policies that weaken the democratic opposition of the left and unions through unemployment. This is a global rather than domestic scene. Schwarzmantel (2005) claims that neoliberalism may be regarded as a hegemonic ideology, but also identifies counter-ideologies present in the discourse. As movements, social democracy and neo-liberalism share the 'passion of the infinite' (Kierkegaad, 1974, p. 181). The present may be subordinated for the sake of future goals. Thus, within a democracy the neoliberal idea of the self has to be negotiated and adjusted and may be able to fit in a more realistic sense to everyday life and to the varying conditions it has to relate and respond to. The measurements of success are exchangeable and open to discourse. Rorty's ontological position discussing the construct of 'truth claims' is that the world as such cannot be regarded as true or false, but our conceptions of the world imply this all the same (Rorty, 1997, p. 26). Rorty adds that idealists desire a certain world where they impose ontological as well as epistemological truth claims. Neoliberalisation – as I prefer to term it – can be regarded as a discourse becoming materialised through promotion of a certain ideas and values. Giroux (2004) is quoted by Schwarzmantel (2005: 85) arguing that;

> Neoliberalism is not simply an economic policy designed to cut government spending, pursue free-trade policies, and free market forces from government regulations; it is also a political philosophy and ideology that affects every dimension of social life.

Neoliberalism rests on epistemologies with scant support from science, humanities or economy – but with a true foundation within common beliefs in the Gramscian sense. Many have become convinced about the necessity of operating within markets, they have even come to regard themselves as an asset to be invested in throughout life, improving their ability to accumulate symbolic, social, cultural and economic capital.

The origins of neoliberalism

While liberalism may have roots in the Enlightenment and the rise of modernity, neoliberalism developed later. Innset (2016) refers to the work of Slobodian (2015) claiming that the neoliberal movement evolved to confront the nationally founded welfare states and their evolving framework to control capital. It was not as much a worldview of 'Man', but a perspective of the functioning of markets and its ability to order the distribution of commodities among people and countries. Dardot and Laval (2013) take up this idea and refer to Foucault's conception of neoliberalism as a political rationality. It does not need to be a conscious and fully expressed and clear system of thought, but a route to governmentality; power is exercised in such a way that it follows the philosophy of Rorty mentioned above – it becomes a truth claim. Dardot and Laval (2013, p. 21) observe that the *real world of liberalism is shot through with tensions. Its unity has always been problematic.*

Neo-liberal ideas were not part of the dominant discourse of the post-war era and surfaced in the 1970s, although a discourse had been evolving in the field of economics. Social citizenship acted as a common project in the post-war era where negative symbols such as poverty and sickness should be eliminated in order to present a proud and successful nation. Science and professionalism would contribute to a society of professional experts who would know what was 'good for everyone'.

According to Harvey (2005) things started to change in the late 1960s. First, our generation did not want the stereotypes we were offered about freedom and equality. The unified and stereotyped *fraternité* collapsed into a multicultural and morally challenging demand for the right to be different and to express multiple selves. Brown (2015) regards neoliberalism as 'an order of normative reason' and as it evolves it takes shape as 'a governing rationality'. It communicates its ideas of 'economic values, practices and metrics to every dimension of human life' (Brown, 2015 in Leibetseder, 2017, p. 64). Leibetseder (2017, p. 65) sees this development in relation to Foucault's idea that *individuals are subjects for investment by the state in the name of furthering economic growth.* People – as machinery – become capital to be developed and requiring investment. In this way, all investments in people, such as social policy, education and health services, become areas of investment with expectations of return, in line with economic investments as such. Foucault's (2010) critique is based on the idea that as economic thinking permeates society it replaces or subjugates external religious or legal principles for organising society. Economy becomes an internal domain pretending to represent reality. The art of liberal government has to comply with an economic representation of the world, and if rulers do not succeed they are not seen as tyrants but rather as clumsy and out of pace with the market and the 'real world' (Innset, 2016).

Neoliberalism challenging the welfare state

A central theme in the discourse on neoliberalism is how it challenges the welfare state. New ideas and paradigms are always pushing history aside as they enter into the dominant discourse or contribute to the 'common sense' (Gramsci, 1971). Lorenz (2005) claims that the welfare state aimed at making citizenship into a lived daily experience of sharing risks and responsibilities. It also included the will to share work and wealth creation, creating bonds across sections of industry and countries. A third domain of interest was culture and education built on nationalism, a glorious past and the need for legitimating of nation-state and territorial claims. These institutions – welfare, work and culture – arranged a social order. Social work made itself available to this project in order to assist in shaping well-adjusted citizens. Lorenz (2005, p. 94) argues that being part of this project aided social work in its striving for professionalism along with its 'anchoring in the scientific project of modernity for the mastering of social problems with rational means'. The welfare project produced welfare regimes to reduce the social tensions and inequality. Following this logic, social work might be at risk with the fall of the welfare state and the critique of the modernist project. This has obviously not happened as social work seems to be expanding, whether we count the numbers of social workers or the proliferation of further education, research and development in the former welfare states as well as in the new democratic regimes in former communist states. The question is to what extent social workers may assume the role of shepherd or 'pastor' in the process of neoliberalisation and to what extent this is a willed and conscious choice. The disciplining of social workers can resemble the ways in which all citizens are disciplined by self-regulation or governance of the soul (Rose, 1999). Discipline does not have to be imposed since the norms and symbolic capital are communicated in our everyday life experiences and *through the unceasing reflexive gaze of our psy-chologically educated self-scrutiny* (Rose, 1999, p. 213). Social workers are among those who are sup-posed to contribute to the fabrication of the autonomous self as the object of expert knowledge – a *system of moral orthopaedics* (Rose, 1999, p. 221). Foucault's idea of the social workers as the shepherd enacting 'pastoral power' is a common metaphor used to illustrate the disciplinary role (Järvinen & Mortensen, 2005). We may thus regard pastoral power as a phenomenon linked to socialisation in general under neoliberal conditions.

Getting into people's heads

Sennett (2005) argues that neoliberalism causes the 'corrosion of character'. Solidarity is replaced by personal responsibility for one's own project of self-development: 'flexible' work practices are devel-oping a 'precariat' (Standing, 2014). Dufour (2008) writes about *symbolic slavery*. His main critique of neoliberalism is that we have left rational sense and all higher goals about social life by succumbing to marketisation in all areas of life. The new human is presented as a consumer and becomes human capital to enhance the competitive power of a nation.

The social democratic ideas of building a just society and happiness for mankind based on redis-tribution and respect is replaced by a market of symbolic goods where everyone may have a share depending on their own agency. The new ideas are founded on personal happiness in a life where ideas of the holy and eternal grace do not play any substantial role any more. Ehrenreich (2010) places American ideology at the fore, focusing rather on personal success supported by a whole industry marketing happiness and wealth (see also Davies, 2016). If you do not succeed, all the blame is with you. If you are sacked, this is presented as a new opportunity. Forås and Vetlesen (2015, p. 78) refer to Bauman's ideas about 'liquid modernity'. Dufour asserts that deinstitutionalisa-tion of society is a trademark of neoliberal society made possible by adjusting to the critique from Foucault (2010) and Bourdieu (1999). *(Capitalism) is destroying institutions and putting an end to primal domination in such a way as to produce individuals who are supple, insecure, mobile and open to all the market's modes and variations* (Dufour, 2008, p. 157). Dufour may resemble Honneth (2017) in his discussion of the need to reinvent our institutions in order to enable human dignity. These common ideas are necessary to enable collectivity and solidarity – values needed for social cohesion as a basis for the social. Dufour claims that morals have no market value, but fol-lowing Bourdieu (1999a) one may challenge that view since moral acts are part of the symbolic capital available for agents. With commodification as the major narrative, there is no limit to the claims a citizen within a society may present, depending on their purchasing power. In neo-liberalist thinking, freedom is with the market, not the worker any more. Commodification has superseded the religious and churches are empty as the malls fill on Sundays. The new 'priests' are the public relations experts and the market is contributing to the creation of subjects – because 'you're worth it!'. Pleasure has become the basis for learning as we demonstrate the art of living through storytelling. Those who are not able to surface and become visible (as interesting or likeable) are according to Dufour caught by depression and we all may end up like a lost character in the David Lynch movie Mulholland Drive (Dufour, 2008, p. 77).

Neoliberalisation and resistance

First of all, within a neoliberal logic, we are economic creatures with an eye for 'symbolic capital'. Seeing exchange value as being more important than use value may be regarded as a human trait, competition and greed regarded as almost embedded in our genetic imprint. Elaborating on his concept of practical sense, Bourdieu (1999a, p. 59) argued that we are situated within a relational field where we cannot avoid becoming aware of ourselves, that we should stand out and play out our distinctive traits – we play the games within the 'social' regulated by hierarchies of taste and prefer-ences. Taylor (1995) operates with the notion of strong and weak values, where strong values represent principles and preferences we do not usually negotiate but see as fundamental. Weak values may be regarded as taste where we allow for differences of a range of possibilities. While Bourdieu saw these mechanisms primarily as human and social traits, within a neoliberal framework these social mechanisms are transformed to operate within a market where everything becomes commodified. Social and cultural capital as commodities transforms into resources that also count for economic accumulation. Our everyday experience as consumers has become commodified to such an extent that everything operates on a market model. Boltanski and Chiapello (2007, pp. 10–11) argue that:

> The spirit of capitalism is precisely the set of beliefs associated with the capitalist order that helps to justify this order and, by legitimating them, to sustain forms of action and predispositions compatible with it. These justifications, whether general or practical, local or global, expressed in terms of virtue or justice, support the performance of more or less unpleasant tasks and, more generally, adhesion to a lifestyle conductive to the capitalist order … we may indeed speak of a dominant ideology …

The common trait was to succumb to market mechanisms and the recommodification of many areas of life that had been kept out of markets, such as education, health and social care. It also led to turning areas of public interest and shared values into business, like transport, power supply and infrastructure as such. Hemerijck (2013) argued that the foundations created for social citizenship during the twentieth century are still resisting neoliberalisation to such an extent that they remain a strong political force within our democratic systems. This created the space for so-called 'Third Way' politics (Giddens, 1994, 2001). Negotiations are thus still an important trait within our political systems, reducing the ability to maximise profits. Since people also make up a huge market, this cannot be ignored and has to be regarded as a counter force in the globalisation of market and politics. Values have also turned into a major commodity with significant symbolic power influencing the distribution of symbolic power – e.g. the growth of green power literally as well as real.

Democratic socialism and social democracy are founded on the central ideas of redistribution and acknowledgement of differentiated capabilities among men, women and groups of people –requiring systems of sharing and shared responsibility for long-term goals (Honneth, 2017). Just as 'Man' has to be tamed by common laws and shared systems of values regarded as just among the majority of people, we have to regulate capital and its inherent finance systems. Today we are witnessing proofs of increasing inequality once again when it comes to ownership and access to wealth (Piketty, 2014).

The emergence of the social investment state

The emerging concept of social investment politics is in my view the main arena where social work seems, in line with Foucault's (2010) notion of biopolitics, to be expected to professionally contribute to the widening idea and practice of 'partnership' within the helping professions. The social worker occupies the space priests traditionally inhabited, exercising what Foucault coined the pastoral effect since there was a normative ideal that had to be communicated to unbelievers. The expert has to comply with official social policy, putting work and the ability to secure personal income and sustainability in the forefront of all help, reducing the need for public spending and redistributive mechanisms.

Hemerijck (2013) discusses the concept of 'social investment state'.[1] First one has to rethink social policy in order to see that the labour market and families are welfare optimisers and a good guarantee that tomorrow's adult workers will be as productive and resourceful as possible. Second, early childhood development is granted new importance, as well as lifelong learning, family reconciliation, vocational training, all kinds of productivity improvements and all that may support these policies to enhance human capital growth. Third, social protection and social promotion become indispensable twin pillars of the new social investment edifice. Finally, social policy has primarily a productive function and the workers the prime source of all productivity growth. Employment contributes to financial sustainability and Hemerijck claims that *countries that have adjusted to a social investment approach in terms of work organization reveal higher levels of social cohesion.* Hemerijck sees these ideas as being in line with Nussbaum and Sen's use of capability – the idea that we all have different access to resources biologically as well as social and cultural, and that this has to considered when you should expect participation and investment in social and work life. This is contrary to neo-liberalist ideas of utility and competition. Hemerijck is not sure if all these ideas are all benign or if we should regard the discourse on *social investment as a cover for stealthy retrenchment and deconstruction or a Machiavellian foil for reconsolidating old social contracts, pressed by the strong and long-established clientelistic networks around the welfare state?* (2013, pp. 36–37).

Hemerijck asks if we are moving towards a 'capacitating social service' – enhancing human capital growth. Regarding the Nordic countries, we may say that 'nudging' is at work in the fashion that Thaler and Sunstein (2009) discuss in their book about improving decisions about health, wealth and happiness. This emerges as objectified governmentality. Leibetseder (2017) analysed EU documents regarding the European turn to social investment as implementation of the human capital theory of social citizenship. While the official publications define social investment as 'strengthening people's current and future capacities' she quotes critics' arguments that such a focus 'cultivates social inequality and dismantles social citizenship' (Leibetseder, 2017, p. 64).

What about social work?

Neo-liberalism often seems to have become the foundation for all ills and is blamed for all that goes wrong. I do not support this interpretation, but acknowledge the subtle nature of the concept as well as the problems of history and context. What seems important beside the commodification of everyday life and all that is related to our social being is to respond to the challenge as to how social work is being structured. The autonomous self is one important concept and new public management (NPM) - as a structure of organisations as well as a way to obtain efficiency - is another one. NPM is supposed to enable efficiency as well as cost awareness and is related to ideas of neo-liberalism through policies of outsourcing of public interests and institutions. Control and monitoring are based on goal attainments, often deploying variables constructed for databases with little relevance for social work efficiency if the quality of social work is to be regarded as better coping and improving quality of life.

As Eskelinen, Olesen, and Caswell (2008) have observed, social work is not a distinct field of work containing any single agreement about how to understand the world or how it should be changed: several paradigms, as well as in other professions, are here in contest. Ferguson (2008) and McDonald (2006) have identified areas where social work seems to be challenged and discuss the extent to which it is able to resist the ills of neoliberalism. Based on social work's own established set of values, they argue that social work is leaning more towards virtues and reflexivity, in line with much of the critique on evidence-based practices (Marthinsen & Skjefstad, 2011; McBeath & Webb, 2002). The radical side of social work may be leaning towards the leftist ideology of Gramsci, although it may not be an easy-to-sell profile these days (Garrett, 2009, 2013, Ch. 6).

Schwartzmantel relies on Gramsci's neo-Marxist analyses that 'ideology was the application of a broad philosophy to practical concrete problems'. Workfare may be such an identifiable trend in neo-liberal social policies, revealing the ontology that seem to challenge social work practices. Workfare underestimates the many reasons for personal failure and the complexity related to different kinds of poverty and its solutions, pushing forward social work practices that may be regarded by some as unethical as well as humiliating rather than dignified and respectful (Høilund & Juul, 2005; Marthinsen & Skjefstad, 2011). The idea of market fundamentalism in neoliberalism as well as the idea of a rational 'Man' puts strain on social work with marginalised people, challenging the complicated professional understanding of why there are 'haves' and 'have-nots' in a society.

Everything is viewed as a matter of personal responsibility and the family and local environment are regarded as the main sites offering care before state and municipal services are engaged. This can only lead to continuing inequality and poverty as personal problems, not social or for society to care about as it used to. Webb (2006) argues that;

> families and communities are afflicted with a huge burden of responsibility in having to sort out their own problems with a little push from the experts. Economic and structural disadvantage is ignored. (Webb, 2006, p. 62)

Social work management and practice have encountered neoliberal ideas and neoliberalisation as governments increasingly adapted the ideas of marketisation. We are adopting economic administration in public services, increasingly identified as NPM. Lawler and Bilson (2010, p. 5) refer to 'managerialism' as *the development of the interests of management in how organizations are managed, stressing the role and accountability of individual managers.* This has increased interest in controlling activities in economic manners, especially cost efficiency based on attempts to develop measurements related to input and output. Another is the attempt to reorganise social work according to purchaser/provider ideas, simulating business exchange within services. The third is an increasing outsourcing of work earlier done by public services to private companies followed by the need for quality assurance in developing work contracts to secure 'best value' for money. All three of these have challenged social work practices as well as ideology and policies due to the value ambivalence embedded in these models. Lawler and Bilson (2010, p. 6) use the concept of 'desocietalisation' to describe the change of focus from wider social concerns to the individualisation or customisation of service provision.

As Lorenz argues, social work was heavily embedded within the ideology of social solidarity concerned with equality, redistribution, respect and decency in working with marginalised and people who encounter hardship in their lives of temporary or lasting character. Social work did not only work from an individual understanding of hardship, but tried to promote an integrated view where the organisation of the social as such, and the power and interests at play within the social, were regarded as a context for working with the individual as well as society. Social work is to a large extent also policy in practice as well as applied social science. Social workers and their organisations have always had a strong voice in arguing for change that may ease the lives of the disadvantaged, the poor, those in pain or unhappiness related to humiliation and misrecognition. In this sense social work seems to represent a libertarian, solidary attitude in Rawls (1999) sense, meaning that rules and regulations made within the 'social' should be made from an 'ignorant position' (referring to the actor being ignorant of own interests due to the fact that principles are based on not knowing when and where you are born or if rules may favour you or not).

McDonald (2006) discusses how a neoliberal context of practice is challenging social work. She writes about a mounting performance crisis, growth in internal and external criticism, increased pressure to innovate, procedural conformity, increased technical specificity or goal clarity and conflicting internal interests. She argues that you find these conditions in state-operated organisations as well as in the non-profit sector. Her intention was to sensitize *social workers to institutional change and to see that macro-level developments had resonating and concrete implications in the daily lives of social workers and their clients* (McDonald, 2006, p. 5). She regards this consciousness as necessary for social workers as knowing actors in an unstable or unfinished new institutional order. Her book discusses three main drivers for institutional change that have consequences for social work. These drivers are the economics of change, the politics of change and the ideas of change – all within the neoliberal framework discussed here.

Following McDonald (2006), Lorenz (2006), Ferguson (2008) and Rogowski (2010) are among many of those who have tried to articulate the challenges this development has represented for social work practices and ideology (see also Garrett, 2009). The insistence of social work in promoting ideas linked to solidarity and collective resistance to capitalism many render it obsolete in today's society, leaving the profession and its agents without any platform. This situation is linked to the change in what count as dominant values and positions defended by the majority of people and political parties. The mere existence of poverty and beggars was for a long time regarded as a collective responsibility and regarded as a shame for society as such. The decriminalisation of begging, vagabonding and homelessness was regarded as removing the guilt and responsibility from the agent/citizen and placing the blame on society and politics in general. The fact that these social problems continued to exist was left to social workers to cope with. The (naïve) optimism embedded within modernity that a good society would not produce social problems is slowly being replaced by the recurring idea of wrong will and evil spirit as Villadsen (2004) so eloquently has shown with his genealogy of social work. This leaves social policy with a simpler task: according to this damaging logic and rationality, it is all about changing the individual and there is no social responsibility or 'society' to alter.

Neoliberal social work in historical perspective

So what values may have changed and how is social work now different from earlier? Lorenz (2006) is more concerned with the big picture and the dominant values influencing social policy and social work as such, while Rogowski (2010) has tried to identify some of the ways social work has changed as a practice. Let us have a closer look at both of them and see if we may be able to better pinpoint some traits that are now evolving as central to social work practice.

Lorenz and Rogowski return to the 1970–1980s community work and social planning seeking to diminish or eliminate social problems through reforming society. While psychoanalysis and family therapy as well as social medicine were part of the early curriculum in social work, the future was viewed through the lens of social change. Social change was *supposed* to have eliminated phenomena like poverty in the post second world war era and social workers were *expected* to remove the remaining social problems and contribute to the civilisation of the new urban life in a modern world (Marthinsen, 2001). The visions and ideals in most helping professions differed substantially from practices that continued much of the traditional tasks. Despite professionalisation, social services and child welfare continued carrying out the historical tasks of the poor office and core child protection, saving children from harmful parents. As professional social workers were replacing sound citizens as those who carried out these tasks, scientific knowledge played an increasing part in legitimising social work practices although practices scarcely were informed by scientific proof (Claezon, 1987).

Social work was *expected* to be efficient and to relieve individuals and families of their asocial traits and normalise their behaviour. Compared to today, the profession was *granted* legitimacy through expectations based on its scientific background. These expectations are now being replaced by *demands* and goals set up by management and policy rather than emanating from within the profession. Expectations and demands of efficiency based on scientifically proved methods (evidence-based practices) emerged around the turn of the century but are still hard to deliver.

Rogowski questions the development of social work in 'the rise and fall of a profession'. He considers the creation of local authority social services departments as an 'enlightenment project in line with modernity' (Rogowski, 2010, p. 17). In Scandinavia, 'social services' were introduced to replace the 'poor offices'. The idea was to eliminate poverty regarded as a public shame and not worthy of a decent and just society. Social work developed based on the use of a 'relationship' to support and encourage change (see also Garrett, 2014). Empowerment did at the outset also mean to rise and speak up against unfair and exploiting conditions. *The focus was on the circumstances ... rather than on the individual as such* (Rogowski, 2010, p. 32). *Market and social justice could coexist ...* remaining social problems could be understood in relation to diagnosis and treatment, making space for social work within this paradigm (Rogowski, 2010, p. 42). Marxist ideas came to play an important role in social work during the 1970s, imposing a move from focusing on private troubles to public issues (Rogowski, 2010, p. 47). This encouraged the ideas of social administration (planning) as well as social policy measures to cope with social problems, but still casework remained the baseline of social work. These lines can be identified in Scandinavia as well as in Great Britain.

The trust given to the profession during the 1970s and 1980s diminished towards the end of the century, and an emphasis on academic acquired professionalism was replaced by demands for competences – a development followed by deprofessionalisation. Casework method focused on individual pathology rather than strengths, but intervention moved from a strong focus on childhood and youth (psychoanalysis) towards systems theory and short-term interventions. Crises intervention, coping with crises as well as behaviour modification, also played an important part in practices and these moved slowly towards the self-focused ideas behind today's solution and coping/motivational therapies.

The downsizing and dismantling of the welfare state in the 1980s would put social work under pressure, moving away from generics and specialising to meet different user groups. Children, particularly, were given new rights and legal protection as well as managerialising the services through new public management measures like deadlines, limited time available, plans to be made and a renewed focus on legal measures as well as user involvement and user rights. The structural explanations of poverty were replaced by postmodern ideas of individual misery and a renewed focus on the individual – the ontology of evil returned to the scene as well as shame and personal responsibility to act (Andersen, 2003; Nussbaum, 2004; Villadsen, 2004). Conscientisation and politicisation evolved with a more critical idea of governmentality and discipline as the right way to understand the clients' – or now 'users' – claims and actions. Rogowski quotes Howe (1992) saying that social workers under neoliberal conditions have become investigators assessing risk, managers design surveillance systems … parents become objects of inquiry and the system moves from therapy and welfare to surveillance and control (Rogowski, 2010, p. 74).

While Rogowski sees the 1970s in relation to the students' motivation when *social work became an ethical career in which to engage with capitalist society* (Rogowski, 2010, p. 52), Ferguson (2008) claims that social workers report dissatisfaction about a growing gap between the values that brought them to social work and their day-to-day tasks. He supports the idea that social work is expanding internationally as well as in Britain, but expresses concern about the problem of neoliberal policies impacting on poverty, inequality and insecurity being wrapped in the language of the 'Third Way' and acting like 'soft cops'. He reminds social workers of Rawls' notion of 'justice as fairness' where the advantage of the least favoured has to be the guiding star. This raises questions about the increasing inequality in neoliberal societies. Social work has been reorganised along with other public services towards multi-agency, cross-cutting structures – action zones, youth offending teams and other ways of addressing regeneration and renewal (Ferguson, 2008, p. 47). Ferguson also argues that there is a silence about context, focusing on the 'active citizen' with a service where not even dementia seems like a decent reason for 'welfare dependency' (Ferguson, 2008, p. 48). He presents evidence-based practice and risk assessment as preferred technologies that are difficult to operationalise in every day practice. The concern with what works aligns with NPM and managerialism. Lawler and Bilson (2010) refer to 'managerialism' as the interest of management is such, stressing the accountability of the individual manager to comply with strict guidelines and achievement of objectives. They relate this development to a complex interplay of politics, economics and culture – much in line with Boltanski and Chiapello's analysis of the new spirit of capitalism. Focusing on the local dimension, Lawler and Bilson claim this results in a desocietalisation and fragmentation of services masked as customisation. Ferguson is also concerned with consumerism as a basis for social development.

There is also a strong move towards more marketisation, outsourcing and private services leaving professionals with a job as negotiator of contracts rather than professional social work practice. The consumerist model transforms into 'user involvement' and is seen as an example of commodification and change of responsibility from state to individuals and communities, leaving the idea of needs assessment to history. (Ferguson (2008, p. 87) also argues that this responsibilisation leads service customers themselves responsible for the choices that they make. In the end Ferguson promotes an idea of radical social work, distancing their work from 'the science of happiness' and rather focusing on the question of inequality, avoiding making misery into an experience of personal depression. In order to reclaim social work (as a radical practice) he suggests we should reclaim social work ethics as central. Social workers should reclaim the relationship and process focus as well as the right to what the social should contain meaning. And last social work has to focus on the structural level and reclaim the political in a struggle for *a more equal, more just society* (p. 136).

Social workers may in different ways respond to the new development of service provision. Skjefstad (2015) operates with four different logics of practice: of pathology, of bureaucracy, of sanction and a logic of inclusion. Using Honneth's idea of recognition as an interpretive grid to respectable practices, she argues that the logic of inclusion corresponds mostly to social work ethics, but the other logics may have moved into practices following the increasing management focus of neoliberal infused practices. Her research seems to correspond to other research dealing with newer forms of practice (Caswell, 2005).

The professional focus should be promoting representation and supporting an authentic subject who should be encouraged to present itself with a personal symbolic capital demanding recognition. Representation and recognition thus become paramount ideas within practice and social policy measures. Innovation and tailor-made solutions are encouraged. On the other side, we have an encroaching managerialism dominated by intrusive control apparatuses often identified with suspicion and humiliation. This makes the system rife with ambivalence. Having a positive social impact is at the heart of what social workers do. In the preface to the second edition of *Good Times, Bad Times -* where the welfare state is debated – Hills asserts:

> More than ever as we enter a period of huge uncertainty, we need to better understand what we are arguing about and who really benefits from and pays for the systems we have designed to cope with risks and uncertainties.

The research Hills refers to questions the construction of 'them' and 'us' where 'us' is the well situated and the precariat and the poor make up 'them'. Here, the prevailing idea within neoliberalism is that the poor cost too much and that welfare has to be restricted. However, Hill's empirical work illuminates that *if anyone got too expensive, it has, in fact, been the rich* (Hills, 2015, p. 45).

Conclusion

In our society social work is one of the expert areas concerned with governing the family, the child and the 'social' in general. The paradox of social work becoming increasingly important is that this task does not seem to have the requisite conditions to perform best practices. This is caused by management of these organisations increasingly being preoccupied with systems drawing attention to parts of the work and activities not necessarily relevant to doing good social work. This seems to leave social work in an ambivalent position. The 'enabling social investment state' could have been a benign construction rather than a rhetoric device merely disguising pernicious austerity politics favouring the 'haves' at the expense of the 'have-nots'.

Note

1. This concept is also discussed by Neil Gilbert (2002) in his book, Transformation of the welfare state, the silent surrender of public responsibility. Oxford University Press.

Acknowledgements

I would like to thank the reviewers for their constructive comments and my fellow editors Paul, Anne and Nina for their cooperation and a special thanks to my colleague Professor Graham Clifford for his comments and support.

Disclosure statement

No potential conflict of interest was reported by the author.

References

Andersen, N. Å. (2003). *Borgerens kontraktliggørelse*. København: Hans Reitzel.

Boltanski, L., & Chiapello, E. (2007). *The new spirit of capitalism*. London: Verso.

Bourdieu, P. (1999). *Moteld*. Stockholm: Brutus Östlings Bokförlag Symposion.

Bourdieu, P. (1999a). *Praktisk förnuft*. Uddevalla: Daidalos.

Brown, W. (2015). *Undoing the demos. Neoliberalism's stealth revolution*. New York, NY: Zone Books.

Caswell, D. (2005). *Handlemuligheter I socialt arbejde – en casestudie om kommunal frontlinjepraksis på beskæftigelsesområdet* (PhD thesis). Roskilde: Roskilde Universitet.

Claezon, I. (1987). *Bättre beslut*. Umeå: Universitetet i Umeå.

Dardot, P., & Laval, C. (2013). *The new way of the world – on neo-liberal society*. London: Verso Books.

Davies, W. (2016). *The happiness industry – how the government and big business sold us well-being*. London: Verso Books.

Dufour, D.-R. (2008). *The art of shrinking heads. The new servitude of the liberated in the Era of total capitalism*. Cambridge: Polity Press.

Ehrenreich, B. (2010). *Livets lyse sider - hvordan den hemningsløse dyrkelsen av positiv tenkning har underminert Amerika*. Oslo: Oktober.

Eskelinen, L., Olesen, S. P., & Caswell, D. (2008). *Potentialer i socialt arbejde*. København: Hans Reitzels forlag.

Ferguson, I. (2008). *Reclaiming social work*. London: Sage.

Forås, P. B., & Vetlesen, A. J. (2015). *Angsten for oppdragelse*. Oslo: Universitetsforlaget.

Foucault, M. (2010). *The birth of biopolitics*. Basingstoke: Palgrave Mamillan.

Garrett, P. M. (2005). Social work's 'electronic turn': Notes on the deployment of information and communication technologies in social work with children and families. *Critical Social Policy, 25*(4), 529–553.

Garrett, P. M. (2009). *'Transforming' children's services? Social work, neoliberalism and the 'modern' world*. Maidenhead: McGraw Hill/Open University.

Garrett, P. M. (2013). *Social work and social theory*. Bristol: Policy Press.

Garrett, P. M. (2014). Re-enchanting social work? The emerging 'spirit' of social work in an age of economic crisis. *British Journal of Social Work, 44*(3), 503–521.

Giddens, A. (1994). *Beyond left and right*. Cambridge: Polity Press.

Giddens, A. (Ed.). (2001). *The global third way debate*. Cambridge: Polity Press.

Gilbert, N. (2002). *Transformation of the welfare state, the silent surrender of public responsibility*. Oxford: Oxford University Press.

Giroux, H. A. (2004). *The terror of neoliberalism. Authoritarianism and the eclipse of democracy* (P. b.). Boulder, CO: Paradigm Press.

Gramsci, A. (1971). *Selections from the prison notebooks*. London: Lawrence and Wishart.

Habermas, J. (1990). *Kommunikativt handlande*. Uddevalla: Daidalos.

Harvey, D. (2005). *A brief history of neoliberalism*. Oxford: Oxford University Press.

Hemerijck, A. (2013). *Changing welfare states*. Oxford: Oxford University Press.

Hills, J. (2015). *Good times, bad times. The welfare state of them and us*. Bristol: Polity Press.

Honneth, A. (2017). *The idea of socialism*. Cambridge: Polity Press.

Høilund, P., & Juul, S. (2005). *Anerkendelse og dømmekraft i socialt arbeide*. København: Hans Reitzels Forlag.

Howe, D. (1992). Child abuse and the bureaucratisation of social work. *Sociological Review, 40*(3), 491–508.

Innset, O. (2016). *Nyliberalisme – filosofi eller politisk rasjonalitet? AGORA nr* 2–3, 16 s. 5–31

Järvinen, M., & Mortensen, N. (2005). Det magtfulde møde mellem system og klient: teoretiske perspektiver. In M. Järvinen, J. E. Larsen, & N. Mortensen (Eds.), *Det magtfulde møde mellem system og klient*. Aarhus: Aarhus Universitetsforlag.

Kierkegaad, S. (1974). *Concluding unscientific postscript*. Princeton, NJ: Princeton University Press.

Lawler, J., & Bilson, A. (2010). *Social work management and leadership. Managing complexity with creativity*. London: Routledge.

Leibetseder, B. (2017). Investing in social subjects. The European turn to social investment as the human capital theory of social citizenship. In S. F. Schram & M. Pavlovskaya (Eds.), *Rethinking neoliberalism. Resisting the diciplinary regime* (pp. 63–83). New York, NY: Routledge.

Lorenz, W. (2005). *Social work and new social order – Challenging neo-liberalism's erosion of solidarity. Social Work & Society*, *3*(1), Retrieved from http://www.socwork.net/Lorenz2005.pdf

Lorenz, W. (2006). *Perspectives on European social work*. Opladen: Barbara Budrich.

McDonald, C. (2006). *Challenging social work – the context of practice*. Hampshire: Palgrave Macmillan.

Marthinsen, E. (2001). *ISA 25 år*. S. 13-23 i Tronvoll, Inger M. og Marthinsen, Edgar 2001: Sosialt arbeid – refleksjoner og nyere forskning. Trondheim: Tapir Akademiske.

Marthinsen, E., & Skjefstad, N. (2011). Recognition as a virtue in social work practice. *European Journal of Social Work, 14*(2), 195–212.

McBeath, G., & Webb, S. A. (2002). Virtue ethics and social work: Being lucky, realistic, and not doing ones duty. *British Journal of Social Work, 32*(8), 1015–1036.

Nussbaum, M. C. (2004). *Hiding from humanity: Disgust, shame, and the Law*. Princeton, NJ: Princeton University Press.

Piketty, T. (2014). *Capital in the twenty-first century*. Belknap: Harvard Univeristy Press.

Rawls, J. (1999). *En teori om rättvisa*. Uddevalla: Daidalos.

Rogowski, S. (2010). *Social work, the rise and fall of a profession?* Bristol: Polity Press.

Rorty, R. (1997). *Achieving our country*. Cambridge: Harvard University Press.

Rose, N. (1999). *Governing the soul – the shaping of the private self*. London: Free Association Books.

Schwarzmantel, J. (2005). Challenging neoliberal hegemony. *Contemporary Politics, 11*(2), 85–98.

Sennett, R. (2005). *Det fleksible mennesket*. Bergen: Fagbokforlaget.

Skjefstad, N. S. (2015). *Sosialt arbeid i overgangen til NAV – utfordringer for en anerkjennende praksis* (NTNU PhD thesis).

Slobodian, Q. (2015). *World federation against the welfare state: Hayek and Röpke think global before 1945*. Tokyo: Hitotsubashi University.

Standing, G. (2014). *The precariat: The new dangerous class*. London: Bloomsbury Academics.

Taylor, C. (1995). *Identitet, frihet och gemenskap: Politisk-filosofiska texter i urval av Harald Grimen*. Gøteborg: Daidalos.

Thaler, R. H., & Sunstein, C. R. (2009). *Nudge. Improving decisions about health, wealth and happiness*. New York, NY: Penguin books.

Villadsen, K. (2004). *Det sociale arbejdets genealogi*. København: Hans Reitzels forlag.

Webb, S. A. (2006). *Social work in a risk society*. Hampshire: Palgrave Macmillan.

Index

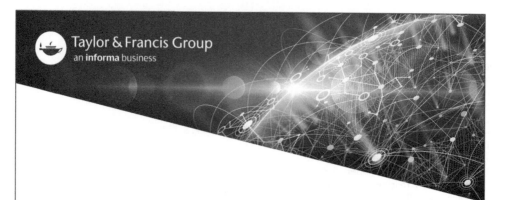
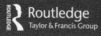
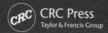